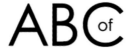
ABC of

Occupational and Environmental Medicine

Third Edition

EDITED BY

David Snashall

Professor of Occupational Medicine, King's College London, London, UK
Honorary Consultant and Clinical Director
Occupational Health and Safety Services, Guy's and St Thomas' NHS Foundation Trust, London, UK

Dipti Patel

Consultant Occupational Health Physician, Foreign and Commonwealth Office, London, UK
Joint Director, National Travel Health Network and Centre, London, UK

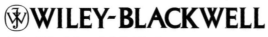
WILEY-BLACKWELL
A John Wiley & Sons, Ltd., Publication

BMJ|Books

Library of Congress Cataloging-in-Publication Data
ABC of occupational and environmental medicine / edited by David Snashall,
Dipti Patel. – 3rd ed.
       p. ; cm. – (ABC series)
    Includes bibliographical references and index.
    ISBN 978-1-4443-3817-1 (pbk. : alk. paper)
    I. Snashall, David. II. Patel, Dipti. III. Series: ABC series (Malden, Mass.) [DNLM: 1. Occupational Diseases. 2. Environmental Exposure.
3. Environmental Health. 4. Occupational Health. WA 400]
    616.9′803–dc23

2012007482

A catalogue record for this book is available from the British Library.

Wiley also publishes its books in a variety of electronic formats. Some content that appears in print may not be available in electronic books.

Set in 9.25/12 Minion by Laserwords Private Limited, Chennai, India
Printed and bound in Malaysia by Vivar Printing Sdn Bhd
Cover image: Ian Casement, Accolade Photography
Cover designer: Meaden Creative

1   2012

ABC of
Occupational and Environmental Medicine

Third Edition

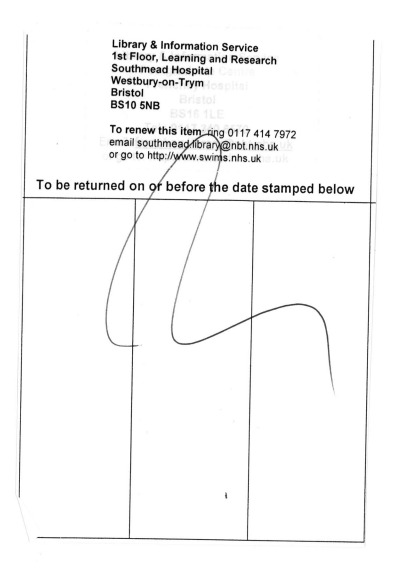

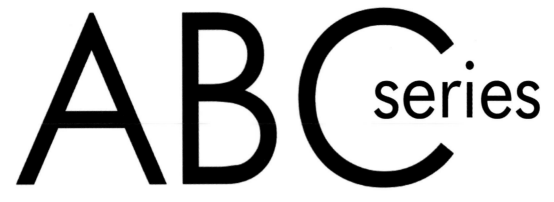

ABC series

An outstanding collection of resources – written by specialists for non-specialists

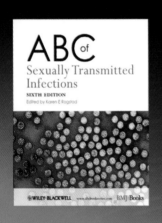

ABC of
Sexually Transmitted
Infections
SIXTH EDITION
Edited by Karen E Rogstad

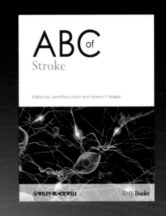

ABC of
Stroke
Edited by Jonathan Mant and Marion F. Walker

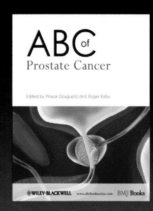

ABC of
Prostate Cancer
Edited by Prokar Dasgupta and Roger Kirby

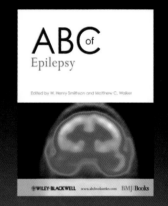

ABC of
Epilepsy
Edited by W. Henry Smithson and Matthew C. Walker

The *ABC* series contains a wealth of indispensable resources for GPs, GP registrars, junior doctors, doctors in training and all those in primary care

▶ **Now fully revised and updated**
▶ **Highly illustrated, informative and a practical source of knowledge**
▶ **An easy-to-use resource, covering the symptoms, investigations, treatment and management of conditions presenting in day-to-day practice and patient support**
▶ **Full colour photographs and illustrations aid diagnosis and patient understanding of a condition**

For more information on all books in the *ABC* series, including links to further information, references and links to the latest official guidelines, please visit:

www.abcbookseries.com

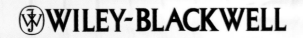

BMJ|Books

Contents

Contributors

Anil Adisesh
Deputy Chief Medical Officer, Centre for Workplace Health, Health and Safety Laboratory, Buxton;
Honorary Senior Clinical Lecturer, University of Sheffield, Sheffield, UK

Kim Burton
Affiliate Visiting Professor, Centre for Health and Social Care Research, University of Huddersfield, Huddersfield, UK

Nicola Cherry
Professor, Department of Medicine, University of Alberta, Edmonton, Canada

David Coggon
Professor of Occupational and Environmental Medicine, MRC Lifecourse Epidemiology Unit, University of Southampton, Southampton, UK

Joanne O Crawford
Senior Consultant Ergonomist, Institute of Occupational Medicine, Edinburgh, UK

Paul Cullinan
Professor in Occupational and Environmental Respiratory Disease, National Heart and Lung Institute (Imperial College), London, UK

Martyn Davidson
Head of Health Operations, Royal Mail Group, Fleet, UK

William Davies
Consultant Occupational Physician, South Wales Fire and Rescue Service, Cardiff, UK

Sarah Harper
Professor, Oxford Institute of Ageing, University of Oxford, Oxford, UK

Samuel B. Harvey
Clinical Lecturer in Liaison and Occupational Psychiatry, Institute of Psychiatry, King's College, London, UK;
School of Psychiatry, University of New South Wales, Sydney, Australia;
Black Dog Institute, Sydney, Australia

Max Henderson
Senior Lecturer in Epidemiological and Occupational Psychiatry, Institute of Psychiatry, King's College, London, UK

John Hobson
Lecturer in Occupational Medicine, University of Keele;
Honorary Tutor in Occupational Medicine, University of Manchester, UK

Nicholas Kendall
Senior Clinical Lecturer, Occupational Medicine, University of Otago, Otago, New Zealand

David Koh
Professor, Saw Swee Hock School of Public Health, National University of Singapore, Singapore;
Chair Professor of Occupational Health and Medicine, PAPRSB Institute of Health Sciences, Universiti Brunei Darussalam, Brunei Darussalam

Peter A. Leggat
Professor and Deputy Head of School (Campus Head), School of Public Health, Tropical Medicine and Rehabilitation Sciences, James Cook University, Townsville, Queensland, Australia

Paul Litchfield
BT Group Chief Medical Officer, London, UK

Ira Madan
Consultant and Senior Lecturer in Occupational Medicine, Guy's and St Thomas' NHS Trust and King's College London, London, UK

Robert Maynard
Honorary Professor of Environmental Medicine, University of Birmingham, Birmingham, UK

Ron McCaig
Consultant Occupational Physician, Advantage: Health at Work Ltd, Chester, UK

Keith T. Palmer
Professor of Occupational Medicine, MRC Lifecourse Epidemiology Unit, University of Southampton, Southampton, UK

Dipti Patel
Consultant Occupational Physician, Foreign and Commonwealth Office;
Joint Director, National Travel Health Network and Centre, London, UK

Andy Slovak
Honorary Senior Lecturer, University of Manchester, Manchester, UK

Derek R. Smith
Professor and Deputy Director (Research), School of Health Sciences, University of Newcastle, Ourimbah, New South Wales, Australia

David Snashall
Professor of Occupational Medicine, King's College London; Honorary Consultant and Clinical Director of Occupational Health and Safety, Guy's and St Thomas' NHS Foundation Trust, London, UK

Judy Sng
Assistant Professor, Saw Swee Hock School of Public Health, National University of Singapore, Singapore

Paolo Vineis
Professor, Imperial College of Science, Technology and Medicine, London, UK

Ian R. White
St. John's Institute of Dermatology, St. Thomas' Hospital, London, UK

Nerys Williams
Independent Consultant Occupational Physician, Solihull and London, UK

Preface

Although work is generally considered to be good for your health and a healthy working population is essential to a country's economic and social development, certain kinds of work can be damaging. Occupational health is the study of the effect – good and bad – of work on peoples' health and, conversely, the effect of peoples' health on their work: fitness for work in other words.

Work places are specialized environments, capable of being closely controlled. Generally speaking, it is the lack of control imposed by employers that is the cause of ill health because of exposure to hazardous materials and agents at work, and of injury caused by workplace accidents.

Working life does not, however, begin and end at the factory gate or the office door: many people walk, cycle or drive to work – a journey that often constitutes the major hazard of the day. Others have to drive or travel by other means as part of their job, live away from home, be exposed to other people, other food, other parasites. Even work from home, increasing in some countries, can have its problems, mainly psychosocial. Occupational health practitioners deal with all these aspects of working life.

A working population consists of people mainly between 15 and 70 years (disregarding for the moment the ongoing scandal of child labour), who may be exposed for 8–12 hours a day to a relatively high concentration of toxic substances or agents, physical or psychological. At least that population is likely to be reasonably fit – unlike those who cannot work because of illness or disabilities, the young, and the very old, who are more vulnerable and spend a lifetime exposed to many of the same agents in the general environment at lower concentrations. This is the realm of environmental medicine of such concern to those who monitor the degradation of our planet, track pollution and climate change, and note the effect of natural disasters and man made ones, especially wars.

This book was first published in 1997 as the *ABC of Work Related Disorders*. In 2003 a much expanded and updated second edition attempted in a compressed and easy to assimilate fashion, to describe those problems of health relating to work in its widest sense and to the environment. This third edition brings these subjects up to date.

The pattern of work is changing fast. There is relatively full employment in most economically developed countries now but low pay and job insecurity remain as significant threats to health manufacturing industry is mainly concentrated in developing countries where traditional occupational disease such as pesticide poisoning and asbestosis are still depressingly common. Occupational accidents are particularly common in places where industrialization is occurring rapidly as was once the case during the industrial revolution in nineteenth-century Britain. Emerging economies often display a mixture of 'ancient and modern' work-related heath and safety problems Modern work is also more varied, more intense, more service oriented, more competitive, more regulated, and more spread around the clock in order to serve the 24-hour international economy. There are more women at work, more disabled people, and a range of new illnesses perhaps better described as symptom complexes which represent interactive states between peoples' attitudes and feeling towards their work, their domestic environment, and the way in which their illness behaviour is expressed.

All occupational disease is preventable – even the more 'modern' conditions such as stress and upper limb disorders can be reduced to low levels by good management and fair treatment of individuals who do develop these kinds of problems and who may need rehabilitation back into working life after a period of disability. These particular disorders now dominate work-related ill health, mainly because their prevalence in the general population is high.

Attitudes to mental health are changing especially to common problems such as mild to moderate depression and anxiety, substance abuse and stress: like asthma, they come and go, can be successfully managed and are generally compatible with work – indeed are often improved by work. For no subject has there been such a revolution in the approach to management than the common musculoskeletal disorders. Medical treatment has its place and so do ergonomic and preventive initiatives in the workplace but wholesale application of the biomedical model has failed and a biopsychosocial approach has to be the answer if disability is to be reduced. These areas are covered in the chapters on musculoskeletal and, mental health (including stress) disorders, frequently intertwined at work. There are chapters also on the traditional concerns of occupational health practitioners such as dermatoses, respiratory disorders, infections, travel abroad and other chapters reflecting occupational health practice covering workplace surveys, fitness for work, sickness absence control issues, ethics and, unfortunately increasing, legal considerations. Genetics and its application to work and the effects of work on reproduction are described in Chapter 17. With a working population moving from providing physical labour to a 'knowledge economy' demanding flexible responses in a complex technology-dominated world, better job design becomes imperative and human factors assume importance – just think of the massive increase in the retail sector and in healthcare and the safety considerations in high speed travel or nuclear energy production (Chapter 16).

Concerns beyond the workplace are covered in the chapters on global issues and pollution. The control of hazards in the general environment presents issues of problem solving at a different level. Ascertainment of exposure is more difficult than in workplaces, and to find solutions needs transnational political will and commitment as well as science to succeed. Many believe that the rash of 'new' illnesses attributed to environmental causes are manifestations of a risk-averse public's response to poorly understood threats in the modern world and an unconscious wish to blame 'industry', or some state institution – agencies that represent irresponsible emitters of toxins, inadvertent releasers of radiation, careless sprayers of pesticides, or well-meaning providers of vaccinations. Chapter 14 addresses this important subject and Chapter 20 looks at what the future has in store.

Occupational medicine can be seen as a subspecialty of public health which itself changes according to the health problems thrown up by a changing environment. Demographic change is a major driver of health and therefore healthcare provision, no more clearly exemplified than by over-population which outstrips resources and an ageing work force typical of present day economically developed countries but also of those huge countries who will soon face this phenomenon (Chapter 18).

In common with the previous edition, this new edition of *ABC of Occupational and Environmental Medicine* will still appeal to non-specialists who wish to understand and practise some occupational medicine; but will also provide all that students of occupational and environmental medicine and nursing will need as a basis for their studies. Each chapter has an annotated further reading list. Most, but not all, of the book is written with an international audience in mind.

David Snashall
Dipti Patel

CHAPTER 1

Hazards of Work

David Snashall

Guy's and St Thomas' NHS Foundation Trust, London, UK

OVERVIEW

- Work has an important influence on health, both public and individual. It brings great health benefits but can also be detrimental to both
- Work related injuries and illnesses take a terrible toll and have massive socioeconomic effects. They are largely preventable
- Occupational disease is particularly poorly reported at a national level. Healthcare professionals need to suspect it and know how to manage it
- The world of work is changing fast and the spectrum of occupational ill health is changing in tune
- 'Traditional' occupational diseases persist in less well regulated industries but mental health and musculoskeletal disorders and hard to define 'symptomatic' illness are the major causes of work-related disability

---

Most readers of this book will consider themselves lucky to have a job, probably an interesting one. However tedious it can be, work defines a person, which is one reason why most people who lack the opportunity to work feel disenfranchised. As well as determining our standard of living, work takes up about a third of our waking time, widens our social networks, constrains where we can live and conditions our behaviour. 'Good' work is life enhancing, but bad working conditions can damage your health.

Global burden of occupational and environmental ill health

According to recent International Labour Organisation (ILO) calculations, every day 6300 people die as a result of occupational accidents or work-related diseases – more than 2.3 million deaths per year (including 12 000 children) – and 337 million people have workplace injuries, causing disability and time off work. Two million workplace-associated deaths per year outnumber people killed in road accidents, war, violence and through AIDS, and

consume 4% of the world's gross domestic product in terms of absence from work, treatment, compensation, disability and survivor benefits, not to mention the human cost (Figures 1.1 and 1.2).

The burden is particularly heavy in developing countries where the death rate in construction, for example, is 10 times that in developed countries, and where workers are concentrated in the most heavy and dangerous industries – fishing, mining, logging and agriculture.

In the United States some 60 300 deaths from occupational disease, 862 200 illnesses and 13.2 million non-fatal injuries with 6500 deaths occur each year.

Environmental disease is more difficult to quantify because the populations at risk are more diffuse than the working population. As an example, it is estimated that lead poisoning accounts for almost 1% of the global burden of disease, most of the exposure affecting children in the developing world. Air and water pollution and extremes of climate also have profound effects on health

Reporting occupational ill health

Occupational diseases are reportable in most countries, but are usually grossly underreported. Even in countries like Finland (where reporting is assiduous), surveys have shown rates of occupational disease to be underestimated by three to five times.

Classifications of occupational diseases have been developed for two main purposes: for *notification*, usually to a health and safety agency to provide national statistics and subsequent preventive action, and for *compensation* paid to individuals affected by such diseases. There are no universally accepted diagnostic criteria, coding systems or classifications worldwide. Modifications of ICD-10 (international classification of diseases, 10th revision) are used in many countries to classify occupational diseases, along with a system devised by the World Health Organization for classifying by exposure or industry.

It is the association of these two sets of information that defines a disease as being probably occupational in origin (Box 1.1). The WHO, in the ICD11 classification, is going to incorporate occupational attribution.

A number of reporting systems exist in the United Kingdom but these are neither comprehensive nor coordinated. After all, they arose at different times and for different purposes.

ABC of Occupational and Environmental Medicine, Third Edition.
Edited by David Snashall and Dipti Patel.
© 2012 John Wiley & Sons Ltd. Published 2012 by John Wiley & Sons Ltd.

Box 1.1 Classification and notification of occupational diseases (WHO)

1 Diseases caused by agents
  1.1 Diseases caused by chemical agents
  1.2 Diseases caused by physical agents
  1.3 Diseases caused by biological agents
2 Diseases by target organ
  2.1 Occupational respiratory diseases
  2.2 Occupational skin diseases
  2.3 Occupational musculoskeletal diseases
3 Occupational cancer
4 Others

Notification

In addition to the diagnosis of occupational disease, additional information should be included in the notification. ILO has defined the minimum information to be included:

a. Enterprise, establishment and employer
  (i) Name and address of employer
  (ii) Name and address of enterprise
  (iii) Name and address of the establishment
  (iv) Economic activity of the establishment
  (v) Number of workers (size of the establishment)
b. Person affected by the occupational disease
  (i) Name, address, sex and date of birth
  (ii) Employment status
  (iii) Occupation at the time when the disease was diagnosed
  (iv) Length of service with the present employer

Classification for labour statistics (ILO)

International Standard Classification of Occupations (ISCO-08) as:

1 Employees
2 Employers
3 Own-account workers
4 Members of producers' co-operatives
5 Contributing family workers
6 Workers not classifiable by status

  – International Classification of Status in Employment (ICSE)
  – International Standard Industrial Classification of all Economic Activities (ISIC)
  – International Standard Classification of Education (a UNESCO classification) (ISCED)
  – Classifications of occupational injuries

Box 1.2 Health and Safety Executive (HSE) statistics

Self-reported ill health 2009–2010

1.3 million workers and 0.8 million former workers reported ill health which they thought was work related. Musculoskeletal disorders and stress formed the most commonly reported illness types.

Reports of ill health by general practitioners (GPs) and specialist physicians

These surveillance schemes which collect reports of new cases of work related ill health confirm that musculoskeletal disorders are the most common type of work related illness but that mental ill health gives rise to more working days lost. Specialist physicians report on musculoskeletal disorders, mental ill health, skin disorders, respiratory disease and audiological disorders.

Ill health assessed for industrial injuries disablement benefit

The number of new cases was 7,100 in 2009. The largest categories were arthritis of the knee in miners, vibration white finger, carpal tunnel syndrome and respiratory diseases associated with past exposures to substances such as asbestos and coal dust.

The trend in numbers is generally downwards except for diseases associated with asbestos.

Labour force survey

The rate of reportable injury from this survey was 840 per 100,000 workers, and falling compared with earlier estimates. When compared with the statutory reporting of injuries (RIDDOR) it is apparent that only about half of such injuries are reported by employers.

Enforcement notices

These detail action taken against employers for health and safety infringements by the regulatory authorities.

The labour force survey is a national survey of over 50,000 households performed each quarter.

Standard industrial classification and standard occupational classification systems are used in UK official statistics.

Industry sectors with ill health rates statistically significantly higher than the rate for all industries, were health and social work and public administration whereas for injuries, agriculture, transport, storage and communication and construction had statistically significantly higher rates than for all industry.

Workers in personal service occupations have statistically significantly higher rates of both injury and ill health compared to all occupations. Associate, professional and technical occupations and professional occupations have statistically significant high rates for ill health but relatively low injury rates. Skilled trades, process plant and machine operatives and elementary occupations have injury rates which are statistically significantly higher than the average.

Occupational injuries are also reportable in Great Britain under the Reporting of Injuries, Diseases and Dangerous Occurrences Regulations 1995 (RIDDOR) and, for purposes of compensation, to the Department of Work and Pensions' Industrial Injuries Scheme (see also Chapter 5). The recording of injuries is generally more reliable because injuries are immediately obvious and occur at a definable point in time. By contrast, cause and effect in occupational disease may be far from obvious, and exposure to hazardous materials may have occurred many years beforehand (Box 1.2).

Occupational or work related?

Some conditions, such as asbestosis and mesothelioma in laggers, and lead poisoning in industrial painters, are hardly likely to be anything other than purely occupational in origin. (About 70 of these 'prescribed' occupational diseases are listed by the UK Department for Work and Pensions.) However, mesothelioma can

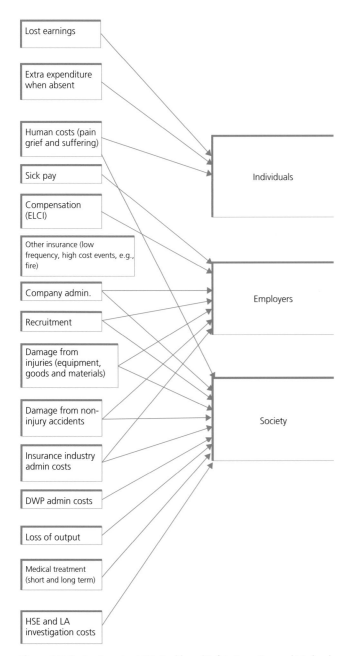

Figure 1.1 Cost categories. HSE, Health and Safety Executive; and LA, local authority.

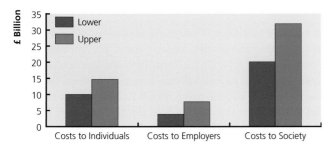

Figure 1.2 Costs to Britain of workplace accidents and work-related illness, 2001/02.

be the result of environmental exposure to fibrous minerals (as in the case of cave dwellers in Turkey), and lead poisoning can be a result of ingesting lead salts from low temperature, lead glazed ceramics used as drinking vessels, mainly in developing countries. In these situations the history and main occupation will differentiate the causes. The situation may be far less clear for conditions such as back pain in a construction worker or an upper limb disorder in a keyboard operator when activities outside work may contribute, as might genetics, psychological factors and symptom thresholds. A lifetime working in a dusty atmosphere may not lead to chronic bronchitis and emphysema, but when it is combined with cigarette smoking this outcome is much more likely. Common conditions for which occupational exposures are important but are not the sole reason or the major cause can more reasonably be termed 'work-related disease' rather than 'occupational disease'.

Some important prescribed diseases such as chronic bronchitis, emphysema and lung cancer are considered work related in an individual case only on the 'balance of probabilities', one common approach being to view occupational attribution as more likely than not if the relative risk exceeds 2.

Certain occupations carry a substantial risk of premature death, whereas others are associated with the likelihood of living a long and healthy life (Table 1.1). This is reflected in very different standardized (or proportional) mortality ratios for different jobs, but not all the differences are the result of the various hazards of different occupations. Selection factors are important, and social class has an effect (although in the United Kingdom this is defined by occupation). Non-occupational causes related to behaviour and lifestyle also contribute

Presentation of work-related illnesses

Diseases and conditions of occupational origin usually present in an identical form to the same diseases and conditions caused by other factors. Bronchial carcinoma, for example, has the same histological appearance and follows the same course whether it results from working with asbestos, uranium mining or cigarette smoking.

The possibility that a condition is work induced may become apparent only when specific questions are asked, because the occupational origin of a disease is usually discovered (and it is discovered only if suspected) by the presence of an unusual pattern (Box 1.3). For example, in occupational dermatitis, the distribution of the lesions may be characteristic. A particular history may be another clue: asthma of late onset is more commonly occupational in origin than asthma that starts early in life. Indeed, some 40% of adult onset asthma is probably occupational. Daytime drowsiness in a fit young factory worker may be caused not by late nights and heavy alcohol consumption but by unsuspected exposure to solvents at work.

The occupational connection with a condition may not be immediately obvious because patients may give vague answers when asked what their job is. Answers such as 'driver', 'fitter' or 'model' are not very useful, and the closer a health professional can get to extracting a precise job description the better. For example,

Table 1.1 Work-related mortality in England and Wales, 1979–2000.

Job Group	Number of deaths from all causes	Cause of death (ICD-9 code)	Excess deaths	Excess deaths per 1 000 deaths from all causes
Publicans and bar staff	12 446	Other alcohol related diseases	263	21.1
		Cirrhosis	98	7.9
		Cancer of the oral cavity	75	6.0
		Cancer of the larynx	64	5.1
		Cancer of the liver	43	3.5
		Cancer of the pharynx	39	3.1
		Total work-related mortality	582	46.7
Coal Miners	24 621	Chronic obstructive pulmonary disease	586	23.8
		Coal workers pneumoconiosis	423	17.2
		Total work-related mortality	1058	43.0
Aircraft flight deck officers	814	Air transport accidents	33	40.1
Steel erectors	3675	Cancer of the bronchus	106	28.8
		Total work-related mortality	139	37.9
Fire service personnel	2643	Cancer of the bronchus	60	22.7
		Motor vehicle traffic accidents	25	9.5
		Total work-related mortality	93	35.3
Managers in construction	5578	Cancer of the bronchus	112	20.0
		Total work-related mortality	128	22.9
Fishing and related workers	1284	Water transport accidents	25	19.1
Metal polishers	970		18	18.4
Moulders and coremakers (metal)	2198		37	16.9
			3	1.4
			40	18.3
Vehicle body builders	1305	Cancer of pleura	15	11.2
		Total work-related mortality	23	17.8
Synthetic fibre makers	204	Asthma	3	17.0
Mine (excluding coal) and quarry workers	1658	Silicosis	13	7.8
		Other lung disorders	7	4.2
		Work-related accidental deaths	7	4.2
		Total work-related mortality	27	16.2

Job groups with largest excesses of work-related mortality as a proportion of total deaths from all causes: men aged 20–74 years, England and Wales, 1991–2000.

Reproduced from *Occupational & Environmental Medicine*, Coggon, D. *et al.* (2010) with permission from BMJ Publishing Group Ltd.

Box 1.3 **How to take an occupational history**

Question 1
What is your job?
or
What do you do for a living?

Question 2
What do you work with?
or
What is a typical working day for you?
or
What do you actually do at work?

Question 3
How long have you been doing this kind of work? Have you done any different kind of work in the past?

Question 4
Have you been told that anything you use at work may make you ill? Has anybody at work had the same symptoms?

Question 5
Do you have any hobbies, like do-it-yourself or gardening, which may bring you into contact with chemicals?

Question 6
Is there an occupational health doctor or nurse at your workplace who I could speak to?

an engineer may work directly with machinery and risk damage to limbs, skin and hearing, or may spend all day working at a computer and risk back pain, upper limb disorders and sedentary stress. Sometimes patients will have been told (or should have been told) their job is associated with specific hazards, or they may know that fellow workers have experienced similar symptoms.

Timing of events

The timing of symptoms is important because they may be related to but not necessarily coincident with exposure events during work. Asthma provides a good example of this: many people with occupational asthma develop symptoms only after a delay of some hours and the condition may present as nocturnal wheeze. It is essential to ask whether symptoms occur during the performance of a specific task and if they occur solely on workdays, improving during weekends and holidays. Sometimes the only way to elucidate the pattern is for the person to keep a graphic diary of the time sequence of events.

Working conditions

Patients should be asked specifically about their working conditions. Common problems are dim lighting, noisy machinery, bad office layout, a dusty atmosphere and oppressive or, almost as bad, inconsistent or 'unjust' management. Such questions not only open up possibilities, but give the questioner a good idea of the general state of a working environment and how the patient reacts to it. A visit to the workplace may be a revelation, and every bit as valuable as a home visit if one wants to understand how a patient's health is conditioned by their working environment and how (both) might be improved. Knowing about somebody's work can help to provide context and insight. Patients are often happy to talk about the details of their work: this may be less threatening than talking about details of their home life and can promote a better relationship between patients and health professionals.

Occupational disease can extend beyond the workplace, affecting local populations through air, water or soil pollution. Overalls soiled with toxic materials such as lead or asbestos can affect members of workers' families if the overalls are taken home to be washed.

Trends in work-related illnesses

Changes in working practices in the industrialized world are giving rise to work that is more demanding in a psychosocial sense but less so in terms of hard physical activity. Jobs are also safer (although this may not be true in those countries where extremely rapid industrialization is occurring) – the result of a shift in many countries from agricultural and extractive industry via heavy factory industry to technology-intensive manufacturing and services, which are inherently safer. Also, most countries have a labour inspectorate that can orchestrate a risk-based strategy of hazard control with varying degrees of efficiency. In those that do not, and where the 'informal sector' dominates, risks are higher for those who have to earn their living that way – there are no health and safety rules when it comes to scavenging in dumps. Life outside work has also become safer, although rapid industrialization and growing prosperity in some countries have meant huge increases in road traffic, with an accompanying increase in accidents and pollution. Traditional occupational diseases such as pneumoconiosis and noise-induced deafness can be adequately controlled by the same strategies of hazard control used to limit accidental injury. However, the long latent period between exposure and the appearance of occupational diseases makes attribution and control more problematic. Thus, the modern epidemics of musculoskeletal disorders and work-related stress reflect new work

patterns and a working population with different characteristics from its forebears, as well as changes in the work environment itself.

Completely new jobs have appeared, with their accompanying hazards – for example, salad composers (dermatitis), aromatherapists and nail enhancers (allergies), and semiconductor assemblers (exposure to multiple toxins). Some ancient crafts have been associated recently with hitherto unrecognized hazards, such as renal failure in traditional Chinese herbal medicine factory workers. Nanotechnology is in its infancy with only a vague appreciation of its hazards. Mesothelioma has yet to reach its peak incidence in the UK, causing over 2000 deaths per year from the major occupational carcinogen, asbestos, significant exposure to which ceased decades ago.

Although working conditions are undoubtedly cleaner, safer and in many ways better than before, work itself has changed. In the economically developed world there has been a shift from unskilled work to more highly skilled or multiskilled work in largely sedentary occupations. There is greater self-employment and a remarkable shift towards employment in small and medium-sized enterprises. More and more people work non-standard hours with consequences to their health. The percentage of women in employment has been growing for decades. Not everyone can cope with the newer, more flexible, less stable, intensively managed work style demanded by modern clients and contractors, and there is an increasing clamour for 'work–home balance'.

Heavy industry and 'dirty' manufacturing have been progressively exported to the developing world where occupational disease is still rife. Public perceptions and an expectation of good physical health and associated happiness, allied to improved sanitation and housing, availability of good food and good medical services, have highlighted those non-fatal conditions which might hitherto have been regarded as trivial but which have large effects on social functioning (such as deafness), work (such as backache) and happiness (such as psychological illness), contributing in turn disproportionately and adversely to disability-free years of life. The public is also more environmentally aware and concerned that some of the determinants of ill health are rooted in modern life and working conditions, giving rise to allergies, fatigue states and various forms of chemical sensitization. The estimation, perception and communication of risk may still, however, be quite primitive even in the most sophisticated of populations. The media definition of risk remains 'hazard plus outrage', and life as a threat has become a reality for many (Box 1.4).

Box 1.4 Annual death risks HSE

Annual risk of death for various causes averaged over the entire population

Cause of death	Annual risk
Cancer	1 in 387
Injury and poisoning	1 in 3137
Road accidents	1 in 16 800
Gas incident (fire, explosion or carbon monoxide poisoning)	1 in 1 510 000
Lightning	1 in 18 700 000

Average annual risk of injury as a consequence of an activity

Type of accident risk	Annual risk
Fairground accidents	1 in 2 326 000 rides
Road accidents	1 in 1 432 000 kilometres travelled
Rail travel accidents	1 in 1 533 000 passenger journeys
Burn or scald in the home	1 in 610

Average annual risk of death as a consequence of an activity

Activity associated with death risk	Annual risk
Maternal death in pregnancy	1 in 8200 maternities
Surgical anaesthesia	1 in 185 000 operations
Scuba diving	1 in 200 000 dives
Fairground rides	1 in 834 000 000 rides
Rock climbing	1 in 320 000 climbs
Canoeing	1 in 750 000 outings
Hang-gliding	1 in 116 000 flights
Rail travel accidents	1 in 43 000 000 passenger journeys
Aircraft accidents	1 in 125 000 000 passenger journeys

Taken from www.hse.gov.uk/education/statistics.htm.

Useful websites

International http://www.who.int/web.org; http://www.ilo.int/web.org; http://www.icoh.int/web.org

Africa http://www.nioh.ac.za

Australia http://www/safeworkaustralia.gov.au

Europe http://osha.europa.eu

Finland http://www.ttl.fi

Japan http://www.jaiosh.go.jp

Poland http://www.imp.ldz.p

United Kingdom http://www.hse.gov.uk; http://www.facoccmed.ac.uk; http://www.som.org.uk; http://www.hpa.org.uk

United States http://www.cdc.gov/niosh http://www.epa.gov/ http://www.acoem.org

CHAPTER 2

Health, Work and Wellbeing

Nerys Williams

Independent Consultant Occupational Physician, Solihull and London, UK

OVERVIEW

- Work is generally good for both physical and mental wellbeing
- Work can help recovery and a return to normal life
- Being out of work has a detrimental effect on physical and mental health
- Health is one of the many factors that influence wellbeing
- Wellbeing has an important influence on productivity at work

Introduction

The links between health, work and wellbeing have been recognized by occupational physicians for hundreds of years but only much more recently by other healthcare professionals, employers and the general public.

There are a number of dimensions to the health–work interface: the health risks of being in and out of work, the health impact of moving between employment and unemployment, and of the effects of work on health, health on work and the role of rehabilitation and of wellbeing.

General health impacts

An independent review of the scientific evidence around health and work by Waddell and Burton (2006) has shown that work:

- can be therapeutic for people with both physical and mental health problems and can help promote recovery
- minimizes the risk of the physical, mental and social effects of long term unemployment
- reduces social exclusion and poverty
- can improve the quality of life and wellbeing

Conversely the review also reported a strong association between worklessness (a term used to describe people who are economically inactive, i.e. of working age but not working, not in full time education or training, and not actively seeking work) and poor physical and mental wellbeing. They also reported that there was strong evidence that unemployment leads to:

- 20% excess mortality
- two to three times the risk of poor general health
- two to three times the risk of poor mental health
- higher medical consultation, medication consumption and hospital admission rates.

The review contained some provisos however – the research which has been undertaken is about group effects – within groups a minority of individuals may experience contrary health effects and that the beneficial effects are dependent on the nature and quality of work undertaken. But overall the authors concluded that work is generally good for health and wellbeing in the majority of cases and that this is true for people with disabilities and for most people with common health problems (such as back pain, stress, anxiety and depression).

It should not be forgotten that work provides more than financial gains – there are also other benefits for specific groups of working age people: for people who are out of work getting back into employment improves their self-esteem and general physical and mental health, and reduces psychological distress and minor psychiatric morbidity.

Effects of work on health

Exposure to workplace agents, badly designed work and work where there is a mismatch between the individual, their capabilities and the demands of the job (be they physical, psychological or both) can harm health. The Health and Safety Executive annual statistics report that in 2009/2010 approximately 28.5 million days were lost overall from workplace injury and ill health, 23.4 million due to work-related ill health and 5.1 million due to workplace injury. There were also 152 deaths and 1.3 million people reported that in the previous year they believed they had suffered from an illness either caused by or aggravated by their work (HSE 2009/2010).

Effects of health on work

Despite the large number of people affected and number of days lost due to work which harms health, it is far commoner that lost

ABC of Occupational and Environmental Medicine, Third Edition.
Edited by David Snashall and Dipti Patel.
© 2012 John Wiley & Sons Ltd. Published 2012 by John Wiley & Sons Ltd.

time results from the effects of health on work, i.e. the person has a health condition which affects their ability to work but which was not caused by their work. Health conditions can result in the person staying at work and working less effectively (sometimes called presenteeism) or lead to their absence from the workplace due to sickness.

Whereas minor illnesses such as colds, flu and headaches are by far the commonest cause of short-term absence, musculoskeletal injuries and back pain are the next commonest for manual workers followed by stress (Chartered Institute of Personnel and Development (CIPD) 2010). Stress remains the second most common cause of short term absence in non-manual workers followed by musculoskeletal injuries and back pain (CIPD 2010). The most common causes of long-term absence are acute medical conditions (e.g. stroke, cancer, heart attacks) followed by musculoskeletal injuries, stress, mental ill health and back pain. Stress and musculoskeletal disorders are particularly common causes of long-term absence in the public sector (CIPD 2010) (Box 2.1).

Box 2.1 **Costs of sickness absence**

The total economic cost of working age ill-health is estimated to be over £100 billion per annum comprising over £60 billion in lost production, £10 billion as the costs of sickness absence from work and between £30 and £56 billion in costs of health and other informal care.

The costs of sickness absence alone we estimate to be in the region of £10 billion, comprising lost production (which effectively falls on employers) and individuals in lost salary. These do not include wider indirect costs to employers (and the additional costs of ill-health to the individual).

Source: Dame Carol Black 'Working for a Healthier Tomorrow' http://www.dwp.gov.uk/docs/hwwb-working-for-a-healthier-tomorrow.pdf

---

Specific risks to health of being out of work

In addition to the general and mental health risks as outlined above, unemployed people are more likely as a group, to smoke, drink alcohol and indulge in sexual risk taking. They also have a higher frequency of usage of GP services, of medication and of admission to psychiatric hospital. In terms of adopting healthy lifestyles people who are unemployed are reported to be less physically active than the employed, to have increased rates of obesity, and to be less successful at stopping smoking.

Unemployment and inability to work due to longstanding health conditions are costly for the individual, their family, for society and for the country. There are over 2 million people of working age currently claiming disability benefits, with mental and behavioural health conditions accounting for around 44% of the total.

Common health problems

Common health problems (CHP) is a term used to describe conditions such as back and neck pain, stress, anxiety and depression (Box 2.2). These are conditions which are very common, cause significant

short- and long-term absence and claims for disability benefits, but which are subjective with very few objective signs of illness. They are not minor or trivial but are often disabling, resulting in social isolation and intensive use of healthcare resources. An evidence review undertaken by Waddell *et al.* (2008) showed that, if identified early and managed correctly by rehabilitation, these conditions need not mean loss of time from work or unemployment.

Box 2.2 **Common health problems**

- Account for about two-thirds of sickness absence, long-term incapacity and early retirement
- Comprise mild/moderate mental health, musculoskeletal and cardio-respiratory conditions
- Have high prevalence rates in the adult population
- Are often subjective, and often have limited evidence of objective disease or impairment
- Are common whether in or out of work, risk factors are multifactorial, and cause-effect relationships ambiguous

Source: Waddell and Burton 2004.

Rehabilitation and obstacles to recovery

Vocational rehabilitation has been defined in the evidence review as 'whatever helps someone with a health problem stay at, return to and remain in work'. The authors concluded that there was a strong evidence base for many aspects of vocational rehabilitation and more evidence on cost benefit than in many other areas of health and social policy. They suggested that common health problems be given priority for a vocational rehabilitation approach because they account for two thirds of sickness absence and incapacity benefit claims and are preventable.

In terms of what action is needed, the evidence suggests that in the first 6 weeks or so, people can be helped to return to work with a few basic principles of healthcare and workplace management. This can be cost neutral. For around 5–10% of workers additional help maybe needed at 6 weeks of sickness absence.

The key message from the review is that what was needed is both a work focussed approach to healthcare and flexible workplaces. A stepped care approach is needed, with early intervention and coordinated communication and coordination between the key players – the employee, the employer and the GP.

The 'fit note'

In the UK, the concepts underlying the evidence base on rehabilitation influenced the replacement of the old style 'sick note' with a new style 'fit note' in April 2010. The 'fit note' differs from its predecessor in that it allows the doctor to certify that a person 'may be' fit for work and recognizes that people can often return to work earlier and safely when they are less than 100% fully recovered, provided they have flexibility in their job and/or their workplace (Department for Work and Pensions (DWP), personal communication, 17 January 2011; DWP 2011). It is hoped that the 'fit note' will encourage conversations about work capability between the individual (the 'patient') and their line manager and so facilitate a return to work and reduce the risk of job loss secondary to prolonged absence.

In order to be effective, a key point is that rehabilitation needs to take place at the right time – if delayed and the person stays away from work then they lose the belief that they can do their job (known as self-efficacy) and move further away from the workplace, thus making it more difficult for rehabilitation to be successful.

Wellbeing

There has recently been a lot of interest in the area of wellbeing. It is increasingly referred to in Government policy and used to capture notions around good health, working conditions, wealth and access to services; it remains an imprecise term as it tries to encapsulate many dimensions of people's lives.

But the challenge for wellbeing is not only its definition but also its measurement. Objective measures such as the United Nations Human Development Index (UNHDI) have been published. This consists of indicators of life expectancy, education and knowledge, and gross domestic product but it has been challenged as to which indicators have been included and how they are weighted against each other.

An alternative approach is that put forward by Layard (2005) which measures 'life satisfaction' or 'happiness'. Here an individual's happiness is determined by the dimensions put forward by Stiglitz *et al.* (2009) which identifies the multidimensional nature to wellbeing and is outlined in Box 2.3, but it is the individual who attaches relative importance and weighting to each factor.

Box 2.3 **Commission on the Measurement of Economic Performance and Social Progress Dimensions of wellbeing**

Material living standards (income, consumption and wealth)
Health
Education
Personal activities including work
Political voice and governance
Social connections and relationships
Environment (present and future)
Insecurity, of an economic as well as of a physical nature

The wellbeing field is developing rapidly as links between employee wellbeing, engagement and productivity emerge.

Conclusion

The evidence underpinning the links between health and work suggests that the right type of work is generally good for both physical and mental health for most people including people with disabilities and common health problems. It also suggests that return to work can improve a person's health condition – for example by ending social isolation.

A key message for doctors is that advice to stay off work can potentially have serious long-term consequences in terms of job loss

and increased health risks. The evidence base on health, work and rehabilitation has influenced the development and introduction of the 'fit note' in April 2010. By including the option of indicating that a patient 'may be' fit for work, the doctor is encouraging communication between the patient and their employer to offer flexible work or working arrangements to allow the person to return before they are fully recovered but when they can safely do so.

Health is only one of many factors which are thought to contribute to wellbeing, that overarching, general state of mind and body which is receiving increasing attention from Government and the research community. The links between work and health and work and wellbeing are clearly established. The challenge for occupational health is to maximize the growing interest in the field and work with other specialities to define and clarify what 'good work' looks like and how it can sustain and support an individual throughout their working life.

The future

The global economy is undergoing substantial change which will impact on the world of work. Economic growth in countries such as China and India, new technologies and globalization will present major challenges to businesses. The removal of the default retirement age and economic pressures will encourage more people to work for longer, and the growing population of older workers may begin to develop conditions such as Parkinson's disease and dementia while in work which were previously only seen in the retired population. At the same time family commitments are likely to increase as people live longer and require care from their family members who may also have children – the so-called sandwich generation

The demographic changes which will occur will bring huge challenges as the need to manage the work–health interface becomes more important and the need to tap into the mental capital of older workers becomes crucial. As yet there is a lot we do not know about what good work looks like, particularly for older workers, and what employers can and should do to make their workplaces and work tasks more older worker friendly.

References

Health and Safety Executive (HSE). *Annual Statistics*. London; HSE, 2009/2010. http://www.hse.gov.uk/statistics/index.htm. Accessed 17 January 2011. *Official Government statistics on accidents and ill health at work in UK*

Chartered Institute of Personnel and Development (CIPD). London Annual Survey Report 2010. *Human resources professionals' annual survey of members*

DWP. Guidance on the 'fit note'. http://www.dwp.gov.uk/fitnote. Accessed 17 January 2011. *Government guidance on how and when to complete a 'fit note'*

Layard R. *Happiness: lessons from a new science*. London: Penguin Books, 2005. *Overview of the concept of happiness and its importance in working life by a leading thinker on the topic*

Stiglitz J, Sen A, Fitoussi J-P Report by the Commission on the Measurement of Economic Performance and Social Progress. 2009. *Economists view of the measurement of business performance*

Waddell G, Burton K. *Is work good for your health and well-being? An evidence review. Review of published literature on the effects of work on health and health on work*. London: The Stationery Office, 2006.

Waddell G, Burton K, Kendall N. *What works, for whom and when? Review of published evidence on what interventions facilitate return to work*. The Stationery Office, London, 2008.

Further reading

Foresight. Mental Capital and Wellbeing Project. *Making the most of ourselves in the 21st century. Final project report–Executive Summary*. London: The Government Office for Science, 2008. *Government commissioned review on mental health and wellbeing*

CHAPTER 3

Assessing the Work Environment

Keith T. Palmer and David Coggon

MRC Lifecourse Epidemiology Unit, University of Southampton, Southampton, UK

OVERVIEW

- Assessment of the workplace is central to the practice of occupational medicine
- 'Risk assessment' involves identifying hazards and gauging the likelihood of harm, so as to plan risk control measures
- Controls follow a hierarchy of effectiveness, with avoidance and substitution (most dependable) at one extreme and measures that rely on employees' compliance (least dependable) at the other
- Sometimes, sophisticated environmental measurements and formal research are needed to identify new hazards or to assess risks
- However, simple common sense observations, systematically made and recorded, can go along way towards preventing ill health at work

---

Understanding of the workplace is as central to the practice of occupational medicine as clinical assessment of the individual patient. It is an essential step in the control of occupational hazards. Moreover, by visiting a place of work, a doctor can appreciate the demands of a job, and thus give better advice on fitness for employment and/or modifications that may assist work after illness (see Chapter 7). Investigations may be prompted in various circumstances (Box 3.1).

Box 3.1 **Circumstances that may prompt investigation of a workplace**

Initial assessment when first taking over care of a workforce
Introduction of new processes or materials that could be hazardous
New research indicating that a process or substance is more hazardous than previously believed
Occurrence of illness or injury in the workforce suggesting an uncontrolled hazard
A need to advise on the suitability of work for an employee who is ill or disabled
Routine review

ABC of Occupational and Environmental Medicine, Third Edition.
Edited by David Snashall and Dipti Patel.
© 2012 John Wiley & Sons Ltd. Published 2012 by John Wiley & Sons Ltd.

Hazard and risk

Managing occupational risks to health requires identification of the 'hazards' in a workplace, and then assessment of the 'risks' that they pose (Figure 3.1). A hazardous agent or circumstance has the *potential* to harm (a hazard of water is drowning); 'risk' is the *likelihood that the hazard will be realized* (nil in a thimbleful of water, high in the open sea). Risk depends on the nature and extent of exposure to the hazardous agent or situation. The art of *risk assessment* (which is a legal requirement in many circumstances – see Chapter 5) is to identify and characterize material risks to health that may require control. In doing this, account must be taken of the seriousness of potential outcomes as well as their likelihood (a low chance of death would merit more attention than a high probability of light bruising). Identification of hazards may be assisted by manufacturers'

HAZARD

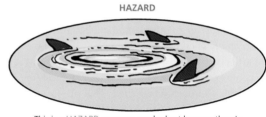

This is a HAZARD - no-one can be hurt becausr there's no-one here.

(a)

RISK

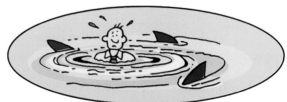

This is a RISK - someone may be harmed.

(b)

Figure 3.1 Hazards and risks. a) A hazard is a *potential* adverse effect of an agent or circumstance. Risk is the probability that harm will occur. Risk assessment involves identifying hazards and characterizing the associated risks. b) After listing the hazards, it is important to consider who might be exposed and in which job(s); how likely this is under the prevailing circumstances of the work (including any precautions followed); and the magnitude of expected exposures and their likely impact on health (the *risks* to health). (See also HSE 2006.).

safety data sheets, but assessment of risk requires an understanding of how work is conducted and of levels of exposure.

Inspecting the workplace

One method of assessment is direct inspection of the workplace. Inspections often take the form of a structured 'walk-through' survey.

Planning a walk-through survey

Industrial processes are complex, and hazards are plentiful. How should a survey be conducted? The arrangements and context are important. The initial visit should be by appointment (an unannounced snap inspection may be revealing, but is practicable only for a health and safety professional who has an established relationship of trust with the employer). Arrangements should be checked beforehand, as pre-planning saves time.

The survey should be structured, but the precise way it is organized is less important. At least three approaches are commonly adopted:

- *Following a process from start to finish* – from raw materials in to finished goods going out. What hazards occur at each stage? What are the risks? How should the risks be controlled? Do the controls actually work? This process-focused assessment aids basic understanding of the work and its requirements.
- *Auditing a single category of activity or hazard (such as dusty or noisy procedures or manual handling)* – wherever it occurs within the organization. Does the control policy work everywhere, or are there special problems or poor compliance (higher risks) in certain groups of workers or sites? This audit trail or hazard-focused assessment is useful for introducing and monitoring new policies.
- *Detailed inspection site by site (Box 3.2)* – What are the hazards in this particular site? How are the potential risks controlled? The inspection moves on only when the geographical unit of interest has been thoroughly inspected. This site-focused approach is appreciated by shop stewards and workers' representatives

with local ownership of the problem. They may accompany the inspection and often provide insight into working practices and problems not apparent during the visit.

Box 3.2 **Arranging a walk-through survey**

Visit by appointment (at least to begin with)
Check whether you will

- be accompanied by someone with responsibilities for safety
- see someone who can explain the process
- have a chance to see representative activities

See documentation on health and safety – e.g. data sheets, risk assessments, safety policy, accident book
Do some preliminary research – identify the sorts of hazard likely to be encountered and legal standards that are likely to apply
If visiting because of an individual's complaint, discuss it first with complainant

---

What to cover in a walk-through survey

The aim is to determine whether risks are acceptable, taking into account both the likelihood of an adverse outcome and its seriousness; or whether further control measures are required, and, if so, what these should be (Table 3.1).

Health and safety professionals use checklists to ensure that all the major types of hazard are considered and to ensure that the control options to reduce risks are fully explored. They seek to verify that these options have been considered in an orderly hierarchy:

- Since prevention is better than cure, can the hazard be avoided altogether? Or can a safer alternative be used (substituted) instead?
- Otherwise, can the process or materials be modified to minimize the problem at source? Can the process be enclosed? Or operated remotely? Can fumes be extracted close to the point at which they are generated (local exhaust ventilation)?
- Have these ideas been reviewed before issuing ear defenders, face masks or other control measures that rely on workers' compliance

Table 3.1 Simple checklist of control measures.

Option	Key questions to ask	Possible controls*
Avoidance or substitution	Does the material need to be used at all or will a less noxious material do the job?	Try using a safer material if one exists
Material modification	Can the physical or chemical nature of the material be altered?	Can it be obtained as a granule or paste rather than powder? Can it be used wet?
Process modification	Can equipment, layout, or procedure be adapted to reduce risk?	Can it be enclosed? Can dust be extracted? If material is poured, tipped, or sieved, can the drop height be lowered?
Work methods	Can safer ways be found to conduct the work? Can it be supervised or monitored? Do workers comply with methods?	Avoid dry sweeping (it creates dust clouds). Be careful with spills. Segregate the work; conduct it out of hours
Personal protective equipment	Have all other options been considered first? Is it adequate for purpose? Will workers wear it?	Provision of mask, visor, respirator, or breathing apparatus suitable for intended use

*A dust hazard is used as an example (see also Aw *et al.*, 2006).

('Do not smoke,' 'Do not chewy our fingernails,' 'Lift as I tell you to')?

- A realistic strategy should always place more reliance on control of risk at source than on employees' personal behaviour and discipline.

What the survey may find

The purpose of the walk-through survey is to be constructively critical. When good practices are discovered these should be warmly acknowledged. Faulty practices arise from ignorance as often as from cutting corners.

We have visited workplaces where expensive equipment, provided to extract noxious fumes from the worker's breathing zone, was switched off because of the draught, or directed over an ashtray to extract cigarette smoke rather than the fumes, or obstructed by bags of components and Christmas decorations.

Local exhaust ventilation may be visibly ineffective –the fan may be broken, the tubing disconnected, the direction of air flow across rather than away from the worker's breathing zone; protective gloves may have holes or be internally contaminated; the rubber seals of ear defenders may be perished with age. Poor house keeping may cause health risks (Figures 3.2–3.6). There may be no audit to check that items of control equipment are maintained and effective. Simple common-sense observations, systematically made and recorded, will go a long way towards preventing ill health at work.

The walk-through survey may prompt improvements directly or highlight a need for further investigation, such as measurements of exposure or a health survey.

Formal assessment of exposures

Formal measurement of exposure may be required if an important hazard exists and the risk is not clearly trivial. Often a specialized technique or sampling strategy will be needed, directed by an occupational hygienist. Two common approaches are static monitoring

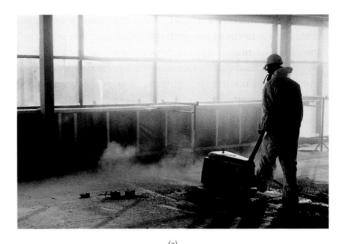

(a)

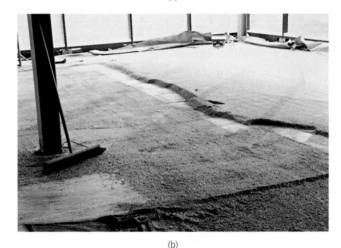

(b)

Figure 3.3 (a) This industrial process (scabbling) generates a lot of dust. Formal measurements revealed that respirable dust and silica levels exceeded those advocated in British standards by several-fold. (b) The highest exposure arose during sweeping up.

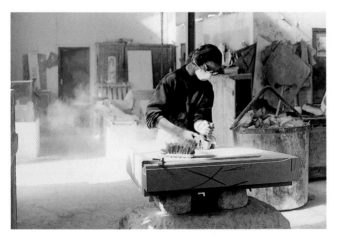

Figure 3.2 Workplace inspection aids understanding of the job demands and risks. This stonemason is exposed to hand-transmitted vibration, noise and silicaceous dust.

(measurement in a fixed worksite location) and personal monitoring (via instrumentation affixed to the worker –e.g. personal noise dosimetry). The former strategy, although more convenient, may be less representative of exposure levels in individuals than the latter. In the UK, the Health and Safety Executive publishes guidance on methods of measurement and acceptable exposure levels for many hazardous airborne chemicals and for some physical agents, such as noise and vibration (Box 3.3). In some cases, legal standards exist. For some chemicals absorbed through the skin or lungs, exposures can also be assessed by blood, urine or breath tests, and biological action levels have been proposed (*see* Further reading).

Action following a workplace assessment

The aim in assessing a workplace is to draw conclusions about prevailing risks and the adequacy of controls. But if this is to have a lasting benefit the results must be *communicated* to senior managers who have the authority to set, fund and oversee workplace policies. A written report is advisable, but a verbal presentation, perhaps at a meeting of the organization's safety committee, may have more impact, as may an illustrative slide show (Figures 3.3–3.6). Feedback on the findings of a workplace health survey can contribute importantly to the promotion of change and a safer working environment.

> **Box 3.3 Some exposure standards for airborne chemicals**
>
> In Britain, the Health and Safety Executive publishes a regularly updated list of exposure standards (EH40); and also advice on measuring strategies (EH42) and techniques (various EH publications)
>
> The listed chemicals are assigned legally binding Workplace Exposure Limits, defined either over the long term (as an 8-hour time weighted average) or the short term (15-minute reference period), or both.
>
> Exposure standards are published also in other countries-for example the threshold limit values (TLVs) established by the American Conference of Governmental Hygienists (ACGIH) (see http://www.acgih.org).

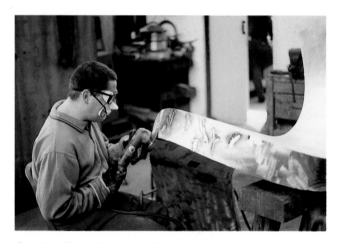

Figure 3.4 The worker is exposed to noise during grinding. He should be wearing ear defenders.

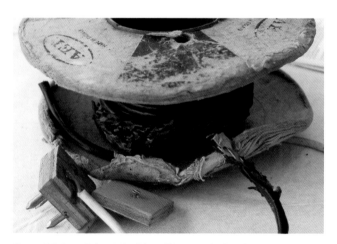

Figure 3.5 Frayed electrical cable and homemade plug discovered at a work site.

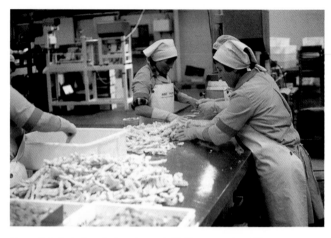

Figure 3.6 A cluster of wheezing and rhinitis occurred on this prawn-processing line. High-pressure hoses (used to free the prawns from the shells) had created aerosols containing crustacean protein.

Investigating new occupational hazards

As well as inspecting workplaces to identify and control known hazards, health and safety professionals should also be alert to the possibility of previously unrecognized occupational hazards. Suspicions may be aroused in various circumstances (Box 3.4). The characterization of new hazards requires scientific research, often using epidemiological methods. The most common types of investigation include cohort studies, case-control studies and cross-sectional surveys (Box 3.5).

> **Box 3.4 Reasons for suspecting an occupational hazard**
>
> Parallels with known hazards – e.g. use of a substance that has a similar chemical structure to a known toxin
>
> Demonstration that a substance or agent has potentially adverse biological activity *in vitro* – e.g. mutagenicity in bacteria
>
> Demonstration that a substance or agent causes toxicity in experimental animals
>
> Observation of sentinel cases or clusters of disease

> **Box 3.5 Commonly used epidemiological methods**
>
> *Cohort studies* – People exposed to a known or suspected hazard are identified, and their subsequent disease experience is compared with that of a control group who have been unexposed or exposed only at a lower level. Cohort studies generally provide the most reliable estimates of risk from occupational hazards, but need to be large if the health outcome of interest is rare.
>
> *Case–control studies* – People who have developed a disease are identified, and their earlier exposure to known or suspected causes is compared with that of controls who do not have the disease. Case–control studies are often quicker and more economical to conduct than cohort studies, especially for the investigation of rarer diseases. However, risk estimates tend to be less accurate, particularly if exposures are ascertained from subjects' recall.

Cross-sectional surveys – A sample of people are assessed over a short period of time to establish their disease experience and exposures. The prevalence of disease is then compared in people with different patterns of exposure. This method is best suited to the investigation of disorders that do not lead people to modify their exposures (e.g. because associated disability makes them unfit for certain types of work). Where a disease causes people to leave a workforce, cross-sectional surveys may seriously under-estimate the risks associated with exposure.

Assessment of disease clusters

One starting point for investigation of a workplace may be the observation of a disease cluster. A cluster of disease is an excess incidence in a defined population, such as a workforce, over a relatively short period (less than a day for acute complaints such diarrhoea to several years for cancer).

Apparent clusters are not uncommon in occupational populations, and investigation sometimes leads to the recognition of new hazards (Table 3.2). For example, the link between nickel refining and nasal cancer was first discovered when two cases occurred at the same factory within a year. On the other hand, excessive investigation of random clusters is wasteful of resources. The extent to which a cluster is investigated depends on the level of suspicion of an underlying hazard and the anxiety that it is generating in the workforce. A staged approach is recommended (Box 3.6).

Box 3.6 **Stages in investigating occupational clusters of disease**

Specify disease and time period of interest. Confirm diagnoses of index cases
Search for further cases. Is the observed number of cases excessive?
What do affected workers have in common? Do their shared exposures carry known or suspected risks?
What is known about the causes of the disease?
Further investigation
Epidemiology
Clinical investigation

Is there a true cluster?
The first step is to specify the disease and time period of interest and to confirm the diagnoses of the index cases that prompted concern. Sometimes no further action is needed. Of three cases of brain cancer, two might turn out to be secondary tumours from different primary sites. If suspicion remains, it is worth searching for further cases. Often, the number of identified cases is clearly excessive, but if there is doubt crude comparison with routinely collected statistics – such as from registers of cancers or mortality – should establish whether the cluster really is remarkable.

Further steps
If an elevated incidence is confirmed the next step is to find out what the affected workers have in common. Do they work in the same job

Table 3.2 Some important occupational hazards that have been identified and controlled through investigation of workplaces.

Hazard	Control measures
Bladder cancer from aromatic amines in the dyestuffs and rubber industries	Substitution of the chemicals concerned by non-carcinogenic alternatives
Lung cancer and mesothelioma from asbestos	Substitution by less hazardous materials such as man-made mineral fibres; dust control and personal protective equipment in asbestos removal
Coal workers' pneumoconiosis from dust in mines	Dust suppression by water spraying
Occupational deafness from exposure to noise	Substitution or enclosure of noisy processes; exclusion zones; personal protective equipment

or building, and do they share exposure to the same substances? If so, what is known about the risks associated with shared activities and exposures? This information may come from published reports, or manufacturers' data sheets. Scientific articles should also be searched to identify known and suspected causes of the disease of interest. Could any of these be responsible for the cluster?

Getting help
At this stage the cause of the cluster may have been identified or suspicions sufficiently allayed to rule out further investigation. If concerns remain it may be necessary to carry out further, more formal epidemiological investigation to assess more precisely the size of the cluster and its relation to work. Help with such studies can often be obtained from academic departments of occupational medicine. Also, patients may need to be referred to specialist centres for investigations such as dermatological patch testing or bronchial challenge.

Conclusion

Over the years, investigation of workplaces has made a major contribution to public health through the identification and control of occupational hazards (Table 3.2) and through improved placement and rehabilitation of workers with illness or disability. While some types of investigation require special technical expertise, all health and safety professionals should be familiar with the principles, and capable of inspecting and forming a preliminary assessment of working environments.

References

Aw TC, Gardner K, Harrington JM. *Occupational health pocket consultant*, 5th edn. Oxford: Wiley-Blackwell, 2006. *This concise textbook explains how to make and interpret measurements of the working environment. It also provides a very good overview of other topics in occupational medicine*
Health and Safety Executive (HSE) *Five steps to risk assessment*. INDG163 (Rev 2). Sudbury: HSE Books, 2006. *This free leaflet suggests a simple five-point plan for assessing the risks in a workplace*

Further reading

Coggon D, Rose G, Barker DJP. *Epidemiology for the uninitiated*, 4th edn. London: BMJ Publishing Group, 1997. http://resources.bmj.com/bmj/readers/epidemiology-for-the-uninitiated/epidemiology-for-the-uninitiated-fourth-edition. *This short primer provides a useful introduction to epidemiological methods and principles*

Coggon D. Epidemiological methods and evidence-based occupational medicine. In: Baxter PJ, Aw T-C, Cockcroft A, Durrington P, Harrington JM (eds) *Hunter's diseases of occupations*, 10th edn. London: Hodder and Stoughton, 2010, pp. 77–88. *A brief overview of epidemiological methods used in occupational medicine*

Health and Safety Executive. Guidance Note EH40/2005. List of approved workplace exposure limits (as consolidated with amendments October 2007). http://www.hse.gov.uk/coshh/table1.pdf. *This HSE publication, which is regularly updated, provides guidance on the permissible limits for exposure to a number of chemicals*

Health and Safety Executive. *Monitoring strategies for toxic substances*. HSG173. Sudbury: HSE Books, 2006. *Assessment of exposure requires a strategy of representative sampling: this priced booklet explains the required approach*

HSE. Working with substances hazardous to health. What you need to know about COSHH. http://www.hse.gov.uk/pubns/indg136.pdf. *The HSE website (http://www.hse.gov.uk) contains many COSHH-related resources, of which this is one example, current at the time of writing. Sample risk assessments by industry, case studies, and worked examples of risk assessment are also provided. (Try entering 'COSHH' as a search term and visiting the guidance pages.)*

Olsen J, Merletti F, Snashall D, Vuylsteek K. *Searching for causes of work-related disease: an introduction to epidemiology at the worksite*. Oxford: Oxford University Press, 1991.

Pittom A. Principles of workplace inspection. In: Howard JK, Tyrer FH (eds) *Text book of occupational medicine*. Edinburgh: Churchill Livingstone, 1987, pp. 91–106. *These two references describe the process of workplace inspection in greater detail*

Verma DK, Purdham JT, Roels HA Translating evidence of occupational conditions into strategies for prevention. *Occup Envion Med* 2002; 59: 205–213. *This review illustrates how evidence on risks and control measures can be used to develop effective preventive strategies in the workplace*

CHAPTER 4

Practising Occupational Health

Anil Adisesh

Health and Safety Laboratory, Buxton, UK

OVERVIEW

- The relationship between health, work and wellbeing is complex and best understood using a biopsychosocial approach
- There are several different models of occupational health service delivery
- An assessment of occupational health needs is key to the delivery of an appropriate service
- Communication is an important aspect of practice and should be conducted within a framework of confidentiality and consent

Introduction

Occupational health (OH) is an endeavour which is contributed to by clinicians, technical specialists and professionals from a range of science backgrounds (Box 4.1). Each will have their area of special knowledge (e.g. a physician will primarily be expert in occupational medicine and therefore the diagnosis and management of occupational disease) and all should have an understanding of the

---

Box 4.1 **Disciplines that may be involved in Occupational Health practice**

- Specialist occupational health physicians
- Specialist nurse practitioners in occupational health
- Other doctors and nurses working in occupational health
- Clinical support workers
- Occupational health technicians
- Psychologists
- Counsellors
- Occupational hygienists
- Health and safety advisers
- Ergonomists
- Epidemiologists
- Toxicologists
- Radiation protection advisers

ABC of Occupational and Environmental Medicine, Third Edition.
Edited by David Snashall and Dipti Patel.
© 2012 John Wiley & Sons Ltd. Published 2012 by John Wiley & Sons Ltd.

beneficial contributions that can be made by other disciplines and the synergies that can result from multidisciplinary working.

There is now a wider understanding of the need to address the complex interaction between work and health as distinct from workplace safety, and this growing recognition is reflective of the increasing maturity of occupational health as a discipline. The World Health Organization (WHO) 1995 statement on OH (Box 4.2) is still valid today, and emphasizes the concept of the wellbeing of workers; a theme that has been further developed in recent years and has been the subject of a national review in the UK, 'Working for a Healthier Tomorrow'. The cause and effect relationship between physical hazard and injury is more readily understood in the context of occupational safety whereas a biopsychosocial approach (Figure 4.1) is required to address the altogether more complex issue of health, work and wellbeing.

Box 4.2 **The World Health Organization (WHO) 1995 statement on Occupational Health**

Occupational health should aim at: the promotion and maintenance of the highest degree of physical, mental and social well-being of workers in all occupations; the prevention amongst workers of departures from health caused by their working conditions; the protection of workers in their employment from risks resulting from factors adverse to health; the placing and maintenance of the worker in an occupational environment adapted to his physiological and psychological capabilities; and, to summarize, the adaptation of work to man and of each man to his job.

Joint ILO/WHO Committee on Occupational Health First Session (1950) and revised 12th Session (1995)

The objectives of an OH service are influenced by statutory requirements for compliance with health and safety legislation, national and other guidance for occupational fitness, and the need for medical advice to inform management action. Looking beyond these fundamental elements, a complementary definition of occupational health might be, 'The value added to workers' health and wellbeing by an employer's activities to realize key business benefits'. One of the challenges for OH practitioners is to demonstrate that benefit by means of meaningful outcome-based metrics or key performance indicators (Box 4.3).

technical occupational safety and medical advice particularly to the HSE.

Provision of occupational health services

There is statutory provision of OH services in many European countries, including France, Spain, the Netherlands, Belgium, Portugal, Germany, Denmark and Greece. In Italy occupational and environmental health services are provided within the national health service. In the UK there is no regulation requiring the provision of OH services by employers, although all employees of the National Health Service (NHS) should have access to an accredited specialist in occupational medicine.

The WHO has formulated a concept of basic OH services which extends the principles of primary healthcare to occupational health (Box 4.4). The 'intermediate level' referred to anticipates a regulatory or inspectorate function provided by an occupational health institution containing both occupational medical expertise and the provision of clinical services. The Occupational Safety and Health Administration (OSHA) in the United States regulates workplaces and enforces health and safety law whereas NIOSH (National Institute for Occupational Safety and Health), a branch of CDC (Centres for Disease Control) conducts research and makes recommendations on matters of occupational health and safety. These twin functions are combined in the UK Health and Safety Executive (HSE), with the Health and Safety Laboratory (HSL) providing

The roots of OH in Germany go back to 1884 when Otto von Bismarck set up a social insurance system emphasizing prevention, rehabilitation and compensation from a single source. This insurance-based system sees the federal technical inspection services of the statutory accident insurers assessing the compliance of employers with regulations and adjusting their premiums based on risk.

The organization of OH services in the UK varies, as does their level of service provision. They may be provided by in-house OH departments, external (outsourced) private OH companies, or a combination of the two. The latter can consist of a small corporate OH (or OH plus safety or plus environment or even plus consumer safety) function procuring certain services from contracting bodies. Access to OH services tends to be universal in the public sector and large private companies, whereas the services available to and/or taken up by small and medium-sized enterprises (SMEs) (defined as those with fewer than 250 employees) tend to be limited.

Multinationals often provide comprehensive in-house OH services which are truly multidisciplinary and can influence population health within the regions or even the countries in which they operate by initiatives such as building local health clinics. However, even these multinational companies tend to outsource their OH services to the private sector, sometimes retaining a Chief Medical Officer as an 'intelligent customer'. In the UK, the public sector is the largest user of OH services, either in-house or contracted. Most NHS OH services are in-house, and many provide commercial OH services to a number of external enterprises (both small local companies and larger industries) as a means of income generation. Large private OH companies tend to focus their activities on large Government or commercial OH contracts.

SMEs, representing a large proportion of the overall UK economy, tend to have limited access to OH services, with the decision to purchase such services often driven either by a need to comply with health and safety legislation, the need for health surveillance or management's occasional need for medical advice in the case of a sickness absence problem. Where SMEs do procure OH services, they tend to be from smaller private OH companies, individual practitioners, NHS OH services, or local general practices. To address this variability, access to a government-funded OH telephone advice line is now available to all SMEs (and also to GPs who

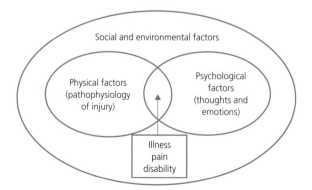

Figure 4.1 The biopsychosocial model: injury, pain and disability.
Source: Dunstan DA, Covic T, Compensable work disability management: A literature review of biopsychosocial perspectives *Australian Occupational Therapy Journal* (2006) 53, 67–77. Reproduced with permission of Wiley-Blackwell.

may need occupational health advice for their patients (Health for Work Adviceline www.health4work.nhs.uk)).

Services can be delivered in a number of ways, and can and should use innovative methods where these enhance occupational health. This increasingly includes the use of telemedicine for remote workers, secure online questionnaires, electronic fitness confirmation to facilitate pre-placement, occupational health assessment, and spirometry with remote over-read by a respiratory physiologist to ensure quality standards and consistent reporting.

In order to make an informed decision about OH provision and how this should be delivered, an OH needs assessment should be undertaken. A needs assessment may simply be based on an organization's health and safety risk assessment; however, an experienced occupational physician is likely to identify pertinent risks to health that may have been overlooked by a health and safety professional, and a workplace visit to inspect the circumstances of work should always be incorporated (Figure 4.2). In addition a thorough assessment would include a consideration of the relevant policies that the company has or should have (e.g. drugs and alcohol, absence management), and relevant occupational health and safety statistics (e.g. workplace accidents, sickness absence data). Also included might be the need for health promotion in that particular work environment (Figure 4.3), and to make recommendations for the involvement of OH in committees such as those owned by human resources, risk management/health and safety, standard setting and communication. The OH needs as perceived by relevant stakeholders (e.g. managers, employees, lawyers, human resources, etc.) should naturally be taken into account

Relationships with others

The procurement, and often the line management of OH services, is usually the responsibility of the human resources function of a business. This can sometimes lead to a skewing of the delivery of OH towards the human resources agenda and away from aspects

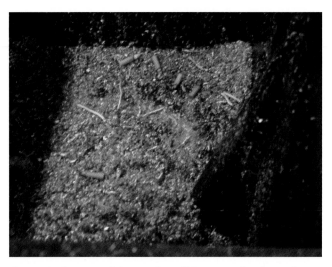

Figure 4.3 Cigarette ends in a metal swarf bin at an engineering works. Targeted workplace health promotion can help reduce the risk of occupational respiratory disease, the medical effects of smoking and fire.

of provision concerned with legislative compliance and the effects of work on health. The OH practitioner may therefore have to make the case for investigative, preventive and health surveillance activities with support from those responsible for organizational health and safety compliance.

The OH service should have a close working relationship with the risk management/health and safety function as accident and other incident data can inform OH activity whereas OH data may contribute to better risk assessment and therefore prevention. Compliance, policy development and mitigation of legal liability may also be aided by cooperation. There may be other specialist functions within an organization where an interdependency with the OH service should occur such as infection prevention and control in a healthcare setting. The senior management of any organization is probably the most important influence on organizational health as through its actions and policies does the organizational culture develop. It is therefore important that the lead OH clinician has good access to key senior managers, who will act as champions for occupational health. Generally a holistic approach to occupational health is aligned with organizational aims, since the health of the workforce is assured and individuals feel secure and valued at work

The Government's role in occupational health in the UK had until about 2006 been limited to that of enforcement and guidance through the efforts of the HSE, although greater emphasis was given to safety. This has in part been redressed by the current HSE strategy in which one of the aims is 'To specifically target key health issues and to identify and work with those bodies best placed to bring about a reduction in the incidence rate and number of cases of work related ill health'. The HSE's parent body, the Department of Work and Pensions (DWP) has done much to highlight the role of OH. With the Department of Health, the DWP commissioned Dame Carol Black's seminal review, and the Government's response has included some useful initiatives in the health and work sector. Examples are the introduction of 'Fit notes', the inclusion of work-based outcomes in guidance from the National Institute for Health and Clinical Excellence, and educational projects for GPs

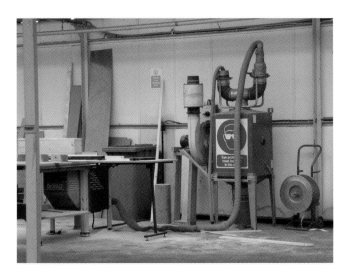

Figure 4.2 Performing a workplace visit allows the circumstances of work to be observed. Wood workshop: note the crushed ventilation exhaust tubing on the floor. Wood dust is a recognized respiratory sensitizer and hardwood dust can cause sinonasal cancer.

designed to increase their confidence in dealing with work-related matters. However, although the HSE publishes annual statistics on health and safety, these relate to its activities rather than the 'occupational health of the nation', and at a local level workplace health is not a matter normally to be addressed in the reports of Directors of Public Health. Furthermore, although GPs have been encouraged to become more aware of work and health the recording of a patient's occupation is not often done and may therefore inhibit the recognition of work-related issues and informed advice on a return to work (Figure 4.4).

Communication

The introduction of the fit note (Statement of Fitness for Work) in the UK has been successful in changing the focus of a GP consultation towards what a person may be able to do and when they may be able to do it rather than the negative connotations of inability. Furthermore, it has allowed direct communication with employers and their OH professionals aimed towards finding suitable work (even if only on a temporary basis) while full resolution of residual medical symptoms occurs. This change has engendered a culture of active rehabilitation rather than passive waiting for full fitness, and has allowed the recognition that the latter is more likely to be achieved sooner with the engagement of the employee, employer, OH and primary care services.

The first indications of a medical condition may be manifest at work through changes in performance, communication with colleagues, or attitudes to work in the case of common mental health problems. In a supportive work environment this may lead to contact with OH services through management referral and access to counselling services. Where an OH service is involved, communication with an employee's GP may be made with the employee's consent. In other cases a medical condition that is thought to be caused by work may be recognized through statutory health surveillance activities (which for example is required for workers with known respiratory sensitizers that may cause occupational

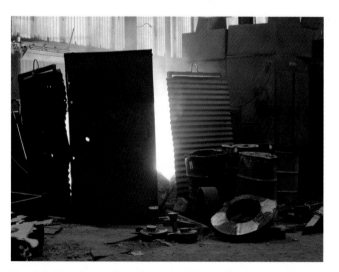

Figure 4.4 To advise on fitness for work a doctor would need to know at least the patient's job. A welder in a foundry uses air arc gouging, note the fume, intense light including UV, heat and several trip hazards.

asthma, e.g. paint sprayers working with isocyanate paints). The OH service should be able to initiate preliminary investigations; however, if further referral to secondary care for formal diagnosis is needed, their GP would need to be aware of the symptoms, medical findings and results of any investigations in order to make an appropriate hospital referral.

Communication between an employer and an employee's treating doctor is usually initiated by the OH service requesting information from the doctor. Occasionally a request may come directly from a manager or human resources department. The request should be accompanied by appropriate authorization to disclose medical details to an employer or their medical representative. In the UK this requirement for consent is a provision of the Access to Medical Reports act 1988 (Box 4.5).

Box 4.5 Medical Reports Act 1988

The act established a right of access by individuals to reports relating to themselves provided by medical practitioners for employment or insurance purposes and to make provision for related matters.

The act gives patients certain rights. The patient may:

- refuse to allow a medical report from their treating doctor
- allow the report to be sent unseen
- see the report during the 6-month period after it was written
- see the report before it is sent to the employer (a 21-day period is allowed)
- ask their doctor to change any part of the report which they consider to be wrong or misleading before consenting to its release
- append their own comments
- refuse to let the doctor send the report

When asked to provide a report it is important for the corresponding doctor to establish whether the report is intended to go to a doctor retained by the company or to a lay person (e.g. a manager). The latter may not fully understand a report containing medical jargon, which could be misinterpreted or give rise to unnecessary concern to the detriment of the patient (Boxes 4.6 and 4.7). Reports to an OH department, however, will be held in medical confidence and medical terminology may aid communication. The work-related implications can then be explained to management with advice based upon a knowledge of the working environment. It is in everyone's interests (patient, family doctor, hospital doctor, employer, occupational physician, society as a whole) to get patients back to suitable work as safely and quickly as possible and to prevent their premature return to work beyond their current capacity. Rapid, accurate communication is essential, but the biggest delay occurs when the treating doctor fails to answer a request for information from the OH service. Delays often cause difficulty to the patient, sometimes financial loss due to inability to work, pending a decision on fitness for work. Opinions, on the part of the treating doctor, regarding fitness to work may be unhelpful when not specifically asked for, particularly if the patient is aware of the opinion. For example, a family doctor may consider a 'process worker' who is undergoing investigation for syncope, as fit to work.

The safety of the individual and others in the workplace may be at risk if the doctor is not aware of their duties, e.g. working alone in a control room, wearing breathing apparatus, etc. Doctors may also create a legal liability for themselves in providing a specific opinion on fitness when not aware of all relevant information and without sufficient expertise.

Box 4.6 **Example 1**

An employee is absent from work certified as having 'back pain' and medical advice is requested about the likelihood of a return to work.

Letter from a doctor acting as medical adviser to a company to a manager, containing too much medical information and terms. There is also a lack of advice about work capabilities and rehabilitation.

Dear Mrs Smith,

You requested a report on Mrs. ... She was seen by her GP the day after a fall at home 3 months ago. She was initially treated with analgesics and given advice to remain active within the limits of her pain. Unfortunately her symptoms progressed with sciatic type pain in the right leg. Owing to the onset of symptoms of urinary incontinence she was referred urgently to the general hospital. She underwent an MR scan which confirmed a large L5, S1 disc prolapse causing a cauda equina syndrome. As a result she had a surgical decompression which was successful. She is expected to make a good recovery. I would hope that she would be able to resume employment as a domestic supervisor in the near future. I hope this is of some assistance to you in organizing your plans.

Yours sincerely,

Box 4.7 **Example 2**

This reply from an occupational health department is more informative for a manager.

Dear Mrs Smith,

You requested a report on Mrs ... , who works as a domestic assistant and has been absent from work for 3 months due to a back condition. Mrs ... back pain progressed and required admission to hospital for urgent surgery. It is now 6 weeks after her operation and she is able to do all her usual activity at home although slower than usual. She is able to walk for 30 minutes before needing to rest.

She is likely to find it easier to return to work starting with some mornings initially, then increasing the length of the working day in discussion with you so that over a period of 6 weeks she resumes her usual hours. She may have more difficulty with tasks involving lifting and bending such as cleaning inside low cupboards or emptying a mop bucket. She tells me that she also has supervisory responsibilities and these would be easier for her to manage at first. She has been given a copy of 'The Back Book' which should help reassure her that a return to work within her capability is appropriate. She is also attending physiotherapy on a weekly basis, and may require time during the working day for these appointments. It is likely that the disability provisions of the Equality Act would apply to her medical condition and the above measures should be considered as possible adjustments.

Kind regards,

The General Medical Council has recently issued helpful clarification on confidentiality and consent when providing reports relating to employment. The essential principle is that there should be 'no surprises' for the patient concerned about the information to be sent (see Chapter 6) (Box 4.8).

Box 4.8 **Faculty of Occupational Medicine advice to minimize the difficulties in complying with GMC advice on confidentiality (Published February 2010)**

- Having clarity of purpose about the assessment being undertaken and whether it is necessary to process information in a way that involves a disclosure
- Ensuring that the patient receives comprehensive information about the whole process at the outset and provides consent for the entire sequence of activity
- Emphasizing the duty of the occupational physician to be impartial and to build trust with every patient contact
- Making it explicit to the patient and the commissioning body that this is a consensual process in which consent can be withdrawn at any time but not seeking renewed consent at every stage
- Considering copying all reports to patients as a routine when sending them out
- Seeking to identify the nature of a patient's concerns about the provision of a report – often these relate to perceptions of their employer's actions rather than the report itself. Signposting the patient to sources of advice (e.g. trade union, Citizens Advice, etc.) may be helpful
- Developing simple procedures to offer to show or provide an advance copy of a report to the patient when such access is requested
- In cases where the patient asks to see a copy of the report before it is sent, allowing a reasonable period between providing the report to the patient and sending it to the commissioning body and advising the patient of these timescales
- Taking account of any factual errors highlighted by the patient and reviewing their impact on the professional judgement provided but making it clear to the patient and the commissioning body that stated opinion will not be altered as a result of lobbying
- Reminding patients that if consent to release a report is withdrawn the employer will have to act on whatever information is available to them and that this may not be in the best interests of the patient
- Where consent to release a report is withdrawn, retaining a copy of it within the occupational health record but marking it clearly to indicate that it has not been and will not be released
- Advising patients that in some cases, such as where there is a legal requirement or a public interest justification, disclosure may be made without their consent

---

The issue of payment for reports can also cause difficulties, and it is helpful for doctors providing reports to agree any fee before writing with a particular expectation. Generally speaking, when the reporting doctor has been asked for an opinion on matters such as fitness for work a higher fee would be attracted; simply reporting factual information such as previous diagnosis, current and proposed treatment does not require the exercise of specific judgement. Prompt payment to medical colleagues on receipt of a report should always be ensured by an OH service as a matter of good practice and professional courtesy. It is perhaps noteworthy that the NHS and other public sector rules may not permit payment before receipt of a report, which some doctors request because of previous experiences of late payment.

The OH practitioner will make an assessment of the information available and the employee's functional capacity to advise a manager whether there should be a restriction of specific duties, e.g. a building facilities assistant (portering duties) with a resolving back strain may have particular difficulty in performing heavier manual handling tasks such as bending and pushing loads for a while. However, he/she may be able to return to work to help staff in the facilities' call centre and assist with job allocation. Even if this activity could not be undertaken, there may still be a wide range of useful work to be undertaken. It is the skill of the manager to accommodate such advice (see Chapter 7). If there is doubt, a telephone conversation between the treating doctor and the OH service may help clarify the options available in managing a return to work. Furthermore there may be a duty on the employer to make a 'reasonable accommodation' to facilitate work under the disability provisions of the Equality Act 2010 (see Chapter 5).

In the rare event of a disagreement between occupational physician and family doctor on an individual's fitness for work, legal authorities tend towards the specialist occupational physician's opinion. They regard the occupational physician as being in fuller possession of all the facts, both clinical and relating to the actual work to be done, and thus in a better position to make a balanced and independent judgement.

Ill-health retirement

Sometimes medical conditions will preclude a return to work, because of permanent incapacity for a particular job – or any job. Information will often be requested in order to support ill-health retirement or it may be necessary to explain why an employee's job is to be terminated due to incapacity (where a person has not attended work for an excessive period because of sickness absence, whether or not eventual recovery of fitness is envisaged), the latter being a managerial decision. The pension fund's criteria for ill-health retirement may be explicit and leave little room for clinical opinion or may be quite open. A number of pension schemes have changed the criteria for award of medical retirement recognizing the impact of an ageing workforce (see Chapter 18) and the pressure on pension funds that follows. The employer is also required to consider whether retraining or redeployment are reasonable options whether under the Equality Act provisions or not. Although in the current economic climate these are becoming infrequently available options, it is preferable that views are discussed openly and an equitable decision made. If work has been a causal factor in the illness then civil litigation may arise against the employer.

The interface between OH and other healthcare providers should therefore be open and two-way, initiated by either party whenever discussion of patient care in relation to employment could be advantageous.

Governance

In common with other medical specialties occupational health has recognized the need for a clinical governance framework. However, unlike other areas of healthcare, in the UK there is no specific regulation of OH services. In the UK, the Faculty of Occupational Medicine is responsible for professional standards in the specialty and has recently issued *Safe and Effective Quality Occupational Health Services* – a document outlining standards for accreditation of good practice. These standards cover six areas : business probity, information governance, people (OH staffing), facilities and equipment, relationships with purchasers, relationships with workers. Currently the accreditation process is voluntary and open to all providers of OH services, whether in the public or private sector. Although the accreditation process is run by the Faculty of Occupational Medicine, it is not restricted to OH services led by occupational health physicians since nurse-led OH services should achieve the same standards. The UK professional registration body the Nursing and Midwifery Council registers qualified occupational health nurses as specialist community public health nurse (Occupational Health). The training a nurse undertakes in occupational health is in addition to general nurse education.

Audit and research

The support for clinical audit in occupational health, even within the NHS, has been poor and often not seriously considered. This has been partly addressed by the establishment in 2007 of the Health and Work Development Unit at the Royal College of Physicians. This unit was initially funded to undertake two national audits of NHS OH practice but now has an ongoing programme of audits and has produced a number of evidence-based guidelines. Audit within OH health services and within industry sectors occurs but is of variable quality and rarely leads to publication.

The UK research base in occupational medicine is small and has diminished over recent years but has been complemented by academic input from related disciplines with an interest in workplace health (e.g. respiratory physicians, organizational psychologists, etc.). The HSE funds most of the research, with some other government departments supporting specific projects. Other significant funding comes from a few charitable sources. Worldwide there has been a variable increase in OH operational research if the profusion of papers submitted to OH journals is any thing to go by (Box 4.9).

Box 4.9 **Research needs**

- Effective methods of health surveillance
- Evaluation of exposure intervention approaches on health outcomes
- Work implications of changes to workforce demographics (age, part time work, sex, disability, outsourcing)
- Organizational culture, leadership and workforce wellbeing
- Health effects of changes to processes and materials, e.g. emerging energy technology, waste recycling, nanomaterials
- OH service delivery models e.g. telemedicine and online data capture

Conclusion

OH is delivered through a variety of models and to a wide range of industrial sectors but the majority of the UK workforce still has no access to OH services. The present economic climate and other factors have focused attention in many countries on the reorganization of OH services to meet the needs of business. Such reviews are being carried out in the UK; in France, since at least 2004, changes have been made to a largely physician-based model with a reform act for occupational medicine recently passed by the Senate. One of the challenges of OH practice is to make the business case for services. This is facilitated by good-quality information, not only on activity but on outcome. The collection and analysis of these data provides a foundation for clinical audit and service-based research which can help build the evidence base that competent practitioners will incorporate into their practice. The importance of the evaluation of interventions was made clear in Dame Carol Black's report, 'if organizations are to form their own business case and share the value of health and well-being programmes with their directors, shareholders and other organizations, then it is imperative that they measure the outcomes of these programmes'.

Further reading

Agius R, Seaton A (2005) *Practical occupational medicine*, 2nd edn. London: Hodder Arnold. A *useful introductory text with many case examples to assist the reader*

Working for a healthier tomorrow. London, TSO, 2008. *Dame Carol Black's Review of the health of Britain's working age population. This report identifies factors that prevent good health for people of working age and identifies practical interventions and changes in attitudes, behaviours and services that are likely to be of benefit*

Occupational health service standards for accreditation. London. Faculty of Occupational Medicine. 2010. *Standards and minimum requirements that apply to occupational health services that participate in the UK voluntary accreditation scheme and to provide occupational health services with a framework for quality assurance. They are organized in six categories: Business probity; Information governance; People; Facilities and equipment; Relationships with purchasers; and Relationships with workers*

Guidance on ethics for occupational physicians, 6th edn, May 2006 and Revised Text for Articles 3.37–3.40 in the light of GMC Guidance on Confidentiality (October 2009) Faculty of Occupational Medicine. Published February 2010. *Addresses the major ethical questions which face occupational physicians and other occupational health professionals it provides an authoritative reference and guidance*

French reforms of occupational medicine. http://www.travail-emploi-sante. gouv.fr/actualite-presse,42/communiques,95/loi-portant-reforme-de-la-medecine,13719.html. *This speech outlines the discussions that are being undertaken to change the practice of occupational medicine in France; analogous reviews have taken place in the UK*

CHAPTER 5

Legal Aspects

Martyn Davidson

Royal Mail Group, London, UK

OVERVIEW

- The law is not a simple set of rules; judgement is required against a background of understanding
- Understanding the legal duties on the employer will ensure that occupational health advice will aid compliance
- Occupational health advice in employment cases must be fair and justifiable, not least because the practitioner can be called to a tribunal
- Recruiting people with a disability can be challenging. Managing them in the workplace means occupational health advice needs to be underpinned by a thorough understanding of relevant law
- Fear of litigation or concerns that when things go wrong there is automatically negligence can drive poor decisions

---

Introduction

Health and safety in the workplace is underpinned by legal duties upon employers to protect the workforce. Many elements of health and safety law fall within the expertise of the occupational health professional (OHP). There has also been a shift towards advising management about human resource issues, which makes an OHP's understanding of employment law and disability all the more important. These legal matters are technically complex, so it is important for OHPs to have a good understanding of relevant areas.

The UK legal system

The UK has a common law jurisdiction, which means that court decisions set precedent, binding future decisions and developing the law. Most civil law, including the area of tort (a civil wrong), has been built in this way. Opinions of higher courts (the highest being the Supreme Court from 2009, previously the House of Lords) are binding on those below. By contrast most criminal law is laid out in statute (Table 5.1). Acts of Parliament tend to be enabling, in that details will be developed beneath in regulations (statutory

Table 5.1 Civil and criminal law.

Civil law	Criminal law
Developed by court decisions	Statute from Parliament
Disputes between individuals	State prosecutes individuals
Corrects using compensation	Punitive
On the balance of probabilities	Beyond reasonable doubt

instruments). Codes of Practice often accompany which, whilst not themselves the law, will be regarded as a breach of the law if not followed.

Health and safety law

Current UK health and safety law has developed from the 1974 Health and Safety at Work Act. This 'umbrella' statute lays out general duties and the foundations for a risk based approach to managing workplace hazards (Box 5.1).

Box 5.1 **Major provisions of the 1974 Health and Safety at Work Act**

The Act sets out the general duties which employers have towards employees and members of the public, and employees have to themselves and to each other.

Section 2 'It shall be the duty of every employer to ensure, so far as is reasonably practicable, the health, safety and welfare at work of all his/her employees', with specific reference to:

- safe systems of work
- provision of information, instruction, training and supervision
- maintenance of the workplace and safe access and egress
- a working environment that is safe, without risks to health, and adequate as regards welfare.

Section 3 generates a duty toward other persons, e.g. contractors, visitors, the general public and clients.

Section 7 requires all employees to:

- take reasonable care for the health and safety of themselves and others
- cooperate with their employers.

ABC of Occupational and Environmental Medicine, Third Edition.
Edited by David Snashall and Dipti Patel.
© 2012 John Wiley & Sons Ltd. Published 2012 by John Wiley & Sons Ltd.

Table 5.2 The influence of Europe.

Legal act	Effect upon member states	Relationship with domestic legislation	Example
Regulations	Immediately in force	Override any conflicting domestic measures	REACH (Registration, Evaluation, Authorisation and restriction of Chemicals)
Directives	Must comply within specific timeframe	States have discretion as to how they achieve the requirements	1989 Framework Directive, generating manual handling, display screen regulations and many others
Decisions	Rulings in individual cases	Not binding	Grimaldi (1990): a miner denied compensation in Belgium since Dupuytren's is not a prescribed disease; appealed to European court

Table 5.3 Key Health and Safety Executive data 2009/10.

	Mortality/morbidity		
	Number	Rate per 100 000 in employment	Commonest cause
Fatalities	152	0.5	Falls
Injuries	12,430	473	Slips/trips
Self reported occupational ill health cases	1.3 million		Musculoskeletal disorders/Stress
Deaths from occupational illness	2249		Mesothelioma

Enforcement

Prosecutions	Completed/convicted	Enforcement notices	Fines total/average
1033	922/737	15 881	£11.6 million/£15 817

European influence
Adoption of the Single European Act in 1987 allowed the European Union (EU) to issue directives on, among other things, health and safety standards. This has since generated considerable UK domestic legislation, with regulations covering work equipment, noise, manual handling and display screens (Table 5.2).

Duty of care
The general principle is that those who generate risk as a consequence of work activities have a duty to protect anyone who may be affected. The extent of this duty in statute is commonly 'so far as is reasonably practicable'. This allows the employer to balance the degree of risk against the cost and difficulty of controlling it. A small employer with modest resources may reasonably argue reduced action in comparison with a large multinational. However, it is for the employer as the defendant to convince the court that he could not have done more; a reversal of the normal burden of proof in criminal cases.

'Reasonably practicable' has been defined more narrowly as a term than 'physically possible'. The risk must be real rather than hypothetical, and an employer can use industry standards and his own experience as a guide.

Prosecution
In the UK, the Health and Safety Executive (HSE) and Local Authorities are responsible for enforcing the 1974 Act. Inspectors have powers to issue improvement or prohibition notices, or prosecute. Prosecution generally results in a fine (Table 5.3).

Larger fines, intended to reflect the severity of the incident, tend to be the only ones to reach public awareness. For instance, the Buncefield fire in 2005 (Figure 5.1) resulted in prosecution by the HSE of five companies. Of these, Total UK was fined £3.6 million plus £2.6 million costs.

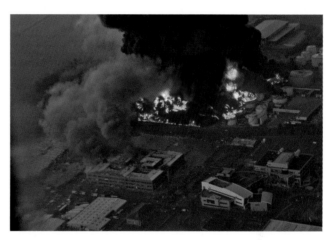

Figure 5.1 Fire at the Buncefield fuel depot. With permission from Chiltern Air Support Unit.

Where cases involve fatalities, they are referred to the Crown Prosecution Service.

Occupational injury and disease
Fatal and major injuries and occupational disease are reported to the HSE under the Reporting of Injuries, Diseases and Dangerous Occurrences Regulations 1995 (RIDDOR). Only medical conditions that are listed are reportable, and then only if the affected worker is involved in a relevant activity and the diagnosis is confirmed by a doctor.

Corporate manslaughter
The Corporate Manslaughter and Corporate Homicide Act 2007 introduced the concept of 'management failure', if the way in which the business was organized fell well below that which was reasonably to be expected and resulted in a fatality. This replaced the requirement to identify the 'controlling mind' within a company who could be held personally liable. The latter principle had proved impossible to apply to large businesses, such as P&O following

the Herald of Free Enterprise disaster. Smaller companies fared differently, as with the 1993 Lyme Bay kayaking tragedy in which four teenagers drowned. Peter Kite, one of the company's directors, was sentenced to 3 years imprisonment as a result.

The new Act removes the requirement to find all the blame in one person; however, this has not resulted in any great change and the Centre for Corporate Accountability, an organisation committed to monitoring activity in this area, closed because of funding difficulties in March 2009. A number of fatalities have occurred since the introduction of the Act in April 2008, and lesser charges brought. In February 2011, Cotswold Geotechnical Holdings Ltd and its managing director became the first company to be convicted of the new offence of corporate manslaughter. This case concerned the death in 2008 of Alex Wright, a junior geologist crushed when an excavation collapsed upon him.

The Health and Safety (Offences) Act 2008 also allows senior management or directors to be given custodial sentences for non-fatal offences.

Civil law

An employee may obtain compensation for the tort, or wrong, that has occurred, if their employer is found to have negligently allowed him to suffer injury or illness.

The applicant employee has to show that:

- the employer owed him a duty of care
- the employer negligently breached that duty
- the employee suffered damage caused by that breach.

Only an estimated 10% of claimants are successful. Damages are generally modest, especially when legal fees and clawback of certain previously paid state benefits are taken into account.

Conditional fee arrangements (no win no fee) make it easier to pursue such a claim, since failure will not incur legal costs. However, this does mean that law firms will tend only to take on cases which stand a good chance of success.

Issues

Duty of care. The duty of care upon the employer is roughly equivalent to that in the criminal courts. The court will take a number of factors into account, including the vulnerability of the individual employee; the employer has a greater duty to safeguard that person (Table 5.4). It may also be that at the time that the harm was caused, the risk of the condition was genuinely not appreciated. The court will set a 'date of knowledge' from which a reasonable employer would have been expected to be aware.

Work-related stress cases. These tend to be of concern to the employer. The landmark decision was *Walker* v. *Northumberland County Council* in 1995. The key point concerning Mr Walker, a social worker, was that following an acute mental illness and prolonged absence, he returned to work with assurances of changes in work design to support him. When these failed to materialize he suffered a second episode of mental illness. It was the failure to foresee and prevent the second episode for which the council were found liable. The law has developed only slightly since then (Table 5.5).

Compensation; government scheme

The industrial injuries scheme administered by the UK Department of Work and Pensions 'prescribes' a number (currently about 70) of occupational illnesses for compensation as well as injuries sustained at work. The claimant must also have worked in an occupation recognized to carry a risk of that particular condition. Their claim

Table 5.4 Employers duty of care in the civil courts.

Issue	Case	Details
Extent of duty	*Stokes* v *GKN* 1968	'The overall test is still the conduct of the reasonable and prudent employer, taking positive thought for the safety of his workers … '
Increased duty toward vulnerable workers	*Paris* v *Stepney Borough Council* 1951	This fitter suffered a penetrating eye injury. He was already monocular, and the employer was negligent in not providing goggles, which were not felt necessary for the rest of the workforce since the risk was small
Volenti non fit injuria is the phrase used when an employee elects to put themselves at risk in the workplace and forgo the right to claim compensation in the event of loss, harm or injury	*Smith* v *Baker and Sons* (1891)	The courts are unlikely to judge in favour of an employer when loss, harm or injury does occur, as they would need to show that the employee: • volunteered • agreed to accept the risk • and made those choices in full knowledge of the nature and extent of the risk. Smith was a quarryman working beneath a crane, although the crane was not always operating. The crane dropped a rock on to Smith injuring him. It was suggested that Smith knew about the danger, but the judgement was in Smith's favour when it was revealed that he was threatened with dismissal if he refused to work under the crane. Lord Hershell, obiter: ' … that where a servant has been subjected to risk owing to a breach of duty on the part of his employer, even though he knows of the risk and does not remonstrate, does not preclude his recovering in respect of the breach … '

Table 5.5 Work-related stress cases of note.

Case	Detail	Legal point
Sutherland v *Hatton* (2002)	Mrs Hatton was a French teacher who was retired on ill-health grounds in 1996. She argued that teaching is intrinsically stressful and that the school governors should have had better support measures in place. Three other cases of work-related stress were brought in the same appeal	Sixteen 'practical propositions' were handed down by the court. Among them was the view that if a confidential advice service, with appropriate counselling or treatment services, were in place, the employer would be unlikely to be found liable
Barber v *Somerset County Council* (2004)	One of the four cases in the above judgement was referred to the House of Lords. Mr Barber was a mathematics teacher who became ill with depression and panic attacks in 1996. This culminated in him physically shaking a pupil	Approved the Court of Appeal propositions, but disagreed in respect of Mr Barber. Their conclusion was that after his first sickness absence, his employer should at least have made 'sympathetic enquiries' and considered what could have been done to help
Intel v *Daw* (2007)	Tracy Daw was promoted shortly after her return to work following childbirth (and her second episode of postnatal depression). Soon after that there was a organisational restructure. Her reporting lines were confused and she had a breakdown in 2001, arguing that her workload was excessive and employer gave her insufficient assistance	Her employer argued that she could have used their confidential counselling service but did not. The Court of Appeal held that where an employee is experiencing stress relating to excessive workloads, the presence of a workplace counselling service will not automatically serve to discharge the employer's duty of care in stress claims
Dickins v *O2 plc* (2008)	Following an office move and change of work, Susan Dickins found herself with a long and stressful commute and stressful job. Her request for a transfer or sabbatical was not acted upon, and she went sick with stress and was dismissed	She should have been referred to occupational health and properly assessed, which should then have guided management actions

will be assessed and paid on the basis of the percentage disablement. Rates vary up to a maximum (100% disability) of £127.10 weekly benefit (2006 figure).

Employment law

The fundamental positions of the two parties – employer and employee – in the contract of employment are consolidated in the Employment Rights Act 1996. There are also influential relevant codes of practice, such as those produced by the Advisory, Conciliation and Arbitration Service (ACAS).

Enforcement

Complaints are heard by Employment Tribunals (ETs). These consist of three members: a legally qualified chair and two lay members who represent employers associations and employee organisations. ETs were established in 1964 so that employment disputes could be settled rapidly without the expense of court proceedings. They are now extremely busy (Table 5.6).

Appeals from the ET are made to the Employment Appeal Tribunal and thence to the Appeal Court.

Compensation paid by ETs for unfair dismissal is capped at £65 300. Disability related claims however are unlimited, the maximum award in 2009/10 being £729 347.

Table 5.7 Reasons for (potentially) fair dismissal.

Capability	'Skill, aptitude, health or any other physical or mental quality', including qualifications
Conduct	Behaviour in, or sometimes outside, the workplace
Redundancy	The role within the organisation has been removed
Illegality	Cannot continue at work without breach of statutory duty (loss of driving licence for instance)
Some other substantial reason (SOSR)	Must be sufficient to justify dismissal

ETs hear claims on many areas of employment, but the commonest reason is unfair dismissal. The 1996 Act allows for the employer to dismiss for a fair reason (Table 5.7), and in general the employee must have been in employment for one year (the qualifying period) to bring an unfair dismissal claim. This does not pertain in disability or health and safety-related claims.

Issues (relevant cases in Table 5.8)

Medical certification. In the UK, the Form Med 3, which in April 2010 changed from the familiar 'sick note' to the 'fit note', is given

Table 5.6 Employment Tribunal (ET) and Employment Appeal Tribunal (EAT) activity 2009/10.

	Claims accepted	Claims disposed of		Of which withdrawn	Settled via ACAS	Successful
ET	236 100*	112 400		32%	31%	13%
	Appeals	Disposed	Rejected	Withdrawn	Full hearing	Allowed
EAT	1963	1848	839	284	403	219

*An increase of 56% on 2008/9.

Table 5.8 Important cases in employment law.

Issue	Case	Details
Medical certification	*Hutchinson* v *Enfield Rolling Mills* 1981	Signed off with sciatica; 2 days later witnessed in a union demonstration. EAT: 'if they [employees] are doing things away from the business which suggest that they are fit to work, then that is a matter which concerns him'
Fraud	*Bailey* v *BP* 1980	Self-certificated absence; worker witnessed on holiday in Majorca; summary dismissal upheld as fair
Long-term absence	*McAdie* v *Royal Bank of Scotland* 2007	Off sick with 'stress' after complaints about manager. ET found dismissal unfair, but this reversed by Court of Appeal
Attendance	*Wilson* v *Post Office* 2000	Confirmed that dismissal for repeated absences is for SOSR

Table 5.9 Definition of disability.

A person is considered to be disabled if they have a *physical or mental impairment*, and the impairment has a *substantial* and *long-term* adverse effect on their ability to carry out *normal day-to-day activities*

Physical or mental impairment	No diagnosis necessary
Substantial	More than trivial
Long term	Has lasted, or is likely to last, at least 12 months, or the rest of the persons life
Normal day to day activities	No longer defined in such detail
Other relevant elements in the Act	
Likely to recur	Treated as continuing to have adverse effect despite having ceased
Severe disfigurement	Act applies
Effect of medical treatment	But for the measures being taken to correct the condition, it would have substantial etc. effect (not visual acuity)
Certain conditions constitute disability from the time of diagnosis	Cancer, HIV, Multiple Sclerosis
Progressive conditions	Act applies once the condition has an adverse effect, which does not have to be substantial
Past disability	The Act may include a condition which occurred prior to the Act coming into force

to the employee by (usually) the GP, after 7 days of absence from work. Often it must be submitted to justify the absence as due to sickness and allow payment of contractual sick pay. Occasionally an employer may have grounds to 'look behind' the note.

Genuineness of illness (malingering). Employers may suspect that the reason given for absence is not genuine. Receipt of sick pay by an employee who is not sick constitutes fraud on the part of the employee. In order to challenge an employee if this is suspected, the employer must have good quality evidence. Suspicion or hearsay does not suffice.

Long-term absence. There will generally be some ongoing, underlying medical reason for long-term absence. The employer would be expected to assess the situation fully before making a decision to dismiss. This would normally include an OH opinion on the individual, and, if relevant, consideration of duties under equality legislation (see below). The employer does not need to have details of diagnosis, and the decision on whether to dismiss is management rather than the OHP. The cause of the ill health is irrelevant to whether the decision is fair, even though it may have resulted from current work activities.

Poor attendance. Recurrent spells of short-term absence are very disruptive to a business, and an employer is entitled to expect a reasonable level of reliable attendance from an employee. Poor attendance may justify dismissal for some other substantial reason (SOSR), although a clear absence policy and adherence to fair procedure are vital. It is also common for an OH opinion to be sought, in case there is an underlying illness unknown to the employer (in which case the reason for dismissal would be capability).

Disability legislation

The UK Equality Act came into force in Oct 2010 to simplify, harmonize and strengthen discrimination law. It gives greater protection from unfair discrimination and makes it easier for employers to understand their responsibilities. The Act unifies the existing discrimination legislation concerning sex, race, disability, sexual orientation, religion or belief, and age. The Disability Discrimination Act 1995 (DDA) is therefore repealed, and the bulk of that existing law directly transferred into the new Act.

The Act introduces the 'protected characteristic', which includes disability. The definition remains unchanged from that in the DDA (Table 5.9) although the detailed descriptions of those activities that could be considered part of 'normal day to day' activities have been removed. A clinical diagnosis is not required, only that the individual can demonstrate that they cannot undertake normal activities.

Discrimination

The Act includes a new protection from discrimination arising from disability – namely that it is discriminatory to treat a disabled person less favourably because of something connected with their disability (e.g. a tendency to make spelling mistakes arising from dyslexia). Less favourable treatment can be proved without reference to a comparator, often a complex area under the old DDA. The Act includes some new forms of discrimination (Table 5.10) and allows for positive discrimination.

Past case law (Table 5.11) will strictly speaking be irrelevant to interpretation of the Act, however some decisions under the DDA will no doubt be used as precedent given the similarity of the two laws.

Issues

Pre-employment health screening. The Act prohibits an employer asking about a candidate's health, including the absence record,

Table 5.10 Types of discrimination under the Equality Act.

Type	Explanation
Direct	Treat less favourably because of disability
Associative	Discriminate against someone because they associate with a disabled person; e.g. they care for a disabled relative
By perception	Discriminate because they think that the person is disabled
Indirect	A rule which applies to everyone but disadvantages the disabled
Harassment	Behaviour that is found offensive even if not directed at the complainant
Third party harassment	Employer may be liable for harassment by people who are not their employees (e.g. customers, clients)
Victimisation	Treat an employee badly when they have made or supported a complaint under the Act

before offering them work. Questions may only be asked to establish whether

- adjustments may be necessary for the applicant to complete the assessment process
- a candidate will be able to carry out a function that is intrinsic to the work concerned (e.g. driving).

Once a conditional job offer is made, health questions may be asked, but only those relevant to the role.

Medical records

OHPs are under the same duties of confidentiality as any other medical professional. Guidance from the General Medical Council and Faculty of Occupational Medicine detail specific circumstances in relation to third parties, including employers. The Data Protection Act (DPA) imposes duties on the data controller to ensure data security, especially when sensitive (health) data are held.

The DPA gives the data subject the right of access to any information about himself. There are provisions for exemption to this general rule where disclosure may put the subject or any other person at risk.

The Access to Medical Reports Act 1988 gives rights of access and consent to the report subject where a report is commissioned by an employer from a physician involved in clinical care. It is not usually held to apply to reports *from* OH Physicians, though this is contentious.

The future

There is a view that health and safety considerations have become overly onerous upon businesses, and that enthusiasm for compensation is detrimental to normal activities. This has resulted in the review, Common Sense, Common Safety, in October 2010. Aspects of claims procedure, insurance arrangements and the plethora of health and safety laws should be 'consolidated into a single set of accessible regulations'. Recommendations within the review which are relevant to the workplace centre around reducing the

Table 5.11 DDA decisions of note.

Is the person disabled?	Early debates about specific conditions moved on, quite correctly, to consideration of the individual and the impact on them. *Ministry of Defence* v *Hay* EAT [2008], in which a series of respiratory problems, some without clear diagnosis, could together constitute a disability under the Act Should not be an issue under the Equality Act given that it does not require the diagnosis of a specific condition
Who decides whether a person is disabled?	Ultimately the judgement is up to the courts, who focus on what the person cannot do rather than what they can do; a recognition of the way that people develop coping or avoidance strategies. The Employment Tribunal was criticized in *Abadeh* v *BT* (2001) in that it appeared to have accepted the OH physician opinion regarding disability rather than considering the issue for themselves
What constitutes a reasonable adjustment?	Employers must maintain a dialogue with absent employees, obtain OH advice as necessary and fully explore all possibilities of returning the employee to work. *Beart* v *HM Prison Service* 2003 concerned a case in which OH recommended transfer to an alternative prison. This was not acted upon and the Court of Appeal found that employment would have been possible and that the employer had discriminated unfairly
When disability discrimination conflicts with health and safety, which is more important?	In theory the statutory health and safety duties upon the employer, if absolute, override the duty not to discriminate; but this is open to abuse. Very often the duty will be so far as reasonably practical, and there will be ways of managing risks that may arise. *Lane Group Plc* v *Farmiloe* 2004 concerned the dismissal of an employee whose psoriasis meant that he was unable to wear safety footwear; dismissal was held to be justified
When does the employer know of a disability?	It used to be held that if an employer's OH department was aware of a relevant disability, then that inferred that the employer 'had knowledge'. However, *Hartman* v *South Essex Mental Health NHS Trust* (a Court of Appeal decision) held that although OH knew of Mrs Hartman's past psychiatric history, that this was confidential to OH, and that the employer could not be aware
What does 'likely to recur' mean?	The 2009 case of *SCA* v *Boyle* has defined this as 'may well happen', a change from the previously accepted 'more likely than not'

duties on employers when workplaces might be regarded as 'low hazard'. It remains to be seen whether any of these recommendations will be actioned.

Further reading

Kloss D. *Occupational health law*. Oxford, Wiley-Blackwell, 5th edn, 2010.
Lewis J, Thornbory G. *Employment law & occupational health*, 2nd edn. Oxford: Wiley Blackwell, 2010

http://www.hse.gov.uk/
http://www.legislation.gov.uk/ukpga
http://www.bailii.org/
http://www.justice.gov.uk/guidance/courts-and-tribunals/
tribunals/employment-appeals/judgments.htm

CHAPTER 6

Ethics

Paul Litchfield

BT Group Chief Medical Officer, London

OVERVIEW

- The principles of autonomy, 'do no harm', 'do good' and justice underpin all medical ethics and apply equally to occupational health
- Occupational health professionals often owe a duty to multiple parties but clinical care has primacy
- Obeying the law does not guarantee that behaviour is ethical and acting ethically does not ensure legal compliance
- Worker confidentiality must be respected unless there is consent for disclosure or an overriding public interest justification
- Occupational health professionals should act with integrity in business and have an additional duty to promote the health and wellbeing of workers

The principles of ethical practice

Ethical behaviour is a cornerstone of good medical practice. The relationship between a healthcare professional and a patient is one where power lies predominantly with the healthcare professional. Patients are, by definition, vulnerable and have little option but to place their trust in the knowledge and skills of the healthcare professional that they consult. The potential for the healthcare professional to abuse that trust has been recognized since antiquity and societies around the world have drawn up behavioural codes to mitigate that risk. The benefits for the patient are self evident but such an approach also benefits the healthcare professional. Clinicians can generally only operate effectively where patients are willing to disclose relevant information and to cooperate with examination and treatment. A healthcare professional who does not command the trust of patients will be less successful professionally and commercially. The moral imperative to act ethically is therefore supplemented by market forces.

Modern ethical codes and guidance derive both from the deontological strand of moral philosophy, where actions are driven by duty, and from utilitarianism, where consequences are the driver.

However, there are four key principles that underpin all medical ethics:

- respect for autonomy of the individual
- non-malfeasance (Do No Harm)
- beneficence (Do Good)
- justice (Fairness and Equality).

In some situations the principles can be opposing, and each healthcare professional must decide on the right course of action in those circumstances and be accountable for their decision. Material is available to help deal with such dilemmas and in the United Kingdom the General Medical Council (GMC), the British Medical Association (BMA) and the Nursing and Midwifery Council (NMC) produce comprehensive guidance. Cultural and societal differences can lead to varied views on what is ethically acceptable and global guidance issued by bodies such as the World Medical Association is particularly useful as both healthcare staff and patients become more mobile internationally. The International Commission on Occupational Health (ICOH) has produced a code of ethics that applies to all occupational health professionals and which is particularly helpful for those with international responsibilities; the current (third) edition is under review and a revised version is expected in 2012.

Exactly the same principles apply in occupational health as in other branches of healthcare. The widespread use in ethical guidance of the term 'patient' for all people with whom a healthcare professional interacts may not be helpful because it implies a therapeutic relationship. Such relationships may occur in occupational health but, certainly in the United Kingdom, are not the norm and usually relate to specific tasks (such as vaccination) which generally constitute only a small part of an occupational health professional's practice. Occupational healthcare staff occupy a similar position of power in relation to workers, whether or not treatment constitutes part of the service provided. In a clinical context a worker is far more likely to divulge confidential information to an occupational health professional than to someone without a healthcare background (such as a line manager or a human resources (HR) professional). Similarly, management is far more likely to accept guidance on health matters from an occupational physician or nurse than from someone who is not qualified in medicine or nursing. Occupational physicians and nurses enjoy authority and

---

ABC of Occupational and Environmental Medicine, Third Edition.
Edited by David Snashall and Dipti Patel.
© 2012 John Wiley & Sons Ltd. Published 2012 by John Wiley & Sons Ltd.

status – they must therefore apply the same ethical principles as others in the healthcare profession.

Duties to multiple parties

It is more common in occupational health than in many other specialties to have dual or even triple responsibilities in relation to a single case (Box 6.1).

Box 6.1 **Examples of dual responsibilities**

- Mixed primary care and occupational health
- Armed forces practice
- Advice on capability for employment
- Advice on medical retirement pension eligibility
- Advice on insurance or State benefits
- Advice on statutory health surveillance

It is becoming unusual in the UK for a situation to arise where GPs provide occupational health services to an organization employing many of their patients; in such circumstances doctors must be unambiguous about which role they are fulfilling and make that absolutely clear to the patient, because the risk for a breach of trust is high. More commonly clinicians will be asked for employment advice in relation to a patient they are treating. In such circumstances they must be clear not just about the clinical aspects of the case but also about the employment issues and be sure that they are competent to provide the advice requested. Treating clinicians may have a clear view on the harm to health that can result from undertaking certain activities but they should also consider the harm to health that arises by excluding individuals from paid work. They must take a balanced view when discussing such matters with their patients and respect the autonomy of the individual to make their own decisions; if the consequences of that decision have a potentially serious impact on health or safety they will need to consider public interest disclosure to the employer or regulator.

It is more usual for an occupational physician to be engaged to provide an impartial opinion on a worker's capability and any measures which might be indicated to adjust the work or rehabilitate the individual. The employer and the worker may have different aspirations for the outcome of the assessment and the doctor must resist inappropriate pressures from either party to sway their objective and evidence-based judgement. Similarly an occupational physician's report may often be the gate to financial benefits for the worker from pension schemes, insurers, etc., and this can influence behaviours – both prejudice and naivety are to be guarded against. Opinions provided must be based on a suitable and sufficient assessment of health status and capability. The process, particularly in activities such as medical retirement benefit assessment, may not include the opportunity to interview or examine the worker and the occupational physician should ensure that the evidence base is as comprehensive as practicable, taking particular care not to rely on material that could be biased or misleading.

Balancing these multiple responsibilities according to ethical principles is consistent with the injunction to 'make the care of

your patient your first concern'. That does not mean taking the side of the worker regardless of the circumstances but rather ensuring that clinical issues are given primacy. The key to operating ethically in this potentially contentious area of practice is the consistent application of fairness, openness and probity.

Ethics and the law

Practising within the limits of the law does not guarantee that behaviour will be ethical and acting ethically does not ensure legal compliance. In general, there is reasonable concordance between medical ethics and the law, at least in democratic societies, but it is risky to try to apply a 'rule book' approach to ethics. Codes and guidance are a useful adjunct to the ethical analysis of a situation but cannot be a substitute for that process.

Most law is specific to a jurisdiction (usually a nation state) but some has its roots in global initiatives (such as the United Nations Human Rights Convention) or in transnational agreements (such as European Union Directives). Legal issues are the subject of another chapter (Chapter 5) but some of the UK legislation impacting on ethical issues in occupational health is shown in Box 6.2.

Box 6.2 **UK* legislation potentially impacting on ethical issues**

- Health and Safety at Work, etc Act – 1974
- Police and Criminal Evidence Act – 1984
- Access to Medical Reports Act – 1988
- Access to Health Records Act – 1990
- Human Rights Act – 1998
- Data Protection Act – 1998
- Public Interest Disclosure Act – 1998
- Equality Act – 2010

*Not all legislation applies in Scotland and Northern Ireland.

Confidentiality and consent

The collection, storage and processing of information is the area that prompts most ethical enquiries in occupational health. In many countries these issues are subject to legislation that may be specific to medical records or which may be encompassed within laws concerning sensitive personal information. In the UK the prime legislation is the Data Protection Act for which the Information Commissioner has produced specific guidance relating to workers' health and this is supplemented by guidance from the GMC on disclosure in the context of employment.

Disclosure

- A disclosure is only made when information *obtained in confidence* is passed on to a third party.
- The consent of the worker to whom the confidential information relates must be obtained.
- The consent must be 'informed' – i.e. the worker must understand what is to be released, to whom, and the likely consequences.

- Consent may be 'implied' for purposes such as sharing information within a healthcare team or clinical audit, but information about these activities should be readily available to workers.
- Refusal of consent may be overridden if required by law or in the public interest – such action requires careful consideration and full justification.

Collecting information

Assembling the evidence base from which to formulate an opinion is generally undertaken by a clinical assessment, which may be face to face or remote using communications technology, and/or by the procurement of reports from the worker's own medical advisers. In either case the worker should give informed consent to the process. Ideally, the worker's written consent should be obtained for a clinical assessment but if this is not practicable (e.g. a telephone consultation) recording verbal consent contemporaneously in the occupational health record should suffice. If reports are sought from a third party then written consent must be obtained in accordance with UK law. Increasing use is being made, particularly in benefit and personal injury cases, of covert surveillance which may be filmed. Occupational physicians should not be party to commissioning such evidence, since (by definition) it is obtained without consent, and should resist pressure to comment on it as a substitute for a properly constituted assessment.

Box 6.3 **Occupational health records should be:**

- contemporaneous to the assessment
- recorded against a pre-determined structure
- suitable and sufficient for the purpose
- accurate reflection of consultation
- relevant to the issues at hand
- legible
- signed and dated

Occupational health professionals should remember that the prime purpose of clinical records is to facilitate good-quality healthcare both at the time of their creation and in the future (when another health professional may seek to rely upon them) – their value for medicolegal purposes is a secondary (though important in practice) consideration (Box 6.3).

Storing information

Occupational health records, whether paper or electronic, must be stored securely and access must be limited to named authorized persons on a 'need to know' basis. In determining 'need to know' the interests of the person to whom the records refer must have primacy. All authorized persons should receive training and instruction in data security and those without a professional duty of confidentiality should have the requirement included in their contract of employment. Occupational health professionals will not normally be 'data controllers' as legally defined; nevertheless,

they retain the ethical duty to ensure the confidentiality of medical records. Requests for access to clinical records for administrative purposes, such as business audit or the generation of management information, should be resisted and alternative means of achieving the required result suggested. All individuals and organizations holding occupational health records should have a written policy (Box 6.4).

Box 6.4 **Occupational health records policy**

- Security
  Paper records – locked storage, clear desks, double bagging in transit
  Electronic records – password protection, screens in public areas, file encryption
- Access
  Authorized persons, 'need to know', release procedures
- Archiving
  Schedule for transfer, physical arrangements, recall procedures
- Retention
  Statutory requirements, non-statutory period, justification for period
- Transfer
  Worker consultation arrangements, consent procedures, 'opt out' provisions
- Destruction
  Pulverization/shredding of paper, disposal, electronic 'wiping'

There are some statutory retention periods relating to health surveillance records but generally it is for individual organizations to determine how long records should be kept. The National Health Service, as a very large custodian of medical records, has a code of practice which may be helpful to others. The guiding principle is that information should not be held for longer than is necessary and any decision may have to be justified to the Information Commissioner (UK) or equivalent authority.

Processing information

In most cases an occupational health assessment will result in a report about a worker to a commissioning body (employer, pension scheme, insurer, etc.). That report may be a simple statement of fitness or a detailed report on capability and work adjustments. Whatever the nature of the report, the occupational physician has a duty to ensure that the worker understands what is being said and consents to its release. There are various means by which this ethical duty can be discharged but for doctors registered in the UK the GMC has prescribed that they should offer to show or give the worker a copy of the report before it is sent. A worker can withdraw consent for the process of an occupational health assessment, including the release of a report, at any stage and this can cause difficulties for the commissioning body, particularly if there are issues like fitness for safety critical work (Box 6.5).

> **Box 6.5 Minimizing the risk of worker non-cooperation**
>
> - Having clarity of purpose
> - Explaining issues in a way the worker is likely to understand
> - Stressing impartiality
> - Building trust with every clinical contact
> - Justifying opinions reached
> - Acting in a reasonable manner

Workers should be reminded that in the absence of occupational health input the commissioning body will have to act on whatever information is available to it and that may not be in the worker's best interests. If consent to release a report is withdrawn after it has been written, a copy should be held in the occupational health record with a clear marking that it has not and will not be released. In some circumstances disclosure may be warranted without consent on the basis of the public interest or a legal requirement; workers undergoing assessment should have this explained to them and if the circumstances arise the occupational physician should make every reasonable effort to obtain consent before breaking confidence.

Promotion and prevention

Health promotion in the workplace is seeing a resurgence after many years of decline. Some employers now view it as an integral part of raising business performance rather than as an employee benefit or a philanthropic activity. Occupational health professionals need to be wary of being complicit in programmes that use compulsion rather than voluntary participation. Programmes that incorporate well person screening should be evidence based and should satisfy established criteria such as those published by the UK National Screening Committee. Immunization programmes need to be similarly well thought through and a clear distinction must be made between programmes designed to protect the worker and those implemented for the protection of others. In neither case is compulsion acceptable ethically but the consequences of refusal must be clearly explained to the worker.

Pre-employment health assessment is a contentious area. The law in Great Britain has recently changed to prevent enquiries about health or disability being made before the offer of employment. Generic pre-employment health questionnaires, even if introduced after a job offer has been made, are considered by many to be unsound ethically because a great deal of information is gathered which has no bearing on capability for a particular post. If questionnaires are used, they should be specific to a role, evidence based, clearly marked as 'medical in confidence when completed' and scrutinized only by occupational health staff. Consent forms seeking blanket access to health records, such as the entire GP record, cannot be justified. A number of organizations now simply ask future employees if they have a health problem or disability with which they would like assistance and refer to occupational health for an individual assessment geared to identifying reasonable adjustments; the British Medical Association has produced such a specimen health and capability declaration. Genetic testing

is not yet well developed but there are isolated instances of testing being used to discriminate against job applicants. This may well run counter to Article 6 of the Universal Declaration of the Human Genome and Human Rights; more information is available from the UK Human Genetics Commission.

Health surveillance programmes may be established either as a part of workplace hazard controls or to ensure workers can meet special requirements for a type of work. Occupational physicians setting standards should ensure that the criteria are based on the best available evidence and regularly reviewed so that workers are neither placed at undue risk nor unfairly denied employment. Drug and alcohol testing programmes can present ethical problems though this is less likely for those introduced for safety critical tasks than those put in place to enhance corporate image. In general, alcohol is easier to deal with because consumption is lawful in most jurisdictions and the pharmacokinetics are relatively predictable. The illegal nature of many recreational drugs, the potential for confusion with prescribed medication, the lack of easily demonstrable dose effect relationships and the persistence of some substances create practical problems as well as potential civil liberties and human rights issues that must be considered. No programme should be introduced without a detailed policy that sets out the reasons for testing, the procedures to be followed and the role of occupational health staff. This issue is the subject of detailed guidance that has been produced by the Faculty of Occupational Medicine. Many organizations employ specialist contractors to conduct testing programmes since this avoids potential conflict of interest for occupational health staff and removes confusion among workers about the role of the service.

Professional relationships

Many occupational physicians work in multidisciplinary teams. Some work in teams which are purely clinical with nurses, physiotherapists, psychologists, etc., while others work in a broader context with safety professionals, occupational hygienists, HR professionals, etc. The qualities and values that an occupational physician should display with colleagues are set out in the Faculty of Occupational Medicine's publication *Good Occupational Medicine Practice*. Sharing information within a clinical team for the benefit of a worker's health is invariably good practice but the 'need to know' principle should be applied and it should be clear to those accessing a service that this is the unit's way of working. Sharing clinical information within a wider team, without specific informed consent, is unlikely to be acceptable ethically. Occupational physicians may manage teams and, if so, should be conversant with guidance such as that prepared by the GMC; they should not also fulfil an occupational health role for their team members and should make suitable alternative arrangements. Team management may be vested in another health professional or a lay manager; nevertheless, an occupational physician is expected to show professional leadership not least in giving ethical guidance.

Communicating with a worker's own healthcare advisers is an important part of clinical occupational medicine practice. Increasingly that contact does not just relate to requests for reports but also in the sharing of information gleaned in the workplace and sometimes even shared care. The principle of informed consent applies regardless of the direction of flow of the information and it must not be assumed that a worker will want confidential material copied to their GP or other healthcare professional. The occupational physician may consider it desirable or prudent to pass information in this way, and may seek to persuade the worker, but should not make an unauthorized disclosure unless that can be justified ethically or legally.

Commercial considerations

Occupational health professionals are more often exposed to commercial matters than colleagues in many other specialties. Much occupational health is delivered by contract and staff may find themselves in the role of either purchaser or provider; the latter may be a direct relationship with the client or through a third party. Occupational health professionals should conduct their business dealings with integrity, which implies not only honesty but also fair dealing and truthfulness. They additionally have a duty, which is over and above non-clinical business colleagues, to promote the health and wellbeing of workers. If they find themselves in a position where they believe that the activities of their employer or their client is causing harm then they have a duty to take action. Concerns should be raised through their management chain and advice should be taken from their defence organization or legal adviser; as a last resort disclosure to an external party (such as the Health and Safety Executive in Great Britain) should be considered and in certain circumstances this may attract legal protection.

Occupational health providers will wish to advertise their services but occupational physicians and others should be mindful of professional constraints which limit such activity to the provision of factual information about professional qualifications and skills. They must only undertake work for which they are competent and this applies not just on a personal basis but also in relationship to others for whom they have professional responsibility. In tendering for contracts they must take care not to denigrate competitors, offer inducements or disclose commercially sensitive information to a competitor. When handing over or taking on an existing service the abiding principle should be to safeguard the health, safety and welfare of those for whom the service is being provided. In such circumstances, transferring clinical records to the new provider is likely to be the most beneficial course for workers and resource implications should be addressed in tender documentation. Consent for transfer may be sought on an individual basis but, if this is not practicable, workers should be informed of the intention and given a reasonable time to make alternative arrangements.

Conclusion

Occupational physicians rarely encounter 'life and death' ethical dilemmas that can be issues in some other branches of medicine.

Difficulties usually relate to the multiple responsibilities inherent in much of the work carried out and in maintaining appropriate levels of confidentiality. Practitioners frequently work either in isolation or as the sole physician in a multi-disciplinary team. Extra effort is therefore required to discuss potential problems with peers and with senior colleagues in the specialty. Comprehensive guidance is published by the Faculty of Occupational Medicine and should be kept close at hand.

Further reading

General Medical Council – *List of ethical guidance.* http://www.gmc-uk.org/guidance/ethical_guidance.asp *This site gives a current list of all the GMC's ethical guidance*

British Medical Association – *Medical ethics.* http://www.bma.org.uk/ethics/index.jsp *This is the BMA's home page on ethics giving access to published guidance, tool kits and learning modules*

International Commission on Occupational Health – *International Code of Ethics for Occupational Health Professionals.* http://www.icohweb.org/site_new/multimedia/core_documents/pdf/code_ethics_eng.pdf *This is the authoritative international code of ethics for occupational health professionals. The current code from 2002 is being updated and the new document is expected late in 2012*

Employment Practices Data Protection Code: Part 4 – Information about workers' health. http://www.ico.gov.uk/upload/documents/library/data_protection/practical_application/coi_html/english/supplementary_guidance/information_about_workers_health.html *This gives guidance from the Information Commissioner's Office about compliance with the Data Protection Act in relation to workers' health. It usefully cross references with other documents including the Faculty of Occupational Medicine Guidance on Ethics*

NHS Code of Practice: Records management. http://www.dh.gov.uk/en/Publicationsandstatistics/Publications/PublicationsPolicyAndGuidance/DH_4131747 *This guidance is specific to the management of records in the NHS but is useful as a model of good practice for others*

UK National Screening Committee – *Programme appraisal criteria.* http://www.screening.nhs.uk/criteria. *These criteria usefully update the WHO principles first articulated by Wilson & Jungner and published by the WHO in 1968*

Human Genetics Commission – *Genetics and employment.* http://www.hgc.gov.uk/Client/Content.asp?ContentId=123 *This site has comprehensive guidance on issues related to genetics and employment*

Faculty of Occupational Medicine – *Guidance on alcohol and drug misuse in the workplace.* ISBN 1-86016-281-9. *This document sets out the practical issues associated with establishing a drugs and alcohol policy and operating a programme in the workplace*

Faculty of Occupational Medicine–*Good Occupational Medicine Practice.* http://www.facoccmed.ac.uk/library/docs/p_gomp2010.pdf *This guidance translates the GMC's 'Good Medical Practice' into the context of an occupational medicine setting*

Faculty of Occupational Medicine – *Guidance on ethics for occupational physicians.* ISBN 1-86016-280-0. *This is the definitive guidance on ethics for occupational physicians practising in the UK. The current (6th) edition is being revised and the new guidance is expected to be published in late 2012*

CHAPTER 7

Fitness for Work

William Davies

South Wales Fire and Rescue Service, Cardiff, UK

OVERVIEW

- As a result of social and legal developments the process of determining fitness for work has become increasingly important
- Guidance on the medical aspects of fitness for work is plentiful; guidance on fitness decision-making is scarce
- Core knowledge, common sense and cooperation between medical advisor, employer and job applicant or employee should produce a positive outcome in the majority of cases
- When significant fitness issues arise, clear understanding of roles and a structured approach is essential
- An agreed process and full participation of the key players is the best way to ensure sustainable decisions and fair outcomes.

Assessments of fitness for work can be important for job applicants, employees and employers. Unfitness because of an acute illness is normally self-evident and uncontentious, but assessing fitness in other cases may not be straightforward and can have serious financial and legal implications for those concerned. Commercial viability, efficiency, health and safety and legal responsibilities lie behind the fitness requirements of employers, and it may be legitimate to discriminate against people with medical conditions on these grounds. Unnecessary discrimination, however, is counterproductive and may be costly if legislation is breached. Employers tend to rely on occupational health practitioners when specific fitness advice is required and on general practitioners and hospital doctors for advice provided via certification. Evidence-based standards for physical fitness, eyesight, hearing, etc., may apply to some occupations. But for most medical conditions, prescriptive standards and blanket restrictions that existed before the advent of anti-discrimination legislation have been replaced by the need for individual assessments, adjustments and decisions on a case-by-case basis. As a result of this and the associated lack of easy-to-apply screening measures, the process of fitness determination and the responsibilities of the participants have become increasingly important.

ABC of Occupational and Environmental Medicine, Third Edition.
Edited by David Snashall and Dipti Patel.
© 2012 John Wiley & Sons Ltd. Published 2012 by John Wiley & Sons Ltd.

Outline

The issue of an individual's fitness for *specified* work is the focus of this chapter and it arises in a variety of employment situations (Box 7.1). Common to all is the broad aim of ensuring as far as is possible the productive and safe employment of the job applicant or employee. Key requirements act as driving forces behind this aim and underpin the process of achieving it: these are statutory and common-law duties, ethical obligations, prevailing social policy and employers' business needs. There are key roles for medical advisors, employers and the subject, i.e. the job applicant or serving employee. In principle, the assessment and decision-making process involves assessing the subject's medical and functional status against the job requirements and deciding on the acceptability of any enabling options and residual fitness issues. In practice this process may involve three or more substantive components or steps, depending on the circumstances of the case. For a framework with general application that integrates the key roles, nine potential steps are identified and explained. This outline is set out in Figure 7.1 and it provides a template for the chapter's format and headings.

Box 7.1 **When fitness assessments may be required**

- Before making an offer of employment, placement or redeployment
- Routine surveillance in safety critical jobs
- During or after sickness absence
- To identify adjustment needs
- When attendance or performance issues arise
- If health and safety concerns arise
- To examine ill-health retirement issues
- If required by statute
- To determine entitlement to state benefits

The issue of fitness or unfitness for *all work* is the basic determinant of entitlement to some UK state benefits and some occupational pension scheme benefits. Responsibility for the processes required to deal with this broader issue rests with the Department for Work and Pensions (DWP) or the relevant pension scheme administrators.

Figure 7.1 Fitness for work outline.

Key requirements

Equality Act 2010

This replaces the Disability Discrimination Act 1995(DDA) and consolidates all discrimination legislation, making it unlawful for employers to discriminate against individuals on grounds of disability, age, sex and other protected characteristics unless the discrimination is a proportionate means of achieving a legitimate aim. The central requirement to make reasonable adjustments remains. Advancing the spirit of the DDA, it has removed unnecessary medicalization of recruitment processes by only permitting occupationally-relevant medical questioning directly relating to questions immediately at issue.

Employment Rights Act 1996

Requires procedural standards of fairness before any decision to dismiss an employee can be taken.

Heath and safety at work etc. Act 1974

Places a far reaching responsibility on employers to reduce risk so far as is reasonably practicable. The related responsibility to undertake suitable and sufficient assessment may create the need for pre-employment and in-service medical questionnaires and

examinations, particularly in occupations involving safety-critical activities. The concept of *reasonable practicability* allows for consideration of socioeconomic factors and the use of a cost-benefit balance for resolving conflicting objectives of risk-reduction and equality of opportunity.

Common law duties

Impart responsibilities of care to prevent reasonably foreseeable risks which mirror or supplement the above legislation. The financial penalties of successful claims for occupational injury and diseases or for wrongful dismissal add to the importance of an effective and equitable assessment process. Cases have established important precedents relevant to fitness assessment and decisions (see Chapter 5).

Ethical obligations

The Faculty of Occupational Medicine affirms that doctors should not presume to decide for others whether risks are acceptable. The General Medical Council recommends that informed consent should be obtained from the job applicant or employee before any report on fitness is given to the employer, and that subjects should be given the opportunity to see and comment on reports in draft. Disclosure without consent is limited to exceptional situations and subject to strict conditions (see Chapter 6).

Social policy

Over the last decade, rehabilitation back to work, and an emphasis on capability rather than limitations, have continued as central themes behind government policies and guidance on health and safety and occupational health. There is increasing acceptance that work is good for the vast majority of people in a majority of jobs, and that the benefits of work should not be overlooked or subordinated within an unduly risk-averse ideology (see Chapter 2). Building on these developments, in 2010 the DWP fundamentally changed the certification process. Hospital doctors and general practitioners are now required to issue 'fit notes' instead of 'sick notes', encouraging adjustments and early rehabilitation. Pathways back to employment have also been incorporated into state benefit assessment processes (see WCA Boxes 7.2 and 7.3).

Box 7.2 **Work Capability Assessment (WCA)**

- Introduced in Oct 2008 replacing personal capacity assessment
- Determines entitlement to Employment & Support Allowance
- Process and criteria set in social security legislation
- Assesses limited capability for work and work-related activity
- High rates of unsuccessful claims and successful appeals
- Aspects of assessment have been called into question
- First independent review in November 2010*
- Review identified clear and consistent criticisms
- Review's 25 recommendations all accepted by Government

*An Independent Review of the Work Capability Assessment – Professor Malcolm Harrington, Nov 2010 (via DWP Home page)

Employers' business needs

The job applicant's or employee's productivity in terms of attendance and performance must meet the levels necessary for commercial success in the private sector or for the equivalent *best-value* criteria in the public sector. There will be limits to the productivity concessions that an employer can accommodate and this may be the basis for a legitimate and lawful decision of incapability for the job from unfitness.

Key roles and responsibilities

Of the many potential contributors to fitness assessments, the key roles fall into three categories, Employer, Medical Advisor and Applicant/Employee. Management representation for the employers' role may include human resources, health and safety, and operational staff. Occupational health practitioners may take on all the responsibilities of the medical advisor role. GPs and hospital practitioners (HPs) may follow the same approach but with a more limited input. The subject of the assessment will either be a job applicant or a serving employee, and from a GP or HP perspective, maybe a recovering patient. As treating clinicians, GPs HPs and other healthcare professionals involved with a case may have an important supporting role in supplying relevant clinical information, with the patient's consent. The key roles and responsibilities are outlined below.

Employer

- To provide job description, person specification and employment details.
- To identify any pre-determined standards.
- To supply occupationally relevant questionnaire if required.
- To explore enabling options identified by GP, Medical Advisor, Employee or Applicant.
- To duly consider medical advisor recommendations.
- To take the decisions if or when fitness issues arise.

Medical advisor

- To assess the subject against the job requirements and work environment.
- To identify enabling options if needed.
- To identify any residual fitness issues.

- To apply any pre-determined standards.
- To consider the prognosis of any health problem, and its clinical management to date.
- To make recommendations on fitness or unfitness when applicable.
- To liaise with the treating clinicians to get further information for assessment, or advise on management.
- To advise on management issues (optional).
- To present assessment report.

Applicant/employee

- To consider the job description, person specification and employment details.
- To complete and return questionnaire if needed.
- To attend medical assessment if needed and supply information for assessment.
- To identify any preferred enabling options.
- To provide personal views on any residual fitness issues.
- To submit evidence or comments for assessment report.
- To consent for making assessment report available to management.

Process in principle

How should the above requirements, roles and responsibilities be consolidated into a process that can be readily applied to most cases and clearly understood by all the participants? Although guidance on the *assessment* and *medical aspects* of fitness for work is plentiful (see Further reading and Useful websites), little has be published on the *decision-making* and *management aspects* of the process. This absence of an established end-to-end process, and consequent confusion of roles, was identified in a systematic review of the subject in 2006 (see Signpost 1).

Previous editions of this chapter proposed a nine-step framework beginning with three steps: *assessing medical and functional status, considering occupational factors* and, if necessary, *exploring enabling options*. Any residual fitness issues are then identified in up to three more steps which represent the core fitness criteria of *attendance and performance, health and safety risks to others* and *health and safety risks to self*. Three further steps provided options for reporting the outcome to management.

The 2006 systematic review began its analysis with reference to the original ABC Fitness for Work chapter and the three core fitness criteria advanced within it. In this edition we build on these foundations, giving more attention to the integration of the key roles and the practicalities of the process.

Process in practice

The practical aspects of each of the nine steps, from the perspective of the medical advisors' role, are outlined below. Figure 7.2 provides a practical framework by identifying the nine potential steps together with the key roles and responsibilities. This should be used as a flexible guide as the number of steps needed, their precise sequence, and the inter-play of roles may vary depending on the circumstances of the case.

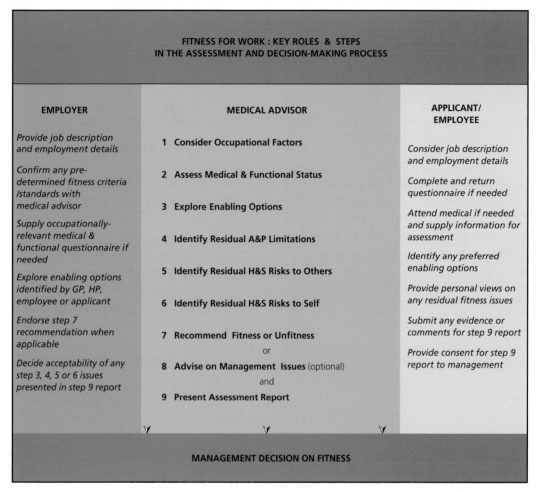

Figure 7.2 Practical framework.

Step 1: Consider occupational factors

Knowledge of the physical and mental demands of the job, the working environment and the associated hazards is the obvious starting point for a fitness for work assessment. Basic details should be given in the job description and the person specification, and the employer may provide additional information. An applicant may supply details given to him or her that are not in the pre-employment documentation. An employee's direct experience of what the work entails will be important in some cases. From this information, relevant questions for the assessment of medical and functional capacity to be undertaken in step 2 may be formulated. If any medical or functional issues are identified in step 2, the detail of relevant occupational factors could be very important and it may be necessary to revisit step 1 issues to obtain the further information needed for an accurate assessment of potential limitations or risks (see Boxes 7.4 and 7.5).

Step 2: Assess medical and functional status

In accordance with established good practice and now a requirement of the Equality Act 2010, pre-employment screening and medical fitness assessments should not take place before an offer of employment is made unless necessary to confirm an essential

requirement of the job or for other precise reasons specified in the Act. When permitted, a medical questionnaire and health declaration is the simplest form of assessment and will be sufficient to enable medical clearance in many categories of employment. Medical questions and any tests should be limited to those necessary for a competent assessment. Pre-determined, evidenced-based standards for physical fitness, eyesight and hearing, may be applicable, e.g. firefighters (see Signpost 2), police (see Signpost 3), armed forces, etc. Some occupations have statutory standards (e.g. UK seafarers)

Box 7.4 **Occupational factors: importance of detail**

- In teaching, healthcare and many other occupations, the perceived hazards of epilepsy are often found to be negligible when the potential for harm to others is properly assessed
- If diabetes is well controlled, the risk of injury from hypoglycaemia may be found to be very remote when the true frequency and duration of hazardous situations are taken into account
- A subject may be able to show satisfactory ability in a job simulation exercise despite a physical impairment that might have affected fitness, for example a work-related test of manual dexterity for an assembly line worker with some functional loss resulting from a hand injury

Box 7.5 **Occupational factors**

Ability in the workplace: consider actual effect of physical or medical condition on performance

- Confirm job requirements such as perception, mobility, strength and endurance
- Ask employee what the work entails
- Review job description or inspect worksite
- Perform field tests of specific abilities or structured job simulation exercises
- Consider trial of employment with feedback from management

Nature of hazards – consider interaction of occupational factors and medical condition

- Harm from:
  - demands (heart attack, back strain, repetitive strain injury)
  - exposures (asthma, dermatitis, hearing loss)
  - situations (seizure in a lone worker, trauma)
  - infections (food handling, surgical procedures)
- How much harm is likely (temporary, permanent, minor, major, fatal)?
- Who may be affected (self, colleagues, clients, public)?

Extent of risk – focus on facts and avoid presumption

- Question employee on relevant details
- Obtain management report on material facts
- Examine documentation such as exposure records, accident reports, etc.
- Observe work, workplace, and working practices
- Identify frequencies and duration of hazardous exposures or situations
- Request technical data from hygienist, ergonomist, etc., if required
- Review relevant literature, journals, and research

Access to Medical Reports Act 1988 or non-UK equivalent

- Details from other specialists such as psychologists or audiologists
- Advice or second opinion from specialist occupational physician
- Advice or second opinion from independent specialists such as cardiologists or neurologists
- Clinical guidelines and evidenced based reviews
- Texts, journals, and research

Work related tests and investigations
Perceptual tests

- Snellen chart: special visual standards may be required for certain occupations such as aircraft pilots, seafarers and vocational drivers
- Colour vision tests such as Ishihara plates or City University test, or matching tests, may be necessary if normal colour vision is essential – for example, for some jobs in transport, navigation and the armed services
- Voice tests, e.g. Pirozzo Whisper Test
- Audiometry: occupations such as the armed services, police and fire service may have specific standards

Functional tests

- Lung function tests (for example, UK regulations require fire service employees to have their respiratory parameters measured before employment
- Dynamic or static strength tests, e.g. hand grip-strength dynamometer
- Physical endurance and aerobic capacity (for example, the fire service or commercial divers)
- Step test
- Bicycle ergometer

Diagnostic (health on work)

- Exercise electrocardiography: needed – for example, for vocational drivers and offshore workers with significant cardiac history
- Drug and alcohol tests may be a requirement in certain safety critical industries

Diagnostic (work on health)

- Haematology, biochemistry, and urine analysis: UK commercial divers will have full blood count and haemoglobin S assessed before employment
- Radiographs: long bone radiographs are a requirement before employment for saturation diving in the United Kingdom

(see Signpost 4) and assessment must include measuring necessary factors. Others have standards set by authoritative recommendations or guidance (for example, the Health Advisory Committee of the UK Offshore Operators Association has drawn up guidelines on the medical standards for offshore work) (see Signpost 5). Drivers would need to satisfy the DVLA standards for the relevant category of licence (see Signpost 6)

A wide range of potential questioning, examination and testing exists (see Box 7.6). In the absence of authoritative guidance or pre-determined criteria confirmed by the employer, doctors

Box 7.6 **Medical and functional status**

History and examination

- Pre-employment/placement questionnaire or health declaration
- Health interview, occupationally relevant direct questions
- Physical examination focusing on job requirements

Functionally specific questionnaires

- Respiratory (MRC questionnaire)
- Pre-audiometry questionnaire

Consultation and research

- Details from general practitioner and medical specialist, under

must judge how extensive the assessment should be by taking account of the type of work, the nature of any relevant medical conditions identified, the reasons for management's request for medical advice, and the precise question at issue (for example, for a pension scheme).

If no fitness issues are identified in steps 1 and 2, a recommendation of fitness can be made by going to step 7. Otherwise the assessment should progress to step 3.

Step 3: Explore enabling options

Where a health problem is identified, a subject's potential fitness often depends on intervention. Under the Equality Act 2010, employers must make reasonable adjustments for applicants or employees who fall within the Act's definition of disability. A public sector employer has extra responsibilities which may go beyond these basic duties. Reasonable adjustments are steps that would be reasonable for an employer to take, to ensure that the disabled person is not at a substantial disadvantage in recruitment or employment. For example, for an arthritic subject, removing a requirement in a job description to undertake occasional lifting may allow a recommendation of fitness with minimal inconvenience for the employer. The Code of Practice (see Signpost 7) provides extensive guidance with many examples. Under the Health & Safety at Work etc. Act 1974, employers must take reasonably practicable steps to eliminate or reduce risks. For example, substituting for a sensitizing or irritant product may, with other sensible precautions, enable an employee with asthma or eczema to continue in their preferred line of work as a paint sprayer or cleaner. There may be other measures, not necessarily required by legislation, such as pursuing unexplored treatments or making reasonable adjustments for applicants or employees not specifically covered by the Equality Act, that might facilitate employment or continued employment.

'Enabling options' is a term which includes *all* the above and therefore *any* measure which would enable the subject to secure, or continue in, safe and productive employment; it applies to *all* applicants and *all* employees (see Box 7.7).

Box 7.7 **Enabling options**

Unexplored treatments

- Drug treatment or surgery
- Physiotherapy or occupational therapy
- Counselling or psychotherapy

Rehabilitative measures

- Graded resumption of responsibilities
- Refamiliarization training
- Temporary reduction of workload
- Management appraisal or progress reports
- Scheduled or self requested medical reviews

Reasonable adjustments

- Modification of duties or working hours
- Redeployment to existing vacancy
- Modifying or providing equipment
- Time off for rehabilitation or treatment
- Providing supervision

Risk prevention and control

- Elimination or substitution of hazard
- Hazard reduction methodology and systems
- Personal protection or immunization
- Information, instruction, and training
- Health and medical surveillance

General

Any other measure or suggestion that would enable the subject to secure, or continue in, safe, productive employment

---

Significantly, with developing legal and social policy, identifying or proposing of enabling options is now open to all participants in the fitness assessment process. Occupational health practitioners should be well versed in this field but their knowledge of all the relevant facts cannot be presumed. In many situations, employers, job applicants and employees may be better placed to see or explore practical ways of overcoming obstacles to employment. Their contribution may therefore be the critical factor that ensures a successful outcome. In view of the limited availability of occupational health practitioners, the new fit note with enabling options at its core has been another positive development. It has established constructive roles for GPs, HPs and employers within the fitness assessment process and should help to extend principles of good practice across the whole spectrum of employment (see Box 7.3)

It follows therefore that if fitness issues arise and create obstacles to employment, enabling options should be fully explored by all the participants as it may be possible to provide a conditional recommendation of fitness that the employer would be willing to adopt.

Steps 1, 2 and 3 should be sufficient produce a step 7 recommendation in most cases, but further steps may be needed if, despite enabling options, there are residual fitness issues. This may occur with one, two, or all three of the core criteria, i.e. attendance and performance, health and safety risk to others, health and safety risk to -self. Dealing with the issues in turn is advisable.

Step 4: Identify residual attendance and performance limitations

Assessments of attendance and performance are the main determinants of employee productivity. From a legal standpoint attendance and performance are covered by the concept of 'capability'. For the purpose of fitness decision-making, they may also be treated as a single entity under one core fitness criterion. Residual attendance and performance limitations may have critical implications for job security and business viability. It is essential therefore that medical advisors provide valid and sustainable advice in clear and meaningful terminology. When empirical data is lacking, 'opinion' advice on prognosis should be based on relevant professional experience and if required, specialty expertise. After surgery, published guidelines (see Signpost 8) may provide a useful benchmark for setting goals. Projections of attendance and performance, should be as positive as possible without misrepresenting the facts, and, as far as possible, agreed with the subject, This should help with motivation and recovery. Feedback from management at a suitable stage of rehabilitation may be required before definitive advice can be given. Open-ended statements such as 'Unfit; review in 3 months' are not favoured by employers – preferring uncertainties to be expressed as probabilities: 'Mr Smith has been incapacitated but is progressing well and is likely to become fit to return to work within 4 weeks'. If social or motivational factors are evident, discuss these with the subject, and advise management accordingly: 'Mrs Jones' absence is due to family commitments that are likely to continue for the foreseeable future. She realizes that her employment could be at risk and would welcome an opportunity to discuss her situation with management.'

Step 5: Identify residual health and safety risk to others

In occupations involving safety-critical activities and responsibilities, medical conditions or functional limitations may pose risks to working colleagues and/or the public despite implementing enabling options to reduce the risks. Then, the residual fitness issue of risk acceptability, has to be resolved. Examples might include; a firefighter applicant with type I diabetes or well-controlled epilepsy; a surgeon with hepatitis B; or nurse or teacher with history of serious mental health problems. The Health and Safety at Work etc. Act 1974 is the overriding statute, and the legal test is whether it would be necessary to prevent employment in order to reduce risk so far as is reasonably practicable. Legal precedent (see Signpost 9) has established that it is the employer not the doctor who bears direct responsibility for the acceptability issue and from first principles it is apparent that a range of responses in a particular case from the *accommodating*, i.e. supporting employment, to the *restrictive*, i.e. prohibiting employment, may be lawful (see Signpost 10). Beyond these generalizations there is no ready formula to apply. However, various approaches to resolving risk acceptability issues have evolved and medical advisors can help employers by providing relevant information. Risks, if quantifiable, may be gauged against established precedents, concepts or conventions. Guidance produced by authoritative bodies or special interest groups or obtained via professional consensus, may be applicable. The merits and limitations of these and other approaches are outlined in Table 7.1. No one approach can be suited to all situations but reviewing their applicability could provide evidence that decisions have been measured and well thought through.

Step 6: Identify residual health and safety risk to self

Where risks would only impact on the subject, particularly where he or she is prepared to accept them, the need to respect autonomy comes into play and here the legal boundaries of acceptability are wider than with *risks to others*. For this reason, risks to self are best dealt with separately in the decision-making process. In some cases, employment may pose a risk of ill health but the employer is satisfied that everything possible has been done to prevent or reduce risks (for example, the risk of relapse in a teacher with a history of work-related anxiety/depressive disorder). To advise that in such cases the subject should always be deemed unfit because of a risk of work related illness is unrealistic. The benefits of employment for the subject, and possibly their employer, may considerably outweigh the risks. On the other hand, there could be issues of liability for both employer and doctor if the risks are overlooked. A pragmatic approach is recommended.

If the subject thinks the benefits outweigh the risks and the doctor agrees, advice should be given in support of employment, provided that the assessment and the judgement of balance between benefit and risk have been competently undertaken and all parties understand and accept the recommendation made.

If the subject thinks the benefits outweigh the risks but the doctor cannot agree, consider seeking a second opinion from a specialist occupational physician before providing management with definitive advice.

If the subject thinks the risks outweigh the benefits and the doctor agrees, then redeployment or early retirement should be considered.

If the subject thinks the risks outweigh the benefits when the hazard and risk seem disproportionately low, then motivational

Table 7.1 Approaches to resolving risk acceptability.

Approach	Example	Merits	Limitations
Defined negligible risk	Risk of less than 1 in a million (1)	Suits risk to others and risk to self	Risk quantification required: may be overzealous/protective
Policy and precedent	<2% annual risk of sudden incapacity for DVLA Group 2 licenses (2) <1% for UK two-pilot airline flights (3)	Well established Risk quantification required	Arbitrary acceptability basis Situation specific
Published consensus	Diabetes UK: Guidelines for Employment in Hazardous Occupations (4)	Covers risk to others and risk to self Quantification not required	Acceptability basis unclear May be potential for bias
Informal consensus	ALAMA Website Forum ANHOPS Discussion Forum	Applicable to all cases Rapid access to opinions	Consensus quality assurance maybe limited
Autonomy model	Legal commentary (5) Case law precedent	Suits risk to self Flexibility of reasonableness	Unsuited to risk to others Subject to employer discretion
Individual propositions	Quantitative/comparative risk equations to assist decision-making (6)	Covers risk to others and risk to self Rational and systematic	Risk quantification required Level of support for criteria uncertain
Comparing accepted risks	I in 16.8 k annual death risk from all forms of road accident in UK (7)	Suitable for risk to self	Not well suited to risk to others as imposed risk is preventable

1 Calman KC. Cancer: science and society and the communication of risk. *BMJ* 1996;313:799–802.
2 At a glance guide: www.DVLA.org.uk.
3 Mitchell SJ, Evans AD. Flight safety and medical incapacitation risk of airline pilots. *Aviation Space and Environ Med* 2004;75:3.
4 Diabetes UK guidelines for employment of people with insulin controlled diabetes in potentially hazardous occupation: www.diabetes.org.uk.
5 Davies J. Reconciling risk and the employment of disabled persons in a reformed welfare state. *Ind Law* J 2000;29:347–377.
6 Donoghue AM. The calculation of accident risks in fitness for work assessments: diseases that can cause sudden incapacitation. *Occup Med (Lond)* 2001;51:266–271.
7 Reducing Risks, Protecting People – HSE's decision-making process, 2001: HSE Home-page/HMSO.

factors (such as a common law claim or ill health retirement incentives) may be relevant. If so, the doctor should proceed cautiously and consider obtaining a second opinion from a specialist occupational physician.

The conclusions should be presented to management in context, indicating the nature of the hazard, the extent of risk, and strength of medical consensus. This will enable the employer to discharge his or her responsibility in a complex area with the benefit of such medical support as the circumstances allow.

Step 7: Recommend fitness or unfitness

A recommendation of fitness can be made if no issues are identified in steps 1 and 2. A conditional recommendation of fitness can be provided if enabling options identified in step 3 are likely to be available. A recommendation of fitness or unfitness can be made if the findings of steps 1 and 2 and any fitness/acceptability issues identified in steps 3, 4, 5 or 6, satisfy, or fail to satisfy, pre-determined criteria, when applicable. If fitness/acceptability issues remain, step 8 advice may be required, before proceeding to step 9.

Step 8: Advise on management issues

Although it is well established that acceptability issues in steps 3, 4, 5 and 6 are a management responsibility, an employer may request the medical advisor's opinion or even try to delegate to the medical advisor responsibility for decisions. Given that specialist occupational physicians and experienced medical advisors may have considerable expertise in this area, such expectations are reasonable. It must be appreciated that the medical advisor would then be acting in a management capacity and that if their opinion or decision comes under scrutiny, it would be judged according to the standard expected of a reasonable and prudent employer. This may be a harder standard to satisfy than the standard for medical care, which takes some account of medical consensus. This means that doctors defending such an opinion or decision could not simply rely on the assumption that their colleagues would have advised or decided in the same way. In practice, therefore, the use of medical advisor opinions or decisions in this context should be conditional on a clear understanding of the capacity in which they are acting and the liability implications for both parties.

Step 9: Provide assessment report

This final step consolidates the assessment findings. Presenting step 7 recommendations for endorsement should be straightforward. Any step 3, 4, 5 or 6 acceptability issues should be set out in terms which are clear to both management and subject. If advice on management issues has been provided in step 8, ensure that its non-medical status is clear. The employee should have the opportunity to see the report, submit comments or evidence, and consent to its release.

Reaching a management decision

A multiplicity of factors may affect the outcome of a fitness assessment, and one employer may reach a different conclusion to another in a similar case. Provided the above roles and responsibilities have been properly discharged, then differences would have to be accepted as arising from a legitimate variation of opinion or approach. Understandably, however, a job applicant's or employee's experience of being treated differently may cause considerable distress. For difficult and potentially contentious cases, establishing a representative panel to consider carefully the issues and reach a collective decision is one way to ensure the process and outcome is both fair and seen to be fair.

Synopsis

The process of establishing fitness for work requires a substantive input from all the participants. In many cases core knowledge, cooperation and common sense will suffice. However, when significant fitness issues arise and there are no pre-determined standards to apply, the benefits of a shared and structured approach are clear. It gives employers terms of reference for the essential part they must play. Job applicants and employees can contribute themselves, helping to ensure fair treatment and job satisfaction. Medical advisors have a firm basis for consistency, comparison and audit, and for banking examples of good practice. Most importantly, the key players can work together from the same brief for the common goal of productive and fulfilling employment with minimal risks.

Signposts

1 Criteria and methods used for the assessment of fitness for work: a systematic review. Consol Serra *et al. Occupational and Environmental Medicine* Vol. 64, Number 5, May 2007. Systematic review of reports published in scientific journals from 1966–2005 identifying 39 reports mostly from Western Europe

2 Medical and Occupational Evidence for Recruitment and Retention in the Fire and Rescue Service. Available via Department for Communities and Local government (CLG) Home page under Fire and Resilience

3 Home Office Circular 25/2003 (Eyesight) and Home Office Circular 59/2004 (Medical)

4 Seafarers Medical Examination System and Medical and Eyesight Standards; Application of the Merchant Shipping (Medical Examination) Regulations 2002 and Medical fitness Requirements for those working on domestic vessels and small commercial vessels – Your Health at Sea 6. Both available via Maritime and Coastguard Agency (MCA) home page

5 Medical Aspects of Fitness for Offshore Work: Guidance for Examining Physicians- issue 6 (CD ROM) or in hard copy available via UK Offshore Operators Association (UKOOA) homepage

6 At a glance Guide to the current Medical Standards of Fitness to Drive (For Medical Practitioners). Available via Driving and Vehicle Licensing Agency (DVLA) home page. Regularly updated prescriptive standards for wide range of medical conditions

7 Equalities Act 2010 Employment Code of Practice: available on-line via EHRC Homepage or from HMSO

8 Information on post-surgery rehabilitation and recovery times for a wide range of procedures is given under patient information on the Royal College of Surgeons and Royal College of Obstetricians and Gynaecologists home pages. Comprehensive user-friendly tables are available on www.workingfit.com

9 *Stokes* v *GKN (Bolts and Nuts) Ltd* [1968] 1 WLR 1776

10 Davies J, 'Balancing disability rights and safety requirements' Health and Safety Bulletin (Vol. 301 September 2001)17–22

Further reading

Palmer K, Cox R, Brown I. *Fitness for work: the medical aspects*, 4th edn. Oxford: Oxford University Press, 2007. *A comprehensive text on medical issues covering background issues, all medical systems and specific occupations*

Kloss D. *Occupational health law*, 5th edn. Oxford: Wiley-Blackwell, 2010. *Authoritative text covering many areas of relevance to fitness for work, including health and safety, employment and equality/discrimination law in the context of occupational health practice*

RCGP, FOM, SOM. *The health and work handbook: patient care and occupational health: a partnership guide for primary care and occupational health teams*. DWP. www.dwp.gov.uk. *On-line publication focusing on the roles of primary carers and occupational health professionals in ensuring and maintaining patients' fitness for work: helpful links for CPD and on-line learning*

Employers Forum on Disability. *A practical guide to health and safety and the DDA*. www.employers-forum.co.uk. *Pragmatic guidance on overcoming some of the potentially conflicting responsibilities of health and safety and equality legislation*

Coggon D, Palmer, KT. *Assessing fitness for work and writing a 'fit note'*. BMJ 2010; 341:C605. *Authoritative and clear guidance for GPs explaining why and how doctors might support patients in their return to work, how to identify helpful modifications and how to frame useful advice on the fit note within the time constraints of a busy clinic*

Useful websites

Legislation: legislation.gov.uk. *Full text of all UK statutes*

Case law: www.bailii.org. *Full text of law reports of UK cases*

Health and Safety Executive: www.hse.gov.uk. *Regulations, codes of practice, statutory medicals, health surveillance, appointed doctor, etc.*

General Medical Council: www.gmc-uk.gov. *Guidance on confidentiality, consent, health clearance for medical students*

Faculty of Occupational Medicine: www.facoccmed.ac.uk. *Guidance on ethics and many important areas of OH practice*

Association of Local Authority Medical advisors (ALAMA): www.alama.org.uk. *Membership access to forum, links and guidance*

Association Of National Health Occupational Physicians: www.anhops.com. *Membership access to forum, links and guidance*

Department of Health: www.dwp.gov.uk. *Hepatitis B and bloodborne virus guidance*

Food Standards Agency: www.food.gov.uk. *Food handlers fitness to work*

Department for Communities and Local Government: www.communities.gov.uk. *Guidance on Local government and firefighter pension schemes*

CHAPTER 8

Musculoskeletal Disorders

Kim Burton[1] and Nicholas Kendall[2]

[1]Centre for Health and Social Care Research, University of Huddersfield, Huddersfield, UK
[2]Occupational Medicine, University of Otago, Otago, New Zealand

OVERVIEW

- Musculoskeletal symptoms are very common, with lifetime prevalence rates of 75% or more for problems such as low back pain. Causes are frequently assumed, but are actually unpredictable and largely unknown. This makes outright prevention unfeasible

- Explanations and diagnostic labels can negatively influence responses to symptoms. Care needs to be taken to reassure and emphasize the benefits of maintaining participation, and avoiding prolonged rest and inactivity

- Clinical management should aim at symptomatic relief with maintenance of activity and work. Most interventions exhibit only weak to moderate treatment effects, and combining or repeating them does not seem to enhance effectiveness

- Effective occupational management depends on communication and coordination between the key players, with optimal intervention being a combination of work-focused healthcare and accommodating workplaces

- Psychosocial issues contribute most strongly to absence from work. These obstacles can be identified in three main areas: the person, their workplace and the everyday context in which they function. Actively tackling obstacles results in improved outcomes

Musculoskeletal disorders (MSDs) are commonly experienced across the population from childhood to old age, but are most frequently complained of to healthcare services by working-age people. They encompass the everyday aches and pains that are part of life as well as the consequence of specific injuries. MSDs can and do affect capability for work, both short and long term. They are a principal reason for sickness absence, yet they vary inconsistently by occupation. In terms of self-reported ill health, MSDs dominate the conditions that people believe are caused or made worse by their current or past work (despite the lack of evidence for direct causation). The occupational impact of MSDs has been stubbornly resistant to reductions in occupational physical exposures and increased access to healthcare. This suggests that simply focusing

on ever more prevention and treatment is inappropriate. Instead, the ongoing challenge of managing work-relevant MSDs requires innovative and collaborative approaches from both healthcare and the workplace.

What the epidemiology tells us

The musculoskeletal problems most frequently reported in the workplace are low back pain, neck pain and upper limb pain; lower limb problems are less frequently reported.

The lifetime prevalence of bothersome back pain is of the order of 75%, but occasional aches and pains are probably a universal experience. In the general adult population, over 40% can be expected to experience back symptoms during the course of a month, with the daily prevalence being up to 30% (Figure 8.1). The annual incidence rate (those developing a new episode) in the UK adult population is some 36%. Many children also experience back pain, and by adolescence over 50% will have experienced one or more spells. Thus, irrespective of occupational exposure a large proportion of the population will experience an episode of back pain over any given period. Leg pain (in the form of referred pain) will accompany back pain in perhaps 35% of cases, but lifetime prevalence of true radicular pain (sciatica) is only about 5%.

The pattern is similar for neck and upper limb disorders, with a similarly high lifetime prevalence of bothersome pain somewhere

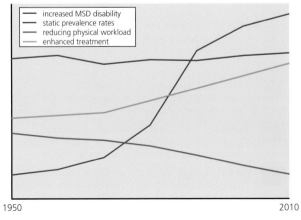

1950   2010

Figure 8.1 Paradoxical increased disability despite enhanced ergonomics and healthcare. MSD, musculoskeletal disorder.

ABC of Occupational and Environmental Medicine, Third Edition.
Edited by David Snashall and Dipti Patel.
© 2012 John Wiley & Sons Ltd. Published 2012 by John Wiley & Sons Ltd.

in the upper limb. The proportion of people who experience some level of upper limb and neck pain during the course of a week is of the order of 44% (24% for neck pain and shoulder pain; 11% for elbow pain; 21% for wrist/hand pain), and most of them (70%) will find normal activities (including work) difficult or impossible. There are a number of conditions affecting the upper limb that, in the UK, are termed prescribed diseases (see Chapters 1 and 5) which is where the strength of the relationship with a particular occupation is considered to indicate an occupational risk for the purposes of certain benefits. Unfortunately, there is considerable uncertainty over classification and diagnosis for upper limb disorders, with inconsistent and inaccurate terminology confounding studies of their epidemiology, treatment, and management. Stated simply, upper limb disorders, whether specific diagnoses or non-specific complaints, are common entities, irrespective of work.

The epidemiological evidence strongly suggests that most musculoskeletal cases are characterized by complaints of symptoms, for which it is often not possible to objectively demonstrate an underlying pathology. Symptoms tend to coexist at numerous anatomical sites, but that is not to imply a common genesis. MSDs tend to be recurrent in nature, describing an untidy pattern of episodes having variable frequency, severity and impact. For most episodes, most people do not seek healthcare and do not require time off work: if they did there would be few people at work! The various presentations of MSDs – presence of symptoms; reporting of symptoms; attribution to work; sickness absence; prolonged disability; wellbeing – are generally independent of the medical condition; rather they are dominated by psychosocial factors – arising from the person, their workplace and the context in which they function (Figure 8.2).

Why people experience musculoskeletal disorders

The onset of symptoms may be sudden and associated with activity, either trivial or strenuous. Onset can also be gradual with no identifiable triggering event. That said, it is common experience that some physical stress, often an everyday action, can precede the onset of acute symptoms. Overall, though, the causative mechanisms

are unpredictable and largely unknown, so strategies aimed at preventing symptoms arising are destined to have limited overall impact. This does not mean they do not have a role, but it does mean that overall reliance on a primary prevention strategy will disappoint. Rather, the focus needs to broaden with adoption of a much smarter approach to prevention: one that meaningfully brings to life the adage 'work should be comfortable when we are well and accommodating when we are sick or injured'.

The ubiquity and natural history make it very difficult to differentiate everyday experiences from work-induced symptoms (Box 8.1). Many musculoskeletal symptoms are perceived as 'work related', but causation is complex and relationships to purported physical risk factors at work remains, in most instances, unsupported by the epidemiology. That is, self-reported attributions are often unreliable and tend to overestimate work as the cause of any musculoskeletal condition. Nevertheless, MSDs are frequently work relevant in that some aspects of the work may be temporarily difficult, painful or impossible. Beliefs that a health condition is work related can be a major obstacle to continuing or returning to that job, irrespective of whether they are correct. The 'injury model' and attribution to work dominate contemporary thinking, a situation generally reinforced by the availability of benefits and compensation.

Box 8.1 Work relevant does not mean work caused

- Primary prevention of musculoskeletal symptoms is largely unfeasible
  - most episodes are not caused directly by work
- Symptoms may affect ability to work
  - symptoms may be more pronounced at work
  - work may be difficult because of symptoms
  - consequences are driven more by psychosocial than physical factors
- Musculoskeletal problems may be work-relevant, irrespective of cause

---

Assessment and classification issues

Depending on the context, common MSDs are variously referred to in terms of symptoms, injury or pathology (Box 8.2). There is a wide spectrum of classification systems, ranging from specific disorders (diagnoses) to descriptive syndromes (non-specific), as well as a plethora of colloquial labels. However, most cases actually fall under the rubric *non-specific*.

From a clinical perspective, there is a distinction between specific musculoskeletal diagnoses (e.g. carpal tunnel syndrome or intervertebral disc prolapse) and 'non-specific' disorders (characterized by an absence of identifiable relevant pathology). Some specific diagnoses may require specific clinical interventions, but the principles of occupational management are largely independent of diagnosis. The terms 'disorder' and 'injury' are not clearly distinguished and are often used interchangeably, although 'injury' is more often used when there is some question of work relatedness and the potential for compensation.

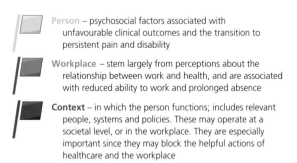

Psychosocial Flags Framework – obstacles to work participation

Person, Workplace, Context

Person – psychosocial factors associated with unfavourable clinical outcomes and the transition to persistent pain and disability

Workplace – stem largely from perceptions about the relationship between work and health, and are associated with reduced ability to work and prolonged absence

Context – in which the person functions; includes relevant people, systems and policies. These may operate at a societal level, or in the workplace. They are especially important since they may block the helpful actions of healthcare and the workplace

Figure 8.2 Psychosocial flags framework: obstacles to work participation.

Box 8.2 **Key messages for tackling MSDs**

Concept messages

- *Musculoskeletal symptoms are a common experience* – although symptoms are often triggered by physical stress (minor injury), recovery and return to full activities can be expected: activity is usually helpful: prolonged rest is not
- *Work is not the predominant cause* – although some work will be difficult or impossible for a while, that does not mean the work is unsafe: most people can stay at work (sometimes using temporary adjustments), but absence is appropriate when job demands cannot be tolerated
- *Early return to work is important* – it contributes to the recovery process and will usually do no harm; facilitating work retention and return to work requires support from workplace and healthcare
- *All players onside is fundamental* – sharing goals, beliefs and a commitment to coordinated action

Process messages

- *Promote self-management* – give evidence-based information and advice – adopt a can-do approach, focusing on recovery rather than what's happened
- *Intervene using stepped care approach* – specific treatments only if required for particular diagnoses (beware detrimental labels and over-medicalization); encourage and support early activity; avoid prolonged rest; focus on participation, including work
- *Encourage early return to work* – stay in touch with absent worker; use case management principles; focus on what worker can do rather than what they can't; provide transitional work arrangements (only if required, and time-limited)
- *Endeavour to make work comfortable and accommodating* – assess and control significant risks; ensure physical demands are within normal capabilities, but don't rely on ergonomics alone; accommodating cases shows more promise than prevention
- *Overcome obstacles* – principles of rehabilitation should be applied early: focus on tackling biopsychosocial obstacles to participation – all players communicating openly and acting together, avoiding blame and conflict

Care needs to be taken when providing any explanation of MSDs: the language used must not inadvertently contribute to the development of psychosocial obstacles to activity and work. An easily recognized example is telling people to avoid effort and rest up when it hurts: this promotes the development of a fear–avoidance cycle leading to inactivity. Reporting an X-ray as showing a degenerate spine is alarmist: a simple explanation that there are normal age-related changes that are probably nothing to do with the pain is more accurate. It is also important to remember the high rate of false-positives that occur with magnetic resonance imaging. More than 30% of asymptomatic people have abnormal findings in the lumbar and cervical spine. Attributing the pain to a work injury will readily provoke absence or impede return: explaining that some aspects of work may well be difficult or painful because of the problem is intuitively acceptable and overcomes uncertainty.

In general, terms to avoid include any that may contribute to development of catastrophizing, e.g. 'ruptured', 'torn' or 'degeneration'. Useful language emphasizes a positive expectation of recovery,

maintaining activity and continuing to participate in daily activities wherever possible. Often, focusing on asking what the patient is doing instead of on the symptom can help to achieve this.

Treatment and rehabilitation

The outcome for MSDs tends to be positive, with or without healthcare. Most people, for most episodes, do not seek healthcare, and only a very small proportion of cases require surgical intervention (for low back pain the estimates range from 0.5% to 5%).

The vast majority of clinical evidence for effective intervention relates to *symptomatic* relief while the natural process of healing and recovery occurs (Figure 8.3). By and large, clinical guidelines tend to recommend consideration of a relatively small range of therapeutic interventions. The common treatments offered fall broadly into the main categories of manual therapy, exercise therapy, medication and invasive procedures. Their effectiveness, and thus indications for use, varies from condition to condition.

Manual therapy includes a variety of techniques and procedures but the cardinal categories are manipulation, mobilization and massage offered by a range of clinicians (physiotherapy, osteopathy, chiropractic and musculoskeletal/orthopaedic medicine). Despite considerable study the effectiveness of manual therapy remains contested. A plausible argument for its use is the provision of symptom relief while natural recovery occurs. This needs to be balanced against the possibility of inadvertently encouraging passive dependence as opposed to participation in movement and activity. The same issue arises with use of therapeutic equipment such as bracing, strapping or splinting. These may be useful to facilitate continuance of otherwise painful activities through support during the initial (acute) stage, but only in the short term. Despite widespread use, evidence does not support their effectiveness, and prolonged use risks muscular atrophy and deconditioning.

Exercise therapy includes a wide variety of specific exercises advocated by particular practitioner 'schools'. There is strong evidence that prolonged rest for more than a few days is counterproductive, and that maintaining movement and activity is beneficial. However, there is little or no evidence to support specific types of exercise. That is, the most important issue is to ensure the individual does participate in movement and activity and does not guard particular parts of the musculoskeletal system: moving and staying active are more important than the type of exercise. As a rule of thumb progress should be evaluated after 2–3 weeks. Only if there is a significant decrease in symptoms after a couple of weeks of consistently adhering to a stretching and strengthening exercise programme is it likely to be worth persevering.

Other treatment modalities include acupuncture, transcutaneous electrical nerve stimulation (TENS), ultrasound, laser, etc. Despite popular appeal, there is little evidence for their effectiveness in musculoskeletal problems, although short-term reductions in symptoms and placebo responses are common.

Nearly everyone with an MSD tries some medication or other. Often this is an over-the-counter product, but those people who see their GP are frequently offered a prescription. Simple analgesics (such as paracetamol) can often provide adequate pain relief. Non-steroidal anti-inflammatory drugs may have a role to play,

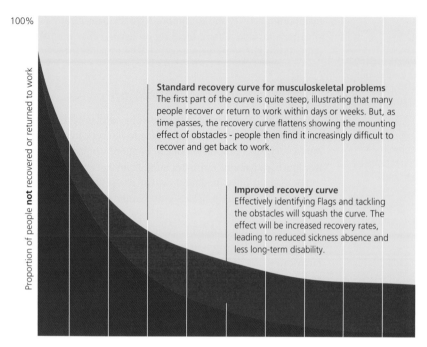

100%

Proportion of people **not** recovered or returned to work

Standard recovery curve for musculoskeletal problems
The first part of the curve is quite steep, illustrating that many people recover or return to work within days or weeks. But, as time passes, the recovery curve flattens showing the mounting effect of obstacles - people then find it increasingly difficult to recover and get back to work.

Improved recovery curve
Effectively identifying Flags and tackling the obstacles will squash the curve. The effect will be increased recovery rates, leading to reduced sickness absence and less long-term disability.

Figure 8.3 Recovery curve. Reproduced with permission from Kendall NAS, Burton AK, Main CJ, Watson PJ, on behalf of the Flags Think-Tank. *Tackling musculoskeletal problems: a guide for the clinic and workplace – identifying obstacles using the psychosocial flags framework*. London, The Stationery Office, 2009 © kendallburton.

although they have little or no demonstrated advantage over simple analgesics but do have the potential for significant adverse effects and may therefore be best kept as a second-line approach or for intermittent use. Strong analgesics such as opioids are not usually required except for acute trauma, with long-term use carrying a risk of habituation and dependence.

Invasive intervention is commonly provided. Injection therapies generally use a mixture of a corticosteroid and local anaesthetic. Aside from short-term relief of acute pain the effectiveness of injection therapy is widely debated, with an overall lack of convincing evidence. There may be grounds for using single injections when there is severe pain and the person is highly distressed (or where there is a clear inflammatory component); however, this does not yield a longer term solution and there is the risk that the person will come to expect such medical intervention repeatedly. There may be a role for other invasive interventions in specific cases and these include radiofrequency denervation, implantable stimulators and pumps, extracorporeal shockwave therapy and a range of percutaneous techniques too lengthy to discuss here. Surgery is an appropriate option for a very limited number of MSDs, and can often be precluded by adequate conservative management.

Overall, the main role for clinical intervention in MSDs is symptomatic relief while natural healing and recovery takes place. This means that ready access to healthcare for advice and treatment is important, but that must be balanced against the risk of medicalizing everyday symptoms and causing iatrogenic disability.

Rehabilitation refers to the process of restoring as much function as possible following injury or onset of disease. Modern understanding of vocational rehabilitation recognizes the need to deliver (work-focused) healthcare and rehabilitation simultaneously, rather than the one before the other. This is of particular importance in the musculoskeletal field since it contributes directly to the important outcomes of activity and work.

Adopting a rehabilitation approach from the outset provides the most useful framework in which to deliver any type of intervention or treatment. The evidence clearly indicates there is a high probability of residual and recurring symptoms. If the only framework used is a treatment one then strong expectation of repeated and additional treatment will be established. However, if expectations are first established for recovery that involves the active participation of the individual there is a natural pathway to progress beyond a treatment mode.

Stepped care and timing

The idea of providing 'only what's needed when it's needed' is commendable, and makes efficient use of healthcare resources. It is based on the observation that more intensive and complex intervention is generally needed only with longer duration of symptoms and inactivity. This needs to be balanced with the adverse effects of providing serial ineffective therapy, which tend to create passivity and inactivity. A 'stepped-care approach' to MSDs should be initiated very early, starting with simple, low-intensity, low-cost interventions, which may start just with accurate information and advice. This will be adequate for many cases, but can be 'stepped up' to more intensive, complex and costly interventions for people who fail to respond and who need additional help (Figure 8.4).

Active and working

There is strong evidence that prolonged work absence is detrimental to both physical and mental health, so it is good clinical practice to encourage early and sustainable return to work. Thus, an essential

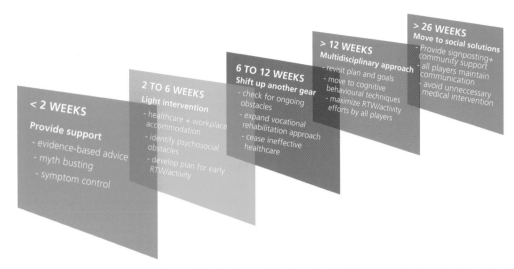

Figure 8.4 Stepped care principles. RTW, return to work. Reproduced with permission from Kendall NAS, Burton AK, Main CJ, Watson PJ, on behalf of the Flags Think-Tank. *Tackling musculoskeletal problems: a guide for the clinic and workplace – identifying obstacles using the psychosocial flags framework*. London, The Stationery Office, 2009 © kendallburton.

component of all clinical care for MSDs should be a focus on work together with individually tailored support. In principle the earlier someone with a musculoskeletal problem can be helped to stay at or return to work the better for the person, the employer and society. Early intervention is most effective when the workplace is involved, usually through temporary provision of accommodation or modified work. This concept of early intervention is central to occupational management, because the longer anyone is off work, the greater the obstacles to return to work and the more difficult it becomes. Therefore, it is simpler, more effective and cost-effective to help people with MSDs avoid progressing to long-term sickness absence. However, too early a return to work that involves stressful activities can exacerbate symptoms, and may be inappropriate in safety-sensitive areas.

Effective occupational management depends on communication and coordination between the key players – particularly the individual, healthcare and the workplace. There is general consensus that successful return to work requires the provision of consistent information and advice (including the correction of unhelpful beliefs and myths) (Box 8.3).

The optimal intervention requires work-focused healthcare *and* accommodating workplaces. Both are necessary: they are interdependent and need to be coordinated. The major role for work-focused healthcare is to ensure that in addition to provision of evidence-informed advice about musculoskeletal problems nothing is done to undermine the goal of being active and working. The major role for workplaces is to facilitate provision of temporary modifications, allowing the person with a health problem to stay at or return to work.

Identical impairments may impact differently. For example, a middle-aged man with shoulder pain who works as a ticket inspector may be impaired but able to stay at work, whereas if he works as a bus driver he is more likely to be both impaired and unable to do his normal work (and may require temporary modified work).

A key role for occupational health providers is to establish, negotiate and monitor both 'stay-at-work' and 'return-to-work' programmes. For graduated return to work programmes there are two key variables: (1) amount and type of job tasks to begin with, and (2) the rate of increase over a specified duration. This is best achieved through careful consideration of the job description and any potential safety issues. It's a question of balance. For the best success, it is important to ensure that the plan supports the returning worker without disadvantaging co-workers and supervisors (Box 8.4).

Fit note

The introduction of the *fit note* (see also Chapters 2 and 7) in April 2010 is the public face of UK statutory recognition that work is generally good for health, that going back to work can actually aid recovery, and that staying off work can lead to long-term absence, job loss and social exclusion. The underlying rationale recognizes the need to emphasize what an individual experiencing an MSD still 'can do', rather than merely focusing on what they cannot or will not do. On this basis, the certifying doctor is expected to give positive messages about work and health, while the fit note itself permits the doctor to state the person may be fit for work where their health condition does not necessarily mean they cannot return to work, recognizing they may need some support from the workplace. The doctor is asked to take account of any obstacles to staying at work or returning to work and to give advice on what can be done to overcome them – the options given are a phased return to work; altered hours; amended duties; and/or workplace adaptations. The fit note is a process intervention that is intended to help shift the culture around the work–health interface, influencing the attitudes of all the key players – health professionals, employers and workers – and provide a tool to encourage and facilitate early sustained work participation.

Box 8.3 **The myths around MSDs**

Myth	Why it needs busting
Pain means serious damage and injury	Believing hurt means harm results in focus on symptoms and activity-avoidance behaviours, which are obstacles to stay-at-work and return-to-work initiatives
	Worrying about 'damage' and 'injury' is an obstacle to active interventions that see work as a therapeutic intervention
Work/activity is the cause: something's damaged	Erroneously blaming work leads to an undue concentration on mechanical causation, which gets in the way of effective interventions
	Undue focus on mechanical workplace factors fosters the restrictive belief that ergonomic interventions are the only solution
Work/activity will make matters worse	Work is generally good for health and wellbeing, so the belief that work is inherently dangerous is unhelpful, and poses a major obstacle to helping people get back to work or stay at work
Medical treatment is necessary	The beliefs of health professionals can fuel over-cautious behaviours, which are powerful obstacles to recovery and return to work
	Reliance on medical treatment alone negates the possibility of involving the workplace in helping people back to work
Musculoskeletal problems must be rested	Using rest as a treatment is a major obstacle to modern management strategies that encourage and support return to activity/work.
	Advising patients to take unnecessary rest can give the disadvantageous impression that the problem is serious
Sick leave is needed as part of the treatment	Helping people stay at work can contribute to their recovery
	Injudicious use of medical certificates reinforces fears and uncertainty, and encourages reliance on rest, whilst fostering fears of activity
Contacting an absent worker is intrusive	Failure to make early contact with people who are off work leaves them isolated and unvalued, thus fostering distress or depression
	Lack of contact means these is no chance to make a return to work plan, and no chance to discuss transitional working arrangements

Box 8.4 **Modified work**

Examples of helpful workplace accommodations to tackle common obstacles:

- Alter the work tasks or physical environment to reduce physical demands – e.g. reduce reaching; provide seating; reduce weights; reduce pace of work/frequency; enable help from co-workers; job enlargement (added task variety)
- Alter the work organization – e.g. flexible start/finish times; reduced work hours/days; additional rest breaks; graded return to work (starting at achievable level, and increase on a regular quota, or start with a short week)
- Change the job – e.g. allow someone who cannot drive or use public transport to work at home during the transitional period, or exchange problematic secondary tasks for part of another employee's job description
- Use a flexible approach – e.g. schedule daily planning sessions with a co-worker at the start of each day to develop achievable goals; allow reasonable time to attend healthcare appointments

Further reading

Australian Acute Musculoskeletal Pain Guidelines Group. Evidence-based management of acute musculoskeletal pain. Brisbane, Australian Academic Press, 2003. *Comprehensive evidence review for assessment and treatment of acute pain (i.e. less than 3 months) arising from the musculoskeletal system*

Burton AK, Kendall NAS, Pearce, BG, Birrell LN, Bainbridge LC. *Management of upper limb disorders and the biopsychosocial model* (RR 596). London: HSE Books, 2008. *Evidence review establishing the role and applicability of biopsychosocial approaches to upper limb pain. Also includes a review and comparison of the effectiveness of biomedical treatments*

Carter JT, Birrell LN (eds) *Occupational health guidelines for the management of low back pain at work.* London: Faculty of Occupational Medicine, 2000. *Seminal evidence review that provides strong scientific basis underpinning the key messages about maintaining activity and work*

European Commission, Research Directorate General. *Low back pain: guidelines for its management.* 2004, www.backpaineurope.org (accessed January 2011). *Comprehensive report from task forces on prevention, acute, and chronic low back pain*

FOM. The Health and Work Handbook. London. The Faculty of Occupational Medicine, 2005 www.facoccmed.ac.uk/pubspol/pubs.jsp (accessed January 2011). *Emphasizes the role both primary care teams and occupational health professionals can play and the major contribution they can make to helping keep people in work, with all the advantages that brings*

FOM. Upper Limb Disorders: Occupational Aspects of Management. The Faculty of Occupational Medicine, 2009 www.facoccmed.ac.uk/pubspol/pubs.jsp (accessed January 2011). *This guideline offers evidence-based advice on the management of four upper limb disorders in the workplace: carpal tunnel syndrome, non-specific arm pain, tenosynovitis and lateral epicondylitis (tennis elbow). Useful summary leaflets accompany it for employers, employees and health care professionals*

Kendall NAS, Burton AK, Main CJ, Watson PJ, on behalf of the Flags Think-Tank. *Tackling musculoskeletal problems: a guide for the clinic and workplace – identifying obstacles using the psychosocial flags framework.* London, The Stationery Office, 2009 www.tsoshop.co.uk/flags (accessed January 2011). *Definitive guide to identifying and managing psychosocial issues with all types of musculoskeletal problems. Contains useful practical material for clinicians, workers, line managers and employers*

Waddell G, Burton AK, Kendall NAS. *Vocational rehabilitation—what works, for whom, and when?* (Report for the Vocational Rehabilitation Task Group) London. The Stationery Office, 2008. *Comprehensive evidence review of musculoskeletal, minor mental health, and cardiorespiratory problems that demonstrates the strong scientific basis for helping people stay at work and return to work. Emphasizes the need for both work-focused healthcare and accommodating workplaces*

Information booklets for public and patients: *The Back Book; The Arm Book, The Neck Book; Health & Work*: The Stationery Office www.tsoshop.co.uk/evidence-based

Information and advice leaflets/PDFs on work and health: *Advising patients about work*[practitioners]; *Work & Health*[workplace], *Health & Work*[workers]: The Stationery Office http://www.tsoshop.co.uk/evidence-based

CHAPTER 9

Mental Health

Samuel B. Harvey[1,2] *and Max Henderson*[2]

[1]School of Psychiatry, University of New South Wales and Black Dog Institute, Sydney, Australia
[2]Institute of Psychiatry, King's College Hospital, UK

OVERVIEW

- Mental health problems are common. At any time, around one in six working age individuals will suffer from symptoms suggestive of a psychiatric disorder. Mental ill health is now the leading cause of sickness absence and long-term work incapacity in most developed countries
- Mental health problems can have a significant impact on work performance
- Asking about symptoms of common mental health problems and considering risk should be part of routine clinical practice. Mental health problems often occur together with physical health problems and therefore may not be immediately obvious
- There are effective, evidence based treatments for psychiatric disorders. Most individuals who suffer from mental illness should be able to remain in the workforce
- An adverse psychosocial work environment may act as a risk factor for mental illness, but 'work stress' is not a diagnosis. Being in work has many beneficial effects on mental health

Introduction

Until recently, the most common reasons for sickness absence and disability pensions were musculoskeletal disorders such as back pain and shoulder complaints. However, over the last few decades, the clinical problems faced by occupational health practitioners, GPs and doctors assessing insurance and benefit claims have changed, with mental health problems now being the leading cause of work incapacity. This change is demonstrated in Figure 9.1a. As shown in Figure 9.1b, the trend toward a greater amount of work incapacity being attributed to mental illness has continued, although in recent years this has been in part due to lower numbers of claims for other conditions, with no change in the overall numbers claiming incapacity benefits. Psychiatric disorders now account for around 40% of the total time covered by sickness certification. Within Organization for Economic Cooperation and Development (OECD) countries (comprising much of Europe, the

United States, Canada, Mexico, Australia, New Zealand, Japan and Korea) mental ill health is listed as the primary reason for around 35% of all disability benefits.

There is also increasing recognition that psychiatric disorders can adversely affect work aside from sickness absence. Presenteeism refers to the situation where an individual is unwell, yet remains at work and is less productive as a result of their illness. Presenteeism can be difficult to measure, but the Sainsbury's Centre for Mental Health calculated that the costs arising from mental health-related presenteeism are around double those of sickness absence. For a variety or reasons, such as stigma, delayed treatment and the specific symptom profile, presenteeism appears to be particularly prominent in psychiatric disorders.

As a result of the increasing social and economic consequences of psychiatric disorders, both policy-makers and professional bodies involved in occupational health have become increasingly interested in mental health. However, the relationship between mental health and work is complicated. In the UK, the United States and many European countries, there is a growing awareness that good health, both physical and mental, is unevenly distributed in society. Those at the bottom of society have worse health and are more likely to be workless or have poor-quality employment. In this context mental ill health can be regarded as both an exposure and an outcome. Poor mental health, whether alone or in combination with physical ill health makes sustained employment difficult. In addition, worklessness or adverse working conditions can contribute to the onset and maintenance of mental ill health.

Epidemiology

In the UK the Office for National Statistics has carried out surveys of the prevalence of psychiatric disorders in the general population using objective assessment tools in 1993, 2000 and 2007. The prevalence of all psychiatric disorders has stayed largely static during this time, with around one in six of the working age population meeting diagnostic criteria for a common mental disorder at all time points. The prevalence of more severe mental disorders, such as psychosis was much lower, at around 0.5%. The prevalence estimates for a range of psychiatric disorders obtained using highly structured interviews in community surveys are shown in Table 9.1. As demonstrated in this table, females are at increased risk of

ABC of Occupational and Environmental Medicine, Third Edition.
Edited by David Snashall and Dipti Patel.
© 2012 John Wiley & Sons Ltd. Published 2012 by John Wiley & Sons Ltd.

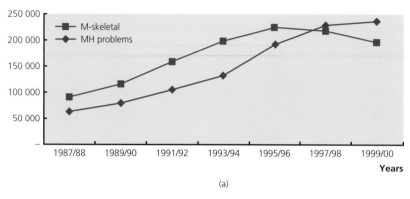

(a)

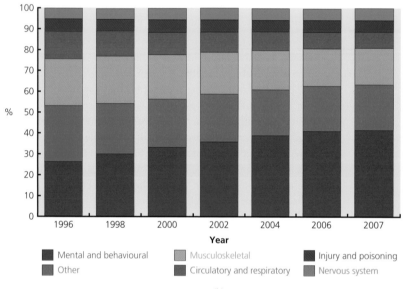

Mental and behavioural

Other

Musculoskeletal

Circulatory and respiratory

Injury and poisoning

Nervous system

(b)

Figure 9.1 (a) The numbers of incapacity benefits in England and Wales throughout the late 1980s and 1990s, demonstrating an apparent change in the 'cause' of occupational incapacity. Source 1% sample of all Incapacity Benefit claims. Similar changes were observed in most developed countries around the same period. (b) Percentage of incapacity benefits in England and Wales by primary condition from 1996 to 2007. MH, mental health; M-skeletal, musculoskeletal problems. *Source:* Black C. *Working for a healthier tomorrow*. London: The Stationery Office, 2008.

Table 9.1 The prevalence of psychiatric disorders in one week of 2000 and 2007 based on a community sample of adults living in England (data from the Adult Psychiatric Morbidity Surveys).

	Rate per hundred in the last week			
	All Adults (in 2000)	All Adults (in 2007)	Women (in 2007)	Men (in 2007)
Mixed anxiety and depressive disorder	9.4	9.7	11.8	7.6
Depressive episode	2.8	2.6	3.0	2.2
Generalized anxiety disorder	4.7	4.7	5.8	3.6
Obsessive-compulsive disorder	1.2	1.3	1.5	1.1
Phobias	2.8	2.6	2.4	1.0
Panic disorder	0.7	1.2	1.4	1.0
Post-traumatic stress disorder	na	3.0	3.3	2.6
Probable psychosis	0.5	0.5	0.6	0.4
Hazardous or harmful alcohol use (in the last year)	na	24.2	15.7	33.2

depression and most anxiety disorders, although men are more likely to use harmful amounts of alcohol.

Despite the prevalence of psychiatric disorder being relatively stable in the population, the extent to which psychiatric disorders are associated with occupational dysfunction has changed dramatically.

The proportion of the UK working age population on long-term benefits has doubled in the last 25 years. Two discrete contributors to this change can be identified. First, a greater proportion of those beginning a claim list psychiatric disorder as their primary illness. As discussed later in this chapter, there are a number of potential reasons for this. Second, those with psychiatric disorder are less likely to leave the pool of benefits recipients than sufferers from other disorders. It has been suggested that this must relate to the configuration of services established to treat psychiatric disorders, especially as effective evidence-based treatments are available for the common mental disorders which affect the vast majority of this group.

How are psychiatric disorders classified?

Common mental disorders

The term 'common mental disorders' does not have a formal definition, but is generally taken to include depression and anxiety disorders. Common mental disorders have a major impact on occupational function and are the biggest single cause of working days lost in most developed countries. Although symptoms typical of common mental disorders may not be as dramatic as those associated with other types of psychiatric disorder, they can be particularly damaging to an individual's ability to work. As a result, the World Health Organization predicts depression will be the leading cause of disability across the developed world by 2020. Within the UK the overall cost of depression is estimated to be more than £9 billion per year.

Depression does not refer to 'normal' or understandable sadness but a psychiatric syndrome consisting of a broad but well-recognized constellation of symptoms. The key features of a depressive episode are shown in Box 9.1. Symptoms must be present for 2 or more weeks and have resulted in significant social or occupational impairment.

Box 9.1 **Key features and symptoms of depression**

Core features
- Depressed mood
- Loss of interest in usual activities
- Fatigue or decreased energy

Other common symptoms
- Difficulty concentrating
- Reduced self-esteem
- Guilt
- Pessimistic view about the future
- Ideas of self harm or suicide
- Disturbed sleep (insomnia or hypersomnia)
- Appetite and weight change (in either direction)
- Agitation or retardation
- Loss of libido

Anxiety is a symptom rather than a diagnosis and can be part of a number of psychiatric disorders. 'Anxiety disorders' is an umbrella term to describe a group of conditions in which anxiety is the predominant symptom. These include generalized anxiety disorder, phobias, obsessive compulsive disorders and panic disorder. Aside from simple phobias, generalized anxiety disorder is the most common anxiety disorder with a prevalence of approximately 5%, although often underdiagnosed. Sufferers report a persistent level of 'background' or 'free-floating' anxiety, present almost all the time. Frequently, they report not knowing why they feel anxious. This presents as worry or tension, often in association with physical symptoms of anxiety such as a dry mouth, 'butterflies', palpitations or sweats. Further symptoms include poor sleep, 'tension' headache and irritability. Within a work setting, anxiety may present as recurrent short episodes of sickness absence, avoidance of responsibility or certain meetings or a loss of productivity. Anxiety can also be a particular problem when a worker tries to return to work after a prolonged period away, regardless of the original cause of the absence.

Severe mental illness

The term 'severe mental illness' is usually used to describe those suffering from schizophrenia, other forms of psychosis or bipolar disorder. Typically these emerge in late adolescence or early adult life and often run a chronic, fluctuating course.

Schizophrenia is a syndrome comprising a number of disturbances of thought, affect, and behaviour. 'Positive' symptoms include abnormal experiences such as thought insertion or withdrawal, delusions (beliefs, firmly held against evidence to the contrary, which are out of keeping with the person's social and cultural background) and hallucinations (perceptions in the absence of stimuli). Often delusions will be unpleasant and persecutory in nature. Auditory hallucinations are the most common in schizophrenia, although hallucinations in other modalities can occur. Positive symptoms respond well to medication, but 'negative' symptoms, such as apathy and social withdrawal, can be more refractory. At times, delusional ideas can focus on the workplace and a psychotic illness may present as ideas about co-workers or entire organizations persecuting an individual. Reports of bullying or harassment are relatively common, but persecutory delusions will differ from such complaints as they are often more bizarre in their nature and will be held with absolute conviction regardless of evidence to the contrary.

Although it used to be thought that the prevalence of schizophrenia is similar among different cultures and countries, it has now been shown that there is wide variation in prevalence between countries, and that that schizophrenia is significantly more common in urban environments and among migrant populations. Occupational outcomes vary somewhat, but across Europe less than 10% of patients with schizophrenia are able to support themselves through work without the need for benefits.

Bipolar disorder is characterized by repeated episodes of disturbed mood. At least one of these episodes must involve elevated mood – mania or hypomania. The differences between mania and hypomania are not well defined and differ between European and American classification systems, but broadly mania is more severe, and often includes psychotic symptoms. Changes in biological function are common to both and include increased energy levels, reduced need for sleep, reduced appetite and increased libido. Attention and concentration are often reduced as the individual copes with an increased volume and speed of thoughts. Although a manic worker may feel they are being very productive and may have grandiose ideas regarding their role in an organization, the reality is that any work produced in a manic or hypomanic state is often disorganized and of poor quality.

The depression of bipolar disorder resembles that of the more common unipolar depression, although some bipolar patients describe increased appetite and increased sleepiness in their depressed phase. While not yet part of all formal classifications systems there is increasing recognition of a subset of patients who may have had only a short-lived or relatively minor episode of mood elevation but whose clinical picture is dominated by recurrent episodes of depression. So called bipolar II patients are important to identify as standard antidepressant medication is often either unhelpful or can worsen symptoms. Alternative treatment strategies are being developed. The prevalence of bipolar disorder is around 1%. Although a return to normal pre-morbid levels of function is much more common in bipolar disorder than other types of severe mental illness, only around 50% of individuals with bipolar disorder are in any form of work. Despite such figures, there are many examples of individuals with bipolar disorder having very successful work careers.

Post-traumatic stress disorder

Post-traumatic stress disorder (PTSD) is a rare psychiatric condition but nonetheless is often discussed within the context of occupational psychiatry. As a discrete condition, it has had a controversial history, and the rise in the number of people being diagnosed has led even some of those who first described the condition to call for a rethink of the diagnostic criteria. Unlike other psychiatric disorders, which are recognized to be multifactorial in origin, the diagnostic criteria for PTSD state that it follows exposure to a stressful event of an exceptionally threatening or catastrophic nature which is likely to cause distress in almost anyone. There are three domains of symptoms.

- The traumatic event is persistently re-experienced, for example as flashbacks or intrusive dreams or thoughts.
- There is persistent avoidance of stimuli associated with the trauma, including an inability to recall some aspects of the trauma and a feeling of detachment from others.
- There is evidence of persistently increased arousal such as hyper-vigilance or difficulty in falling asleep.

These symptoms must last at least a month, cause significant impairment in social or occupational function and strictly need to emerge within 6 months of the traumatic incident. Community studies have shown over 40% of adults report suffering from a major trauma at some point in their life. Although a diagnosis of PTSD should be considered in someone who has suffered a traumatic event, it should be remembered that the majority of those exposed to such events have only transient distress and that other conditions such as depression are a more common response to trauma than PTSD. Many employers are keen to implement debriefing interventions following a potentially traumatic event in the workplace; however, this should be advised against as a number of systematic reviews have shown that such strategies are not of benefit and may even increase the risk of PTSD.

Obsessive compulsive disorder

Obsessive compulsive disorder (OCD) is sometimes seen in the working population, but often undiagnosed. At its mildest, it can be difficult to distinguish from aspects of normal personality, and this is further complicated by around a third of cases beginning in childhood. Obsessions are intrusive and unwelcome thoughts which can be about a variety of topics, for example contamination or safety. These are not just excessive worries about real-life problems but much more disabling concerns which the individual recognizes are not based in reality. Compulsions are behaviours carried out in an attempt to alleviate the distress caused by the obsessions. Hence where the obsessive thought relates to issues of contamination, the compulsive act of handwashing is designed to reduce the distress of this thought. As with all psychiatric disorders the diagnosis requires there to be significant social or occupational impairment. Patients with OCD often take up huge amounts of time in completing their compulsive acts to the point where their anxiety is sufficiently reduced. Such symptoms can make a worker appear to be slow or avoidant of certain tasks.

Cognitive impairment

With an ageing workforce, cognitive function is becoming an increasingly important issue. Cognitive function incorporates a number of domains; attention, language, constructional skills, memory, executive function and others. Dementia is a common cause of cognitive impairment but is by no means the only one. Depression and anxiety are often associated with impaired attention which can in turn present with memory problems. A number of physical disorders (e.g. epilepsy) can also impact on aspects of cognitive function as can both prescribed and non-prescribed drugs. The most common form of dementia is Alzheimer's disease in which memory impairment and confusion are often early signs. In other forms of dementia, such as frontotemporal dementia, personality change and apathy are more prominent. The most obvious occupational impact of cognitive impairment will be impaired work performance, although this is often recognized relatively late due to the very gradual onset of symptoms and ability of previously highly functioning individuals to hide any emerging difficulties.

Alcohol and drug problems

Alcohol problems are widespread in the UK and other developed countries and have a significant impact on both individuals and employers. In England around 250 000 people come to work each day with a hangover. Alcohol is implicated in 20% of all accidents and half of all fatal accidents in the workplace. Up to 15% of days off sick are associated with alcohol. Illicit drug use is also common in most developed countries, with 1 in 10 adults in England and Wales admitting to using drugs at least once in the previous year.

Hazardous drinking describes a pattern where an individual regularly drinks more than the recommended limits (2–3 units per day for women and 3–4 units per day for men). Harmful drinking is hazardous drinking where there is evidence of harmful consequences for the individual. Well-validated tools such as the Alcohol Use Disorders Identification Questionnaire are available to assist health professionals to identify alcohol problems in their patients. Alcohol dependence syndrome consists of a number of symptoms (Box 9.2). It is estimated up to 5% of the workforce in the UK are alcohol dependent.

Box 9.2 **Key features and symptoms of alcohol dependence**

- Strong desire or sense of compulsion to drink alcohol
- Increased tolerance to alcohol
- Withdrawal symptoms when alcohol is not consumed (tremor, anxiety, sweating, nausea, hallucinations, disorientation, seizures, death)
- Relief of withdrawal symptoms by further alcohol consumption
- Salience of drinking behaviour (neglect of other activities or interests)
- Narrowing of drinking repertoire (same type of drink consumed in the same way each day)
- Relapse of alcohol consumption after periods of abstinence
- Persistent use despite evidence of harm

Similar classification systems have been developed for other drugs, with some individuals engaging in episodic use whereas others become dependent. This will depend both on the individual and on what is being consumed, with some substances such as opiates or benzodiazepines being particularly likely to lead to dependence syndromes. Workplace signs which suggest an individual employee may be using excessive alcohol or illicit substances include recurrent short-term absences (particularly on Mondays), reduced work performance, dishevelled appearance, arriving at work intoxicated, mood fluctuations or increased disputes with colleagues.

What is 'stress'?

Stress is not a diagnosis, yet 'stress at work' and 'work-related stress' have become common terms in lay discussion. The term 'stress' is used in many different ways. It can be used to describe an individual's emotional response to their environment or to label a stimulus which may trigger some form of response. The term 'work-related stress' is further complicated by the implicit assumption that the workplace has caused the stress; the basis for such an assumption is not always clear. The European Agency for Safety and Health at Work has adopted the following definition: 'work-related stress is experienced when the demands of the work environment exceed the workers' ability to cope with (or control) them'. Using this definition, it is estimated that around 22% of workers in the European Union are experiencing 'work-related stress'. However, as noted above, this does not mean that these individuals are suffering from a psychiatric illness.

Karasek and Theorell first suggested the job strain model for the psychosocial work environment, where high strain describes the presence of high job demands and low decision latitude (Figure 9.2). An alternative model from Siegrist described an effort reward imbalance where high effort matched with low rewards results in adverse outcomes. Using such measures, an adverse psychosocial work environment has been shown to be associated with biological changes, such as alterations in the autonomic nervous system and the hypothalamic–pituitary–adrenal axis, and, in the longer term, increased rates of hypertension, stroke, coronary heart disease and premature death. Adverse psychosocial work environments have also been associated with sick leave, disability pensions and early retirement and a recent meta-analysis (see Further reading) provides robust evidence that both job strain and effort reward imbalance were independent predictors of common mental disorders. Although such findings highlight the potential importance of work-related stress, it must be remembered that a variety of individual factors, such as personality, coping styles and perceived vulnerability are important in defining how each individual perceives and reacts to their psychosocial work environment.

Both local and European laws now enshrine the notion that employees should have some protection against those elements of their work likely to cause stress. Such laws recognize that employees must accept some pressure in their daily work lives, but that employers must take reasonable steps to reduce unacceptably high or prolonged pressure (e.g. impossible demands) and provide their workers with adequate support and to protect them from bullying and harassment. Case law has also made it clear that if an employer is made aware that an individual employee is more vulnerable to the effects of stress, then their duty of care is increased. The Health and Safety Executive in the UK and the European Commission have both published guidance to advise employers and organizations on how they can meet these obligations (see Further reading). Such advice tends to focus on a risk management approach, with routine assessments of the level of psychosocial hazard and methods to investigate and address problems when they are identified. There are also a variety of individual 'stress management' interventions, although the evidence for most work-related stress interventions is weak.

Although research on the psychosocial work environment highlights the negative impact of 'bad' work, it should not be forgotten that there is also a body of evidence supporting the notion that work is in general good for health, including mental health. In addition to the obvious financial benefits work provides a structure to the day, a sense of purpose and achievement, and the opportunity to engage socially with colleagues. By contrast worklessness is associated with increased rates of common mental disorder, alcohol and drug misuse and self-harm.

What causes a worker to become mentally ill?

Although commonly held views about stress at work might suggest that there is a simple cause-and-effect relationship between work and common mental disorders, the evidence suggests otherwise. As noted above, there is clear evidence that an adverse psychosocial work environment increases the risk of common mental disorders. However, many workers exposed to stressful situations do not become unwell, work factors being only one group of a range of potential risk factors that can interact across the life course. Table 9.2 uses the example of depression to show how a number of biological, psychological and social risk factors may act as predisposing, precipitating or maintaining factors in the aetiology of a psychiatric disorder.

Consequences of common mental disorders

As outlined above, common mental disorders, such as depression and anxiety, can cause considerable distress and place major

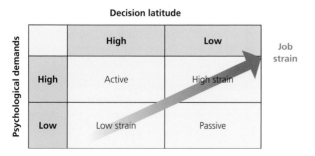

Figure 9.2 The Job Strain model of the psychosocial work environment, as described by Karasek and Theorell.

Table 9.2 Examples of factors which may be involved in the aetiology of a depressive episode.

	Biological	Psychological	Social
Predisposing	Genetic factors Family history	Abuse in childhood Low family cohesion Neurotic personality	Material deprivation Lower socio- economic position
Precipitating	Physical illness Neurobiological changes (serotonin, etc.)	Acute loss	Workplace stress Job loss Other life events
Perpetuating	Changes to the hypothalamic– pituitary axis	Negative automatic thoughts	Lack of social support Financial problems

limitations on an individual's ability to function in the workplace. Individuals suffering from common mental disorders are also more likely to underachieve in education, be less satisfied with life, have greater relationship problems and are at considerably increased risk of suicide or self-harm. However, in measuring the impact of psychiatric disorders it is also important to consider the overlap between mental and physical health. Depression is associated with an increased risk of death from all major disease-related causes. This is thought to be due to a combination of inferior levels of physical health care, poorer lifestyle and a range of biological changes associated with depression (with proposed mechanisms including subtle increases in inflammation, alterations to the autonomic nervous system and dysfunction of the hypothalamic–pituitary–adrenal axis). As a result, the risk of early death associated with depression is similar to that seen with smoking. The relationship between physical and mental health may also work in the opposite direction, with individuals who are already suffering from physical health problems at increased risk of depression or anxiety. Common mental disorders occurring on top of physical health problem can be difficult to detect, but if untreated they are a powerful predictor of poor work outcomes. The reason for psychiatric disorders having such a dramatic impact on occupational function remains unclear. Some symptoms, such as fatigue, lack of motivation, insomnia, impaired social functioning and cognitive impairment appear to be particularly prejudicial to work performance, but there is relatively little association between the overall levels of disease severity and occupational function.

Assessment of an individual's mental state

Given the high prevalence and importance of psychiatric disorders, some assessment of an individual's mental state should form part of all clinical encounters in an occupational health setting. A number of validated self-report questionnaires are available to help in the detection of common mental disorders (as listed in Box 9.3), but these should be used in addition to, rather than instead of, good clinical assessments. Studies have shown that a small number of simple, direct questions about some of the core symptoms of depression and anxiety can be effective screening tools. However, a good assessment of the mental state will require additional, more probing

questions and will need to be combined with careful observation of a variety of non-verbal measures. The types of areas covered by a comprehensive mental state examination are listed in Box 9.4.

Box 9.3 Some examples of screening tools which could be used in an occupational health setting

Depression

- Patient Health Questionnaire (PHQ-9)
- Beck Depression Inventory (BDI)
- Center for Epidemiologic Studies Depression Scale (CES-D)
- Depression in the Medically Ill (DMI-10)

Anxiety

- Beck Anxiety Inventory
- Generalized Anxiety Disorder Screening Tool (GAD-7)

Depression and anxiety

- Hospital Anxiety and Depression Scale (HADS)
- General Health Questionnaire (GHQ)

Alcohol use

- CAGE questions
- Alcohol Use Disorders Identification Test (AUDIT)

PTSD

- Trauma Screening Questionnaire (TSQ)
- Impact of Event Scale (IES)
- The SPAN test
- National Centre for PTSD Checklist (PCL-C)

Box 9.4 The main aspects of a mental state examination and some examples of the questions that should be addressed

Appearance and behaviour

- How are they dressed? Do their appear well groomed or dishevelled? Are their clothes appropriate?
- Do they appear steady on their feet? Are they in any obvious pain or distress?
- Do they smell of alcohol? Do they seem intoxicated? Are there any signs of alcohol withdrawal?
- Are they co-operative? If not, do they seem suspicious or aggressive, or anxious?
- Are they behaving appropriately?
- Are they tearful?

Speech

- Rate, tone and volume of speech. Any slurring?
- Do they talk a lot or is there very little spontaneous speech?
- Do their sentences make sense? Is there any 'thought disorder'?
- Do they stick to the topic, or does their conversation wander?

Mood

- Do they describe feeling low or happy?
- Objectively do they appear flat, elated, blunted, etc?
- Are there other symptoms related to mood, like sleep disturbance?

Thoughts

- Do they appear preoccupied by certain issues?
- Is there any evidence of racing or negative thoughts?
- Are there any delusional or overvalued ideas?

- Any thoughts of suicide, self-harm or violence towards others?
- What role to they think their work has played in their illness?

Perceptions

- Auditory, visual, olfactory or tactile hallucinations

Cognition

- Are they alert and orientated?
- Did they have any trouble remembering events or dates?

Insight

- Do they think they are unwell? If so, what do they think is the problem and are they willing to accept treatment

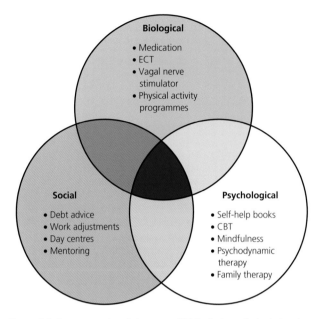

Figure 9.3 Some examples of the types of biological, psychological and social treatments which may be offered.

As outlined above, suicide is a major cause of premature death among those suffering from symptoms of mental illness. The majority of those who harm themselves have been in contact with medical staff in the month prior to their suicide attempt, but they will often not mention their suicidal thoughts unless asked. Asking about suicidal thoughts does not increase the risk of self-harm and should be a regular part of any mental health assessment. If a patient reports thoughts of life not being worth living, other factors such as their past history of self harm, current symptoms and the presence of any specific plans must be enquired about and will be vital in assessing their level of risk. When a risk of harm to self or others is identified, it is important to seek urgent expert advice.

Treatment and prognosis

The early detection and treatment of psychiatric disorders is essential if the occupational consequences of the illness are to be minimized. There are now effective, evidence-based treatments for almost all psychiatric disorders. Many individuals with severe mental illness will be managed by specialized mental health teams, made up of psychiatrists, community psychiatric nurses, social workers, psychologists and occupational therapists. The majority of common mental disorders are managed in primary care by general practitioners and primary care psychology services. Regardless of the setting, the treatment of psychiatric disorders is often most effective when biological, psychological and social interventions are combined. Examples of treatments in each of these categories are shown in Figure 9.3, with a list of treatments known to be effective across a range of disorders listed in Table 9.3.

Unfortunately, the majority of studies examining the effectiveness of different treatments have tended to focus on symptom reduction, with very little attention paid to functional outcomes such as occupational performance. As a result it is difficult to know which interventions have specific work benefits. The Cochrane Collaboration has recently published a systematic review of randomized controlled trials that are available for work or worker-directed interventions for depression. They concluded that although a variety of interventions are effective in reducing symptoms, there was no evidence that any had an impact on the amount of sickness absence taken by depressed individuals. The apparent lack of an effect of standard treatments on occupational outcomes suggests that additional specific interventions addressing return to work

issues may be needed. There is some evidence that work-focused cognitive behavioural therapy approaches may result in employees returning to work more rapidly.

Many companies also provide Employee Assistance Programmes or counselling to provide relatively unstructured psychological support. Workplace counselling may be helpful for some, but at present there is very little good-quality evidence of its effectiveness as a treatment for psychiatric disorders.

Even with effective treatment, many severe mental illnesses tend to have a chronic relapsing course. Common mental disorders, such as depression or anxiety, tend to have a less chronic course and a return to previous functioning should be expected. The risk of relapse in any psychiatric condition can usually be decreased with regular medication, appropriate psychological interventions and ongoing support. For example, in the case of depression there is evidence that continuing to take an effective dose of antidepressant medication for 6 months after recovery may halve the absolute risk of a relapse. All individuals who have suffered from a psychiatric disorder should ideally have a 'relapse prevention plan', which will specify times when they may be at risk of relapse, early warning signs and an agreed action plan if these warning signs are observed. For example, if an employee has been diagnosed with bipolar affective disorder, their relapse prevention plan may note that their relapses tend to occur at certain times of year or when they are experiencing high levels of stress. Early warning signs of a relapse may include symptoms, such as racing thoughts and disturbed sleep, as well as behaviours which may be first detected by work colleagues, such as agitation or decreased quality of work. If an employee agrees, trusted work colleagues may have a role in a relapse prevention plan, such as informing occupational health if they notice agreed early warning signs.

Within mental health services, there is an increased emphasis on the 'recovery model' of treatment, with a focus on improved functionality, rather than just reduced symptoms. This has created

Table 9.3 Some examples of treatments or interventions which have been shown to reduce symptoms or improve functioning.

Disorder	What appears to work	What doesn't work
Common mental disorders	Antidepressant medication (beneficial in both depression and anxiety disorders) Physical activity (for mild depression) Self-help material based on the principles of CBT (for mild depression) Computerized CBT Group or individual CBT IPT Mindfulness-based cognitive therapy Behavioural activation therapy Inpatient care (only needed for a small minority) Electroconvulsive therapy (very rarely used) Behavioural therapy (for some anxiety disorders)	Herbal remedies (although St John's wart has effects similar to antidepressant medication there are a lot of potential interactions with other medications) Benzodiazepines can provide short-term relief from anxiety, but can lead to dependence if used for too long Stigma Avoidance is often unhelpful in anxiety disorders Self-medication with alcohol or other substances Counselling may help some individuals, but does not have a strong evidence base as a treatment for established mental illness
PTSD	Trauma-focused CBT Eye movement desensitization and reprocessing (EMDR) Certain types of antidepressant medication in some specific cases	Post-trauma debriefing Secondary stressors after a traumatic event (e.g. limited practical support)
Drug and alcohol problems	A variety of psychological interventions (such as CBT, MET, 12-step process, etc.) Social network and environment-based therapies Medication to help with abstinence and relapse prevention, such as acamprosate, naltrexone or disufiram Replacement therapy for opioid addiction May need detoxification if dependent Vitamin supplementation (to prevent Wernicke Korsakoff syndrome)	Untreated comorbid common mental disorders (which are very common)
Severe mental disorders	Medication (antipsychotic medication and/or mood stabilizers) Psychological therapies (CBT) Interventions to improve medication compliance Family therapy in some cases Multidisciplinary management Individual placement and support (IPS) shown to improve occupational outcomes	Stigma Substance misuse (e.g. cannabis)

CBT, cognitive behavioural therapy; IPT, interpersonal therapy; MET, motivational enhancement therapy.

an increased focus on work in most mental health services, with many community mental health teams now employing dedicated vocational specialists. With appropriate treatment and support most individuals with mental illness should be able to aim to remain as active participants in the workforce.

Further reading

Lelliott P, Boardman J, Harvey S, Henderson M, Knapp M, Tulloch S. *Mental Health and Work. A report for the National Director for Work and Health.* London: Royal College of Psychiatrists, 2008. *A report produced by the Royal College of Psychiatrists which was published together with Dame Carol Black's landmark review on the health of Britain's working age population. This detailed review brings together much of the literature on how work and mental health are related, including calculations of the costs of mental illness*

McManus S, Meltzer H, et al. (eds) *Adult psychiatric morbidity in England, 2007. Results of a household survey.* Leeds: NHS Information Centre for Health and Social Care, 2009. *The latest round of a general population survey which examines the prevalence and risk factors for a variety of mental health problems*

Health and Safety Executive. Managing the causes of work-related stress: A step-by-step approach using the Management Standards. London: HSE Books, 2007. *The Management Standards approach was developed by the HSE to help employers and managers assess the risk of an adverse psychosocial*

work environment and how to address problems when they are indentified. This booklet (which is available free as a PDF from www.hse.gov.uk) provides detailed notes on the Management Standards and includes lots of illustrative case examples

Henderson M, Harvey SB, Øverland S, Mykletun A. Work and common psychiatric disorders. *J R Soc Med* 2011; 104: 198–207. *A review paper examining the issues around common mental disorders, particularly depression and anxiety, in the workplace*

Nieuwenhuijsen K, Bultmann U, et al. Interventions to improve occupational health in depressed people. *Cochrane Database Syst Rev* 2008; (2):CD006237–. *A systematic review of all trials which have examined the effectiveness of work and worker directed interventions aimed at reducing the occupation disability of depressed workers*

Netterstrom B, Conrad N, Bech P, Fink P, Olsen O, Rugulies R, Stansfeld S. The relation between work-related psychosocial factors and the development of depression. *Epidemiol Rev* 2008; 30: 118–132. *A systematic review of longitudinal studies examining the links between adverse psychosocial work environments and depression. This paper demonstrates moderate evidence for an association between psychological job demands and depression, but also highlights the limitations of many studies*

Michie S, Williams S. Reducing work related psychological ill health and sickness absence: a systematic literature review. *Occup Environ Med* 2003; 60: 3–9. *A systematic review of work factors which may be associated with mental illness, including various measures of 'work stress'. A number of work-based interventions are also discussed*

CHAPTER 10

Skin Disorders

Ian R. White

St. John's Institute of Dermatology, St. Thomas' Hospital, London, UK

OVERVIEW

- The overwhelming majority of occupational skin disorders are dermatitic
- It is a major error to rely solely on the pattern of hand dermatitis when considering a diagnosis
- Understanding the precise nature of a person's job is essential (what do they do and how do they do it?)
- Patch testing is the only objective method of assessing a dermatitis; it should be undertaken when assessing any persistent hand dermatitis
- Delays in diagnosis predispose to chronicity; early referral to a specialist is important

---

Skin disorders are among the most often encountered problems in the occupational health setting, and although there are many dermatoses that have occupational relevance, the overwhelming majority are dermatitic. Occupations considered to be at greatest risk include hairdressing, nursing and similar healthcare, engineering (soluble coolant exposure) and food preparation.

Contact dermatitis

In current terminology, the term 'dermatitis' is used synonymously with 'eczema' and describes inflammatory reactions in the skin with a spectrum of clinical and histopathological characteristics.

A **dermatitis** (Figure 10.1) may be entirely endogenous (constitutional) or be entirely exogenous (contact). The latter consists of irritant and allergic contact reactions. Commonly, a dermatitis has a multifactorial aetiology and may be aggravated by the presence of pathogens (*Staphylococcus aureus*). Assessment of the relative importance (contribution) of the possible factors can be difficult and subjective.

Atopic hand dermatitis and vesicular hand dermatitis are examples of endogenous conditions.

- From the distribution and morphology of a dermatitis on the hands it is not possible to be definitive about the aetiology,

e.g. a vesicular hand dermatitis with a 'classical' endogenous distribution may be mimicked by an allergic contact dermatitis to isothiazolinone biocides or chromate sensitivity.
- It is a major error to rely on patterns of hand dermatitis in making a diagnosis.

An occupational dermatitis is one where the inflammatory reaction is caused entirely by occupational contact factors or where such agents contribute to the reaction on a compromised skin, i.e. they are partially responsible.

In the majority of cases, an occupationally related dermatitis will affect the hands alone. There may be spread onto the forearms. Occasionally the face may be the prime site of involvement (e.g. airborne); other sites may be involved.

Occupational dermatitis may be *suspected* when:

- dermatitis first occurred while employed
- history of aggravation by work
- there may be, at least initially, improvement (or clearance) when not at work
- exposure to irritant factors or potential allergens
- work in an 'at risk' occupation.

Irritant contact dermatitis is initiated by direct chemical or physical damage to the skin. All individuals are susceptible to the development of an irritant contact dermatitis if exposure to the irritant (toxic) agent(s) is sufficient. It occurs particularly where

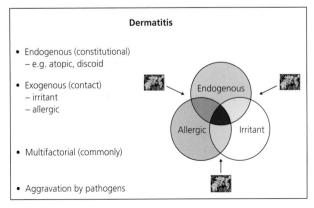

Figure 10.1 Dermatitis.

ABC of Occupational and Environmental Medicine, Third Edition.
Edited by David Snashall and Dipti Patel.
© 2012 John Wiley & Sons Ltd. Published 2012 by John Wiley & Sons Ltd.

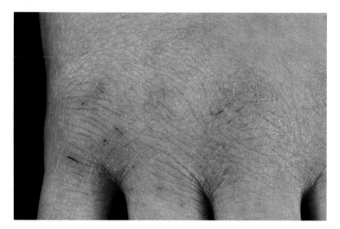

Figure 10.2 Acute dermatitis.
Severity of reaction depends on 'dose' of irritant agent.
'Chapping' can be considered a minor form with a 'chemical burn'
(e.g. cement burn) an extreme event.
Intermediate eczematous reactions are common, minor reactions are very
common.
May occur on the face, e.g. low humidity occupational dermatosis, airborne
irritant vapours.
Once the irritant factor(s) have been removed, resolution is usually
spontaneous without important sequelae.

the stratum corneum is thinnest. Hence, it is often seen in the finger
webs and back of the hands rather than the palms. There are two
principal types of irritant contact dermatitis – **acute** (Figure 10.2)
and **chronic** (Figure 10.3). The former is caused by exposure to
an agent(s) causing early impairment in stratum corneum function
followed by an inflammatory reaction. The latter by repeated
exposure to the same or different factors resulting in 'cumulative'
damage until an inflammatory reaction ensues which persists for
a prolonged period even after further exposure is stopped. Those
with a previous history of atopic eczema, and especially atopic hand

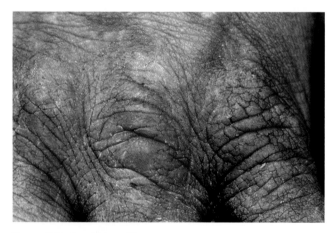

Figure 10.3 Chronic dermatitis.
Persistent dermatitis and the most common cause of continued disability
from occupational skin disease.
Problem continues for long periods even with avoidance of aggravating
factors.
Re-exposure to even minor irritant factors may cause a rapid flare.
After apparent healing there may be a prolonged increased susceptibility to
recurrence of a dermatitis following irritant exposure.

Table 10.1 Examples.

Common irritants	Common occupational allergens
'Wet work'	Rubber accelerating chemicals
Soaps and detergents	Biocides/preservatives
Alkalis	Hairdressing chemicals
Acids	Resin monomers
Metalworking fluids	Chromium
Organic solvents	Plant allergens
Other petroleum products	Fragrance chemicals
Oxidizing agents	
Reducing agents	
Animal products	
Physical factors	

eczema, are at particular risk of developing a chronic irritant contact
dermatitis. A chronic irritant contact dermatitis is particularly
observed where 'wet work' is involved.

Allergic contact dermatitis is a manifestation of a type IV
hypersensitivity reaction. An allergic contact dermatitis will develop
at the site of skin contact with the allergen (Table 10.1) but secondary
spread may occur. Contaminated hands may spread the allergen
to 'non-exposed' sites. Trivial or occult contact with an allergen
may result in a persistence of a dermatitis; some allergens are
'ubiquitous'.

There are two phases to the presentation of an allergic reaction:
induction and elicitation. Even with potent experimental allergens
there is a minimum period of about 10 days from first exposure to
the immunological acquisition of hypersensitivity. The probability
of developing hypersensitivity depends on the sensitising capacity
of the chemical and exposure to it. Exposure is assessed in terms of
dose per unit area applied to the skin. Most potential allergens on
the consumer and industrial market have a low intrinsic allergenic
potential, but there are important exceptions including some biocides (preservatives). Contact allergens tend to be low molecular
weight (<600) and capable of forming covalent bonds with carrier
proteins in the skin. It is not possible to determine an individual's
own susceptibility to the development of contact allergy. Hypersensitivity is specific to a particular molecule or to molecules bearing
similar allergenic sites. Although hypersensitivity may be lost over a
long time, once acquired it should be considered to last indefinitely.

Management of occupational dermatitis

An understanding of the patient's job is essential. A job title is not
sufficient for this understanding; the question to be asked is not
'what do you do?' but 'what do you actually do and how do you
do it?' The title 'engineer' carries a multiple of descriptions from
the desk-bound professional to the lathe worker exposed to soluble
coolants. From the job description, it will be possible to estimate
sources of excessive contact with potentially irritant contact factors
or with allergens. The provision of material safety data sheets
may be helpful in this evaluation although the information that
they contain is often superficial, generic and is that required
for regulatory requirements. A site visit – watching the worker
working – may be necessary.

The *history and anatomical distribution* of the dermatitis may
provide clues as to the aetiology (Figure 10.4).

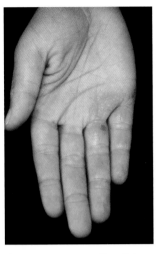
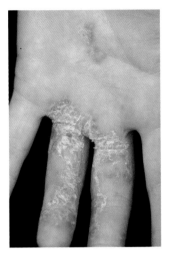
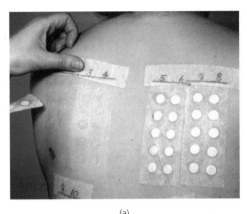

Figure 10.4 Patterns of hand dermatitis.
From the distribution and morphology of a dermatitis on the hands it is not possible to be definitive about the aetiology. e.g., a vesicular hand dermatitis with a 'classical' endogenous distribution may be mimicked by an allergic contact dermatitis to isothiazolinone biocides or chromate sensitivity.
It is a major error to rely on patterns of hand dermatitis in making a diagnosis.

Irritant contact dermatitis may occur as 'epidemics' in a workplace if hygiene has failed. Allergic contact dermatitis is usually sporadic in a workplace.

The *evaluation* of irritant factors is always subjective. Evaluation of allergic contact factors is objective and provided only by diagnostic patch test investigations. Properly performed, patch tests will demonstrate the presence or absence of relevant allergens (Box 10.1).

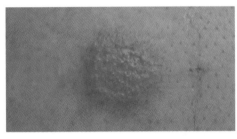

(a)

(b)

(c)

Figure 10.5 Patch testing. a) *Patch testing* is the objective method for the evaluation of a dermatitis. b) There are major pitfalls in the use of this essential tool; proper training and experience is essential. c) Properly performed, patch tests will demonstrate the *presence or absence* of relevant allergens.

Box 10.1 **Exposure factors**

- From the job description, it may be possible to estimate sources of contact with:
  ○ irritants
  ○ allergens
- Personal protective equipment
- Material safety data sheets
  ○ Information is often superficial (that needed to meet regulatory requirements)
- Request information/samples
- A site visit – watching the worker working – may be necessary

Patch testing (Figure 10.5) is the only method for the objective evaluation of a dermatitis. There are major pitfalls in the use of this essential tool; adequate training and experience is essential if it is to be used properly. Ability to assess relevance of allergens is central.

A *competent assessment* requires all of the above followed by recommendations on reducing/stopping exposure to the offending agent(s) and similar ones.

The *diagnosis* of an occupational dermatitis should describe thoroughly the nature of the condition with due regard to any endogenous or aggravating factors. A general practitioner medical record entry in a patient's notes of '*Works in a factory, contact dermatitis. 2/52*' is inadequate as a description of an important disease process and it can have profound implications on the patient's concept of his problem and employment.

Delays in diagnosis resulting in continued exposure to relevant irritants/allergens can adversely affect the prognosis.

Early referral to an appropriate dermatology department is necessary for a comprehensive assessment of a suspected occupational dermatitis; improper assessment can have devastating effects on future employment prospects for the individual with important medicolegal implications. If in doubt – refer.

Immediate sensitivity (type I); contact urticaria

Immediate hypersensitivity occurs to protein fractions present in natural rubber latex used to make gloves and other items.

The problem was particularly seen among healthcare workers but individuals in other industries where 'examination' gloves are used have also been at risk. Affected individuals are usually atopic. They present with a localised urticarial reaction at sites of skin contact or with respiratory symptoms when starch powdered gloves have been used. It was an important cause of occupational morbidity in some settings. A definitive demonstration of hypersensitivity can be made by skinprick testing with water-soluble proteins. Commercial preparations are available. RAST is less sensitive.

Contact urticaria (Box 10.2) is occasionally seen in those handling food products. Non-immunological contact urticaria occurs with diverse chemicals, e.g. ammonium persulphate, cinnamal.

Box 10.2 **Other occupational dermatoses**

- Contact urticaria – type I hypersensitivity reaction-for example, natural rubber latex protein, foods
- Chloracne acneiform eruption caused by certain halogenated aromatic hydrocarbons; a symptom of systemic absorption
- Oil folliculitis (oil acne) – irritant effect of neat petroleum oils localised to hair follicles
- Depigmentation (leukoderma) – caused by hydroquinone and phenol derivatives
- Hyperpigmentation – caused by mineral oils, halogenated hydrocarbons and tar products
- Skin cancer (see Chapter 13)
- Skin infections (see Chapter 12)

Further reading

Nicholson PJ, Llewellyn D, English J. *Contact dermatitis* 2010; 63: 77–186. *Evidence-based guidelines for the prevention, identification and management of occupational contact dermatitis and urticaria. The guideline is relevant to current practice and from the perspective of the UK*

Menné T, Johansen JD, Sommerlund M, Veien NK. Hand eczema guidelines based on the Danish guidelines for the diagnosis and treatment of hand eczema. *Contact Dermatitis* 2011; 65: 3–12. *A similar guideline from a European perspective*

Johansen JD, Hald M, Lasthein Andersen B, *et al.* Classification of hand eczema: clinical and aetiological types. Based on the guideline of the Danish Contact Dermatitis Group. *Contact Dermatitis* 2011; 65: 13–21. *A practical and pictorial guide to the classification of hand eczema*

Rustemeyer T, Elsner P, John S-M, Maibach HI (eds). *Kanerva's occupational skin diseases.* Springer, 2012. *An encyclopaedic review of occupational groups and associated work related dermatoses*

Johansen JD, Frosch PF, Lepoittevin JP (eds). *Contact dermatitis*, 5th edn. Springer 2010. *The standard European text book for contact dermatitis and occupational dermatoses*

The monthly journal *Contact Dermatitis (Cutaneous Allergy, Environmental & Occupational Dermatitis) (Wiley) publishes papers and case reports on matters relevant to occupational dermatology*

CHAPTER 11

Respiratory Disorders

Ira Madan[1] and Paul Cullinan[2]

[1]Guy's and St Thomas' NHS Trust and King's College London, London, UK
[2]National Heart and Lung Institute (Imperial College), London, UK

OVERVIEW

- A detailed occupational history is essential for the diagnosis of occupational respiratory disorders
- Accurate diagnosis of the subset and cause of occupational asthma is essential for optimal management of the employee
- Globally the incidence of pneumoconiosis and byssinosis is increasing as manufacturing industries are being established and/or outsourced to developing countries, where the standard of health and safety at work may be lower than in the developed world
- Most occupational respiratory disorders can be prevented by reducing the exposure of employees to the causative agent

Table 11.1 Estimated number of new UK cases of work-related and occupational respiratory diseases reported by occupational and respiratory physicians to SWORD by diagnostic category 2007–2009.

Diagnostic category	2007	2008	2009
Benign pleural disease	1008	1125	856
Malignant mesothelioma	885	647	519
Asthma	355	362	223
Other	195	147	178
Pneumoconiosis	172	156	183
Lung cancer	104	91	86
Infectious diseases	64	24	49
Inhalation accidents	21	39	37
Allergic alveolitis	19	87	52
Bronchitis/emphysema	17	30	68
Total diagnoses	2840	2708	2251
Total cases*	2812	2658	2175

*Individuals may have more than one diagnosis.
Adapted from the Health and Safety Executive THOR data.

The sharp reduction in the incidence of asbestosis and pneumoconioses in industrialized countries during the past 70 years is attributable to a decline in manufacturing industries and higher health and safety standards. Asthma is now the most common occupational respiratory disorder in the developed world. By contrast, the traditional occupational lung diseases are commonly seen in developing countries, and occupational asthma is reported less often. However, the true prevalence of asthma attributable to occupation in these countries remains unknown.

Since 1989, the understanding of the epidemiology of occupational lung disease in the United Kingdom has been greatly enhanced by the Surveillance of Work-related and Occupational Respiratory Disease (SWORD), which more recently has come under the umbrella of The Health and Occupation Reporting network (THOR) (Table 11.1). Occupational physicians, respiratory physicians and specially trained family doctors systematically report new cases of occupational lung diseases, together with the suspected agent, industry and occupation.

Work-related asthma

Work-related asthma (WRA) refers to asthma that is exacerbated or induced by inhalation exposures in the workplace. Occupational asthma is a subset of WRA and is defined as *de novo* asthma or recurrence of previously quiescent asthma induced by either (a) sensitization to a substance in the workplace (sensitizer-induced occupational asthma), or (b) exposure to an inhaled irritant at work (irritant-induced occupational asthma). Work-exacerbated asthma is another subset of WRA and is defined as pre-existing or concurrent asthma that is triggered by work-related exposures, for example irritants or exercise.

Sensitizer-induced asthma typically appears after a latent period of asymptomatic occupational exposure. Substances that induce occupational asthma ('respiratory sensitizing agents) are classified as either of high (>10 kd) or low molecular weight (Table 11.2). High molecular weight substances are usually protein-derived allergens such as natural rubber latex and flour. They typically cause occupational asthma by immunoglobulin IgE antibody-associated mechanisms. In contrast, some low molecular weight chemicals, such as diisocyanates, act as haptens and combine with a body protein to form a complete antigen.

To date, more than 250 agents capable of causing immunological occupational asthma have been reported. Figure 11.1 illustrates the causes of occupational asthma reported by chest physicians and occupational physicians during 2007–2009 to THOR.

In some jobs, such as farming, workers are exposed to many potential respiratory sensitizers and sensitization may occur through interaction of several agents including an array of potential

ABC of Occupational and Environmental Medicine, Third Edition.
Edited by David Snashall and Dipti Patel.
© 2012 John Wiley & Sons Ltd. Published 2012 by John Wiley & Sons Ltd.

Table 11.2 Examples of high and low molecular weight substances, which may cause occupational asthma.

Substance	Occupational group at risk/industrial use
Low molecular weight chemicals	
Di-isocyanates	Car/coach paint spraying
Foam and plastic manufacture	Glues
Colophony (pine resin)	Electronics industry
Persulphate salts	Hairdressing
Complex platinum salts	Platinum refinery workers
Proteins (High molecular weight)	
Flour/grain	Bakers
Rodent urinary proteins	Laboratory workers
Salmon proteins	Fish processing plant workers
Natural rubber latex	Healthcare professionals

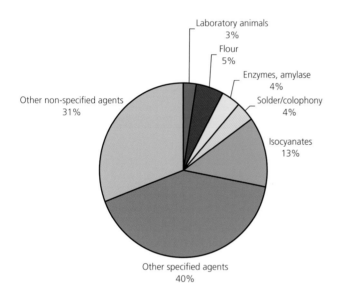

Laboratory animals 3%
Flour 5%
Enzymes, amylase 4%
Solder/colophony 4%
Isocyanates 13%
Other specified agents 40%
Other non-specified agents 31%

Figure 11.1 Occupational asthma: estimated number of diagnoses in which particular causative substances were identified. Reported by chest physicians and by occupational physicians during 2007–2009 (adapted from the Health and Safety Executive THOR data).

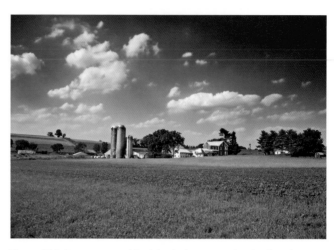

Figure 11.2 Farmers are at risk of developing occupational asthma because they are often exposed simultaneously to an array of potential sensitizers, such as animal-derived allergens, arthropods, moulds, plants and fungicides. Reproduced with permission from Nicholas T, Pennsylvania, USA.

Box 11.1 Diagnostic criteria for reactive airways disease syndrome

- History of inhalation of gas, fume or vapour with irritant properties
- Rapid onset of asthma like symptoms after exposure
- Bronchial hyper-responsiveness present on metacholine (or similar) challenge test
- Individual previously free from respiratory symptoms

---

sensitizers, such as animal-derived allergens, arthropods, moulds, plants and fungicides (Figure 11.2).

Atopic individuals are at increased risk of developing occupational asthma from high molecular weight allergens, but generally not from low molecular weight allergens. Tobacco smokers are at greater risk of developing asthma after occupational exposure to agents such as platinum salts and acid anhydride; the mechanism of this modifying effect is unknown. Tobacco smoking and atopy are common among the working population. These risk factors should not automatically exclude an individual from working with a respiratory sensitizer.

Occupational exposure to high levels of irritant fume – such as chlorine – usually occurs as the result of an industrial accident. Rarely this may induce an asthmatic response, described generally as 'irritant-induced asthma' but known formerly as reactive airways disease syndrome (RADS) (Box 11.1). The condition often resolves spontaneously but can persist indefinitely; it is characteristically resistant to standard asthma treatments.

It is estimated that 15% of cases of new or recurrent asthma in adulthood is attributable to exposures in the workplace. A detailed history of occupational exposures is essential in the assessment of a patient with adult-onset asthma, as is an assessment of any temporal relationship between symptoms of asthma (cough, wheeze and breathlessness) and work. Preceding or concurrent nasal congestion, lacrimation and conjunctivitis may be associated with exposure to high molecular weight substances. Symptoms generally improve at weekends and on holidays, but at advanced stages may persist. Where possible, advice should be sought from the patient's occupational health service, as they will have information on the substances that the employee is exposed to and will know if other workers have developed similar respiratory symptoms.

Patients should record the best of three measurements of peak expiratory flow made every 2 hours from waking to sleeping over a period of 1 month. This period should include at least 1 week away from work. A consistent fall in peak expiratory flow and/or increase in diurnal variability on working days compared with days away from work supports a diagnosis of occupational asthma. An example of the type of peak flow readings found in an individual with occupational asthma is shown in Figure 11.3.

If there is any doubt, the patient should be referred to a specialist centre for further investigation, including a bronchial provocation test with the suspected agent. Evidence of specific IgE sensitization to workplace allergens may be sought through skin prick testing or the measurement of serum specific IgE antibodies. Where there is

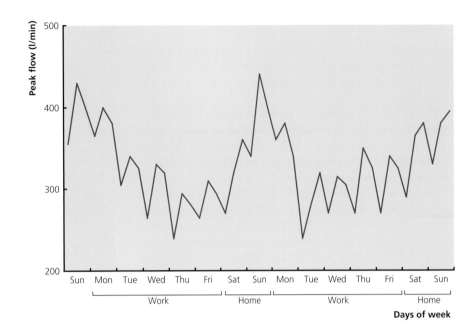

Figure 11.3 Self-recorded peak flow measurements showing a classic pattern of occupational asthma.

any doubt, advice on the choice of appropriate test allergens should be sought (Box 11.2).

Box 11.2 **Specialist investigation of occupational asthma**

a. Identification of atopy: skin prick tests with common allergens, e.g. grass pollen, Dermatophagoides pteronyssinus, and cat fur
b. Skin prick tests with specific extracts of putative sensitizing agent
c. Serology: tests to identify specific IgE antibody
d. Bronchial provocation test with the suspected causative agent

---

Symptomatic treatment of occupational asthma is the same as for asthma generally, but it is important to ensure that further exposure to the causative agent is avoided. As this often means relocation or loss of current employment, it is essential that the specific cause be accurately identified. In sensitized individuals exposure to even minimal quantities of the sensitizing agent may precipitate bronchospasm. If their job entails working with the causative agent, relocation to another area will need to be considered; again the patient's occupational health service (where there is one) will be able to advise on suitable areas for redeployment and will be in a position to liaise with the individual's manager. The employer should review their statutory risk assessments and control measures in the area where the affected employee was working to prevent other workers being similarly affected.

Byssinosis

New cases of byssinosis are very rare in Europe but rapid outsourcing of cotton manufacture to developing countries, where control measures are often poor, means that the disease remains common elsewhere (Figure 11.4). The symptoms of byssinosis occur as a result of hypersensitive airways and an acute reduction in FEV_1

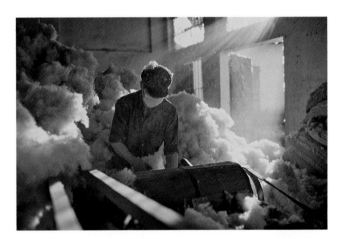

Figure 11.4 Cotton worker in a cotton factory in the developing world. Reproduced with permission from Olivier Epron, Wikimedia Commons.

(forced expiratory volume in one second) in susceptible individuals when they are exposed to dusts of cotton and other vegetable dusts, e.g. hemp and sisal. Characteristically, individuals working with these dusts experience acute dyspnoea with cough and chest tightness on the first day of the working week, 3–4 hours after the start of a work shift. The symptoms improve on subsequent working days, despite continued exposure to the sensitizing agent. As the disease progresses the symptoms recur on subsequent days of the week, and eventually even occur at weekends and during holidays. If workers who develop byssinosis are not removed from further exposure, they go on to develop long-term respiratory impairment.

Endotoxin–heat-stable lipopolysaccharide protein complexes contained in the cell wall of Gram-negative bacteria found in cotton and other vegetable fibres are responsible for the development of byssinosis. Dust control and bactericidal treatment of raw fibres are key measures in prevention of the disease.

Pneumoconiosis

Pneumoconiosis is the generic term for the inhalation of mineral dust and the resultant diffuse, usually fibrotic, reaction in the acinar part of the lung. The term excludes asthma, neoplasia and emphysema.

Silicosis is the commonest type of pneumoconiosis worldwide. It is caused by inhalation of crystalline silicon dioxide, and may affect people working in quarrying, mining, stone cutting and polishing, sandblasting and fettling. Figure 11.5 illustrates a chest radiograph of a tunneller showing simple silicosis.

Silicosis occurs in several different forms depending on the level and duration of exposure. Simple nodular silicosis is the most common form and is frequently asymptomatic. More severe forms present with increasing dyspnoea over several years, restrictive or mixed abnormalities of lung function testing and radiographic changes of (upper lobe) nodular fibrosis; 'accelerated' forms of disease also occur. Acute silicosis (causing alveolar proteinosis) results from a brief but heavy exposure: patients become intensely breathless and may die within months. Chest radiographs show an appearance resembling pulmonary oedema.

Coal worker's pneumoconiosis is caused by inhalation of coal dust, which is a complex mixture of coal, kaolin, mica, silica and other minerals. Globally, it is a common disease. Simple coal worker's pneumoconiosis usually produces no symptoms or physical signs apart from exertional dyspnoea. The diagnosis is made by a history of exposure and the presence of characteristic opacities on chest radiographs. A small proportion of individuals with simple coal worker's pneumoconiosis go on to develop progressive massive fibrosis which, when sufficiently advanced, causes dyspnoea, cor pulmonale and ultimately death.

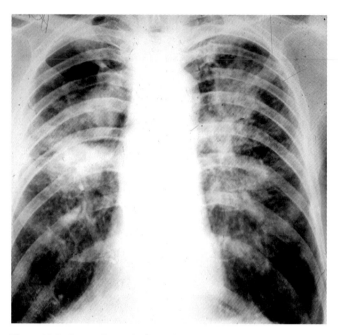

Figure 11.6 Chest radiograph of a coal miner showing typical radiological features of progressive massive fibrosis.

Typical radiological features of progressive massive fibrosis in a coal miner are shown in Figure 11.6.

Asbestos-related diseases

Exposure to asbestos causes several separate pleuropulmonary disorders, including pleural plaques, diffuse thickening of the pleura, benign pleural effusions, asbestosis, bronchial cancer and malignant mesothelioma (Box 11.3). Bronchial cancer and malignant mesothelioma are discussed in Chapter 13. Asbestosis is a diffuse interstitial pulmonary fibrosis caused by high and prolonged exposures to fibres of asbestos, and its diagnosis is aided by obtaining a history of regular exposure to any form of airborne asbestos. The presence of calcified pleural plaques on a chest radiograph indicates exposure to asbestos and helps to distinguish the condition from other causes of pulmonary fibrosis. Asbestos is commonly found in buildings and, provided it is left undisturbed, it is unlikely to pose a risk to health (Figure 11.7).

> Box 11.3 **Occupational groups at greatest risk of developing asbestos-related diseases**
>
> - Carpenters and electricians
> - Builders
> - Gas fitters
> - Roofers
> - Demolition workers
> - Shipyard and rail workers
> - Insulation workers
> - Asbestos factory workers

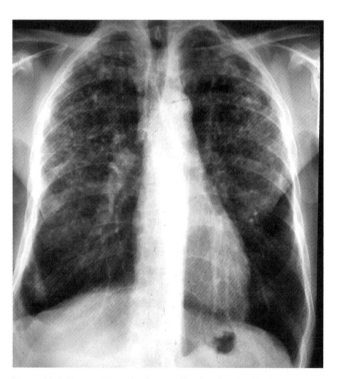

Figure 11.5 Chest radiograph of a tunneller showing simple silicosis.

Table 11.3 Some examples of causes of extrinsic allergic alveolitis.

Disease	Source of antigen	Antigen
Farmer's lung	Mouldy hay and straw	*Micropolyspora faeni* *Thermoactinomycesvulgaris*
Bird fancier's lung	Bird excreta and bloom	Bird serum proteins
Bagassosis	Mouldy sugar cane	*Thermoactinomyces sacchari*
Ventilation pneumonitis	Contaminated air conditioning systems	Thermophilic actinomycetes
Malt worker's lung	Mouldy barley	*Aspergillus clavatus*
Mushroom worker's lung	Spores released during spawning	Thermophilic actinomycetes
Cheese worker' lung	Mould dust	*Penicillium casei*
Animal handler's lung	Dander, dried rodent urine	Serum and urine proteins
Chemical extrinsic allergic alveolitis	Polyurethane foam manufacture and spray painting	Toluene (TDI) and diphenylmethane (MDI)

Table 11.4 Characteristic abnormalities of lung function in extrinsic allergic alveolitis.

Total lung capacity (TLC)	Residual volume (RV)	Vital capacity (VC)	Forced expiratory volume in one second (FEV$_1$)	FEV1/FVC	Transfer factor for carbon monoxide (TLCO)	Gas transfer coefficient (KCO)
Reduced	Reduced	Reduced	Reduced	Normal or increased	*Reduced	Reduced

*Sensitive indicator of the disease.

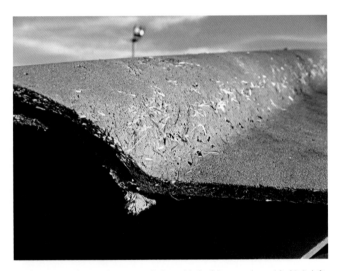

Figure 11.7 Asbestos is commonly found in buildings and provided it is left undisturbed it is unlikely to pose a risk to health. Reproduced with permission from Bill Bradley.

Extrinsic allergic alveolitis

Extrinsic allergic alveolitis (Table 11.3) is a granulomatous inflammatory reaction caused by an immunological response to certain inhaled organic dusts and some low molecular weight chemicals. Farmer's lung and bird fancier's lung remain the most prevalent forms of the disease.

Acute extrinsic allergic alveolitis usually occurs after exposure to a high concentration of the causative agent. After a sensitizing period, which may vary from weeks to years, the individual develops flu-like symptoms after exposure to the sensitizing antigen. Prolonged illness may be associated with considerable weight loss, but symptoms usually improve within 48 hours of removal from the causative agent. Chest radiography in acute extrinsic allergic alveolitis may show a ground glass pattern or micronodular shadows. There is generally evidence of IgG sensitization on serum assay although the test is not specific for disease.

Chronic extrinsic allergic alveolitis is caused either by chronic exposure to low doses of the causative antigen, or as a consequence of repeated attacks of acute alveolitis over many years. It results in irreversible pulmonary fibrosis, and the dominant symptom is exertional dyspnoea. Diagnosis principally depends on a history of relevant exposure and on identification of a potential sensitizing agent at home or at work. Inspiratory crackles may be heard on examination of the chest, and. In chronic extrinsic allergic alveolitis lung shrinkage in the upper lobes is usually apparent. The diagnosis is confirmed by detailed pulmonary investigations.

Further reading

Becklake MR, Bagatin E, Neder JA. Asbestos-related diseases of the lungs and pleura: uses, trends and management over the last century. *Int J Tuberc Lung Dis* 2007; 11: 356–369. *A state of the art, evidence-based review, of disease of the lungs and pleura caused by exposure to asbestos. The review is liberally illustrated with illustrative radiographs*

Girard M, Cormier Y. Hypersensitivity pneumonitis. *Curr Opin Allergy Clin Immunol* 2010; 10: 99–103. *This paper summarizes recent research on the clinical and immunological aspects of hypersensitivity pneumonitis*

Hendrick DJ. Recognition and surveillance of occupational asthma: a preventable illness with missed opportunities. *Br Med Bull* 2010; 95: 175–192. *An excellent overview of the diagnosis and management of occupational asthma in primary or secondary care*

Khan AJ, Nanchal R. Cotton dust lung diseases. *Curr Opin Pulm Med* 2007; 13: 137–141. *A review of the epidemiology, pathogenesis and diagnosis of cotton dust disease*

Ross MH, Murray J. Occupational respiratory disease in mining. *Occup Med (Lond)* 2004; 54: 304–310. *A review focusing on conditions in miners arising from exposure to asbestos, silica and coal*

CHAPTER 12

Infections

Dipti Patel

Foreign and Commonwealth Office; National Travel Health Network and Centre, London, UK

OVERVIEW

- Occupational infections can be easy to miss unless there is a high index of suspicion
- A detailed occupational history combined with knowledge of infectious diseases will often reveal the diagnosis of unusual illnesses due to infectious hazards
- There are no anatomical or pathological differences between infectious diseases arising from work exposures and those arising from non-work exposures
- Immunization, universal precautions, personal hygiene measures, education and personal protective equipment where appropriate are the main strategies for prevention
- Prevention of infection is an important aspect of occupational health practice as it will impact favourably on communicable disease in the general population

Introduction

The pattern of infectious hazards at work has changed over time, and specific occupational infections, while not common, can be serious and easy to miss unless there is a high index of suspicion combined with an understanding of infectious diseases (Box 12.1). Furthermore, infections of predominantly historic interest in the developed world continue to be a significant problem in the developing world, and the changing pattern of travel means that those who visit or work overseas remain exposed (see Chapter 19). Drug resistance, the resurgence of certain diseases and the emergence of new or previously unrecognized organisms further complicate matters, as does the increasing number of immunocompromised individuals. A detailed occupational history is therefore essential, as this will often reveal the diagnosis of unusual illnesses due to infectious hazards.

Occupational infections may be work specific or may be common in the general population, but they occur more frequently in those with occupational exposure. There are no anatomical or pathological differences between infectious diseases arising from

Box 12.1 **Basic concepts in infectious disease**

The traditional model of infectious disease causation is the epidemiological triangle which consists of:

- **an external agent** – the organism that produces the infection
- **a susceptible host** – attributes that influence an individual's susceptibility or response to the agent e.g. age, sex, lifestyle
- **environmental factors which bring the host and agent together** – factors that affect the agent and opportunity for exposure e.g. climate, physical surroundings, occupation, crowding.

An infectious disease is **endemic** if there is a persistent low to moderate level of occurrence. It is **sporadic** if the pattern of occurrence is irregular with occasional cases, and when the level of disease rises above the expected level for a period of time, it is referred to as an **epidemic**. An **outbreak** is two or more cases of illness which are considered to be linked in time and place. A **pandemic** is the worldwide spread of a new disease.

The **chain of infection** is the transmission of infection which occurs when the agent leaves the reservoir or host through a portal of exit, and is conveyed by some mode of transmission and enters through an appropriate portal of entry to a susceptible host.

Reservoir – This is any person, animal, arthropod, soil etc. in which the infectious agent normally resides.

Mode of transmission – This is the mechanism by which an infectious agent is spread from source or reservoir to a susceptible person, i.e. direct (touching, biting, eating, droplet spread during sneezing) or indirect (inanimate objects – fomites, vector-borne) transmission, or airborne spread (dissemination of microbial aerosol to a suitable port of entry – usually the respiratory tract).

work exposures and those arising from non-work exposures. However, if an infection is unusual in the general community and known to be a risk factor in a particular occupation, the connection between infection and work can usually be established reasonably easily. Like all occupational diseases, they are mostly preventable (Box 12.2).

There are several work-related factors that can predispose a worker to contracting an infection. These include:

- intentionally working with micro-organisms, e.g. laboratory workers

- having contact with people who have an increased prevalence of infectious disease, e.g. healthcare workers
- having contact with animals that may be reservoirs for infectious diseases, e.g. agricultural workers
- working in an area where an infectious disease is endemic, e.g. business travellers/expatriates
- having an increased likelihood of a micro-organism gaining entry into the body, e.g. through cuts, sharps injuries or dermatitis.

There are three main categories of occupational infections (Figure 12.1):

- zoonoses
- infections from human sources
- infections from environmental sources.

Epidemiology

No single source of information provides comprehensive data on occupationally acquired infections, and data sources underestimate the true incidence. In the UK, information is collated from a variety of sources including statutory reporting schemes such as the Public Health (Control of Diseases) Act 1984 (as amended by the Health and Social Care Act 2008), the Reporting of Disease and Dangerous Occurrences Regulations (RIDDOR) 1995, and Social Security Industrial Injury (Prescribed Diseases) Regulations 1985, and voluntary schemes such as the Labour Force Survey, and The Health and Occupation Reporting (THOR) network.

The relatively short incubation period (commonly days or weeks) between exposure and onset of disease for most infectious diseases means that the relationship of an infection to work is usually obvious. However, identifying this relationship can be a problem for infectious diseases with longer latencies such as hepatitis C, where the diagnosis may be made several years after exposure and where exposure can occur in occupational and non-occupational circumstances.

Data from UK reporting schemes indicate that the industries with the highest estimated rates of work-related infection are Health and Social Care, Fishing and Agriculture and Forestry. Diarrhoeal illnesses are the most frequently reported work-related infections.

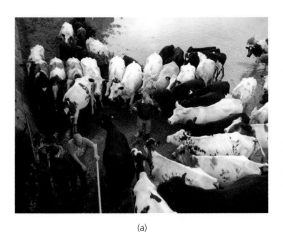

(a)

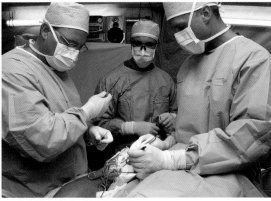

(b)

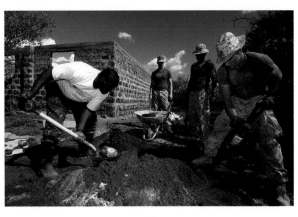

(c)

Figure 12.1 Main occupational groups at risk of infections. (a) Zoonotic infections: Farmers and other agricultural workers, Veterinary surgeons, Poultry workers, Butchers and fishmongers, Abattoir workers and slaughtermen, Forestry workers, Researchers and laboratory workers, Sewage workers, Tanners, Military staff, Overseas workers. (b) Infections from human sources: Healthcare workers, Social care workers, Sewage workers, Laboratory workers, Overseas workers, Archaeologists (during exhumations). (c) Infections from environmental sources: Examples include legionellosis and tetanus, Construction workers, Archaeologists, Engineering workers, Military staff, Overseas workers.

via vectors, such as mosquitoes or ticks (e.g. West Nile fever and Lyme disease).

There are approximately 40 zoonoses in the UK and approximately 300 000 people in a variety of occupations are potentially exposed. Their diagnosis, surveillance, prevention and control require close collaboration between a variety of agencies and disciplines particularly between health and agriculture (Box 12.3, Box 12.4).

Zoonoses

These are infections that are naturally transmissible from vertebrate animals to man. Transmission may occur by direct contact with an animal (e.g. orf), through a contaminated environment (e.g. leptospirosis) and via food (e.g. campylobacteriosis), or indirectly

Anthrax

Malignant pustule, Woolsorter's disease, Ragpicker's disease

This is an infection caused by *Bacillus anthracis* (a spore-forming Gram-positive bacterium); the normal animal reservoirs are grazing

Box 12.4 **Features of some important occupational zoonoses**

Brucellosis (undulant fever or Mediterranean fever) *Brucella abortus B. melitensis, B. suis, B. canis*
Main animal reservoirs: Cattle, sheep and goats, pigs, dogs
At-risk workers: Farmer workers, butchers, abattoir staff, vets
Distribution: Worldwide, endemic areas include Mediterranean Basin, South and Central America, Eastern Europe, Asia, Africa, the Caribbean, and the Middle East. Rare in the UK
Transmission: Direct contact with infected animals, ingestion of contaminated milk or dairy products
Clinical features: Variable incubation period (5–30 days, up to 6 months). Acute or insidious onset with intermittent fever, fatigue, arthralgia, and localized suppurative infection of organs. Splenomegaly and lymphadenopathy occurs in about 15% of cases. Neurological symptoms may occur acutely. Chronic symptoms include depression, fatigue and destructive arthritis/osteomyelitis
Treatment: Doxycycline with rifampicin or streptomycin for 6 weeks. Immunization possible for cattle, but not suitable for humans

Cryptosporidiosis–*Cryptosporidium parvum*
Main animal reservoirs: Cattle, sheep and goats, deer
At-risk workers: Farmer workers, vets
Distribution: Worldwide
Mode of acquisition: Faecal–oral; ingestion of oocysts excreted in human/animal faeces
Clinical features: Average incubation period of 7–10 days, oocysts appear in stool at onset of symptoms, and continue to be excreted in stool for several weeks after symptoms resolve. Often asymptomatic, but symptoms include fever, watery diarrhoea, abdominal cramps, nausea and anorexia. Most improve within 30 days. The immunocompromised may have severe and protracted illness
Treatment: Usually self-limiting. In immunocompromised specialist advice may be required

Vero cytotoxin-producing *Escherichia coli O157* **(VTEC O157)**
Main animal reservoirs: Cattle, Sheep and goats, and wide range of other species
At-risk workers: Farm workers
Distribution: Worldwide
Mode of acquisition: Ingestion of contaminated food, direct contact with infected animals, direct person to person spread, and waterborne
Clinical features: Incubation period generally from 2 to 14 days. Asymptomatic, diarrhoeal illness, haemorrhagic colitis, haemolytic uraemic syndrome (HUS) in up to 10% (particularly in children), and thrombotic thrombocytopenic purpura
Treatment: Usually self-limiting, and clears within a week. Antibiotics are not recommended, and are likely to increase the risk of getting complications such as HUS. Complications require hospital admission

Erysipeloid–*Erysipelothrix rhusiopathiae*
Main animal reservoirs: Fish, wild or domestic animals
At-risk workers: Farm workers, fishermen, butchers, fish handlers, poultry workers, vets
Distribution: Worldwide
Mode of acquisition: Direct contact with infected animal via pre-existing skin wounds

Clinical features: Localized cutaneous skin infection/cellulitis with violaceous tinge (fishmonger's finger). Occasionally fever, articular pain, rarely septicaemia and endocarditis. Usually self-limiting
Treatment: Penicillin, cephalosporins, or erythromycin

Lyme disease–*Borrelia burgdorferi*
Main animal reservoirs: Wild rodents, deer
At-risk workers: Shepherds, farm workers, foresters, outdoor workers
Distribution: USA, Canada, Europe, former USSR, China, Japan
Mode of acquisition: Tick-borne
Clinical features: Erythema migrans generally occurs within 7–10 days after tick bite, in 60–80%, often associated lymphadenopathy, general malaise and arthralgia. Aseptic meningitis, cranial nerve lesions, myopericarditis, AV block, cardiomegaly, and arthritis may occur up to 2 years after infection
Treatment: Doxycycline or amoxicillin. Transmission of infection unlikely within 24 hours of tick attachment therefore prompt removal of tick essential. Prophylactic antibiotics are not routinely recommended in Europe, but may be used in immunocompromised

Newcastle disease–*Paramyxovirus*
Main animal reservoirs: Domesticated and wild birds
At-risk workers: Poultry workers, pet shop staff, vets
Distribution: Rare in UK, occasional outbreaks in import quarantines
Mode of acquisition: Direct contact with eyes or inhalation
Clinical features: Mild systemic illness with conjunctivitis
Treatment: Nil

Orf – Parapoxvirus
Main animal reservoirs: Sheep and goats
At-risk workers: Farm workers, abattoir staff, vets
Distribution: Worldwide
Mode of acquisition: Direct contact with mucous membranes of infected animals
Clinical features: Incubation period usually 3 – 7 days. Solitary maculopustular lesion surrounded by erythematous rim. Lesion dries, and crust detaches after 6–8 weeks with no persisting scar. Secondary bacterial infection may result in cellulitis and regional lymphadenitis.
Treatment: Nil

Psittacosis (Avian chlamydiosis, Ornithosis)–*Chlamydophila psittaci*
Main animal reservoirs: Waterfowl, pheasants, pigeons, psittacine birds
At-risk workers: Poultry workers, pet shop staff, vets
Distribution: Worldwide
Mode of acquisition: Mainly inhalation of aerosols contaminated by infected avian faeces or fomites
Clinical features: Incubation 1–4 weeks. Fever, headache, myalgia, respiratory symptoms. Respiratory symptoms often disproportionately mild when compared with chest radiograph findings. Complications include encephalitis, myocarditis and Stephens–Johnson syndrome
Treatment: Tetracyclines or erythromycin

Ovine enzootic abortion–*Chlamydophilia abortus*
Ovine strains can cause severe septicaemic illness with intrauterine death in pregnant women. Maternal death due to disseminated intravascular coagulation may also occur. Women who are or may be pregnant should avoid exposure to sheep particularly during lambing

Rabies including Australian (ABL) and European bat lyssavirus (EBLV) – lyssavirus in the family Rhabdoviridae

Main animal reservoirs: Domestic and wild animals. Mammals that carry rabies include: bats, dogs, cats, raccoons, skunks, monkeys. Bat lyssavirus occurs in bats and it is unusual for this virus to cross the species barrier

At-risk workers: Workers in laboratories, quarantine kennels, and licensed and unlicensed bat handlers, business travellers

Distribution: Present on all continents except Antarctica, but more than 95% of cases in Asia and Africa. Land mammal rabies does not exist in a many countries including UK, Australia and New Zealand

Mode of acquisition: Usually through saliva via the bite of an infected animal. Dogs are the source of 99% of human rabies deaths, in USA and Canada most cases of human rabies occur in bat handlers

Clinical features: Incubation period is generally between 3 and 12 weeks but rarely can be several years. Rabies, ABL, and EBLV appear to cause similar symptoms. These include headache, fever, malaise, sensory changes around the site of the bite or scratch, excitability, an aversion to fresh air and water, weakness, delirium, convulsions, and coma. Death usually follows several days after the onset of symptoms

Treatment: Nil

Vaccine is available for animals and at risk humans. Effective post-exposure treatment can prevent the onset of symptoms and death

Worldwide, more than 55 000 people die of rabies every year. Since 1977, there have been five human deaths in Europe (three confirmed, two possible) from EBLVs. All cases were the result of a bat bite/scratch in individuals who had not received rabies vaccine pre or post incident. This included a UK case in 2002 when a bat handler was infected following a bite from a Daubenton's bat in Scotland. Only two cases of human infection with ABL have been recorded

Streptococcus suis

Main animal reservoirs: Pigs

Workers at risk: Pig workers, pork processors

Distribution: Worldwide

Mode of acquisition: Direct contact with infected pigs or pork

Clinical features: Primary skin infection with surrounding erythema and associated septicaemia and meningitis. Sequelae include ataxia and deafness in those with meningitis. Infection may, rarely, lead to toxic shock syndrome. Case fatality is extremely high in asplenics. Arthritis, pharyngitis, and diarrhoea may also occur

Treatment: Penicillin

Transmissible spongiform encephalopathies (TSE) – prion disease

These are a group of progressive and fatal neurological disorders occurring in humans and certain animal species. Research suggests that TSEs are caused by infectious proteins (prions) which are unusually resistant to conventional chemical and physical decontamination. They do not appear to be highly infectious and, with the exception of scrapie, do not appear to spread through casual contact

Bovine spongiform encephalopathy (BSE) was first recognized in British cattle in 1986, and in 1996, a previously unrecognized form of Creutzfeldt–Jakob disease (CJD) was identified in younger patients. The Government's Spongiform Encephalopathy Advisory Committee concluded that the most likely explanation for the emergence of this variant CJD (vCJD) was that it had been transmitted

to humans through exposure to BSE as a result of consumption of contaminated bovine food products

A number of measures have now been taken to minimize disease transmission of BSE and vCJD, and while there is no clear evidence of occupational risk, advice on safe working practices has been provided by the Advisory Committee on Dangerous Pathogens. Those potentially at risk include workers in abattoirs, slaughterhouses, rendering plants, farmers, neurosurgeons, pathologists, and mortuary technicians. In the UK, a new registry to find out more about the risk from occupational exposures to CJD and other TSEs among healthcare and laboratory workers has been set up

A major concern now is the risk of transmission in a healthcare setting. To date in the UK, there have been four cases of vCJD infection associated with blood transfusion

mammals such as sheep, cattle and goats (Figure 12.2). Human anthrax is primarily an occupational hazard for workers who process animal hides, hair, wool, bone/bone products, but it also occurs in vets and agricultural workers who handle infected animals. It is rare in the UK, occurring in those who work with infected animal products from epizootic areas. Anthrax has recently received attention because of its potential for use in bioterrorism.

Cutaneous anthrax accounts for 95–98% of cases, and occurs when the organism enters a cut or an abrasion. Following 1–7 days, a small papule develops at this site. Over 24–48 hours, it enlarges, eventually forming a characteristic ulcer (eschar). If not treated it may progress to bacteraemia, meningitis and death.

Pulmonary or gastrointestinal anthrax occur infrequently, resulting from the inhalation and ingestion of anthrax spores respectively. In pulmonary anthrax (Woolsorter's disease) non-specific upper respiratory tract symptoms follow an incubation period of 1–6 days. Rapid deterioration in respiratory function and death generally follow unless treatment is started promptly. Gastrointestinal anthrax is characterized by severe abdominal pain, watery or bloody diarrhoea and vomiting. Progression to bacteraemia is usually 2–3 days. Case fatality in both these forms of anthrax is high.

Most strains of anthrax are susceptible to penicillin, doxycycline and ciprofloxacin. A vaccine is available for at-risk workers, and oral antibiotics and vaccination may be used for post-exposure prophylaxis.

Leptospirosis

Weil's disease, canicola fever, haemorrhagic jaundice, mud fever, swineherd disease

Leptospirosis is a cause of septicaemia due to pathogenic leptospires belonging to the genus *Leptospira interrogans* (*Li*). The most important serovars in humans are *Li hardjo* (cattle-associated leptospirosis), *Li icterohaemorrhagiae* (Weil's disease) and *Li canicola*. The principal animal reservoirs are cattle, rats and dogs respectively.

At-risk occupations include agricultural workers, farmers, vets, miners, abattoir, sewer and canal workers. There are 50–60 cases reported annually in the UK, and of the indigenously acquired infections about 50% are acquired through occupational activities.

Leptospirosis is usually acquired by direct contact with infected animals or their urine, contaminated soil, food or water (a hazard in watersports). The incubation period is usually 5–14 days, and typical symptoms include fever, flu-like symptoms, headache, myalgia, photophobia and conjunctival injection. In severe cases, haemorrhage into skin and mucous membranes, vomiting, jaundice and hepatorenal failure may occur.

Mild infection is often self-limiting, but penicillin or doxycycline are effective treatments. Severe disease requires intensive and specialized therapy.

Immunization of animals is possible for certain serovars, and in some countries a vaccine is available for at-risk workers. For those at high risk for short periods, prophylactic doxycycline (200 mg weekly) may be effective. In the UK, at-risk workers usually carry an alert card provided by their employer to warn their doctors should they develop such symptoms.

Q fever

Q fever is caused by the rickettsia *Coxiella burnetii*. In its spore-like form the organism is very robust and resistant to dessication and common disinfectants. It therefore can survive for long periods and be transmitted in aerosols or by fomites such as wool, straw and dust.

The principal animal reservoirs are cattle, sheep and goats, but it is also present in other wildlife species and arthropod vectors (mainly ticks). Human infection is usually from inhalation through close exposure to infected animals, contaminated fomites or wind-borne aerosols. The latter can occasionally cause large community outbreaks. Rarer routes of transmission include drinking unpasteurized milk from infected animals, tick bites and through cuts or abrasions. Occupational exposures (abattoir workers, farmers, veterinarians, etc.) account for most cases.

The incubation period is usually 2–3 weeks, and most infections are asymptomatic. The most common presentation is a mild and self-limiting flu-like illness. Other manifestations include pneumonia, hepatitis, myocarditis, encephalitis, osteomyelitis and miscarriage in pregnant women. Chronic Q fever is uncommon (<1% of acutely infected patients), presenting as culture-negative endocarditis in patients with a pre-existing valvular disease. Pregnant women and immunosuppressed people are also considered at high risk for developing severe or chronic Q fever.

Most cases of Q fever resolve spontaneously. Doxycycline may be used for severe or prolonged symptoms, or for recurrences. Antibiotics are less effective in chronic disease and prolonged treatment (3 years) is recommended. Even with combination therapy (doxycycline and chloroquine) relapse rates of over 50% are seen.

Prevention and control of Q fever is problematic and principally relies on hygiene and husbandry methods on farms. Careful disposal of contaminated materials (e.g. birth products) reduces the risk of spore formation and subsequent infection of animals and people, and pasteurization of milk and milk products prevents foodborne transmission.

Pregnant women, immunosuppressed individuals and those with valvular heart disease or vascular grafts should avoid jobs which may expose them to Q fever. A human vaccine for Q fever is available in Australia and Canada, but not in the UK – this is currently under review.

Avian influenza

Avian influenza is an infection caused by avian influenza A viruses, and many different subtypes can be found circulating in wild waterfowl (e.g. ducks and geese) often causing little or no symptoms. Other bird species are susceptible to infection with these viruses and sometimes large outbreaks associated with high mortality are seen in domesticated bird species (e.g. chickens, ducks, turkeys). In these instances the term 'highly pathogenic avian influenza' is used.

Although rare, human infection with avian influenza can occur, and confirmed cases from several subtypes of avian influenza have been reported, with most cases occurring following contact with infected poultry or surfaces contaminated with secretion/excretions from infected birds. Workers at risk therefore include poultry farm workers, veterinarians, workers in poultry-associated industries (transport, poultry meat processing, etc.), and workers with other caged birds (aviaries, zoos, etc.). The spread of avian influenza viruses from person to person has been occasionally reported, but has been limited and unsustained.

Symptoms of human avian influenza are dependent on the causative agent, ranging from typical flu-like symptoms to eye infections, pneumonia, acute respiratory distress, and other severe and life-threatening complications.

The avian influenza A subtype H5N1 is a highly pathogenic strain of the virus that has been confirmed in poultry populations across Asia, Russia, Africa and Europe. Although rare, it has caused the largest number of detected cases of severe disease and death in humans to date. In the current outbreak (to June 2012) 606 human cases have been reported (mainly in South East Asia), with 357 deaths. Analyses of available H5N1 viruses circulating worldwide suggest that most are susceptible to oseltamivir.

Infections from human sources

These infections are of most relevance to health and social care workers (Box 12.5). They are important as this group of workers is at high risk of acquiring infections occupationally and, importantly, they are potential sources of infection to their patients, particularly those who are immunologically impaired. In the UK, there is a requirement for healthcare workers to be screened and, where relevant, protected against certain communicable diseases. There is also a requirement to report infections acquired by patients in a healthcare setting.

Box 12.5 **Healthcare-associated infections (HCAIs)**

HCAIs are infections that occur in patients or healthcare workers and are acquired in a hospital or other healthcare setting (e.g. hospices or care homes), or as a result of a healthcare intervention or procedure.

There are many different types of HCAIs. These include infections caused by meticillin-resistant *Staphylococcus aureus* and *Clostridium difficile*, as well as other less well-known infective agents such as norovirus, which causes a relatively mild gastroenteritis but can spread easily in hospitals or other institutional environments sometimes leading to ward closures.

HCAIs have an impact on patients, their carers and relatives, and also on the healthcare system as a whole.

A study funded by the UK Department of Health estimated that

- HCAIs cost the health sector in England almost £1 billion a year
- patients who contracted an HCAI stayed in hospital an average of 2.5 times longer than patients who did not, increasing their inpatient time by 11 days
- the cost of treating a patient with an HCAI was 2.8 times more than treating a patient without one; an average additional cost of £3154
- patients with an HCAI identified in hospital and post-discharge took an average of 17 extra days to return to normal daily activities.

Bloodborne viruses (BBVs)

Occupational exposure to blood or body fluids poses a small risk of transmission of bloodborne pathogens (Box 12.6); those presenting the greatest cross-infection hazard are HIV, hepatitis C virus (HCV) and hepatitis B virus (HBV). Although healthcare staff are at greatest risk, other occupational groups (e.g. police officers) may also be exposed.

Box 12.6 Risk of transmission of BBVs

Percutaneous exposure injuries carry the greatest risk of transmission of BBVs in the healthcare setting.

The risk of infection following a percutaneous injury, especially deep penetrating injuries involving a hollow bore needle or a device visibly contaminated with blood has been estimated at 1 in 3 for HBV, 1 in 30 for HCV and 1 in 300 for HIV.

In the UK there have to date (August 2011) been 5 documented cases of occupationally acquired transmissions of HIV and 31 probable cases.

In the US, there have been 57 documented cases and 147 possible cases.

There have been 14 occupational HCV seroconversions in healthcare workers reported since 1997.

Post-exposure prophylaxis (PEP)

A. HIV

- A case control study in 1997 suggested that the use of Zidovudine as PEP resulted in an 81% reduction in risk of acquiring HIV in healthcare workers following an occupational exposure to HIV-infected blood.
- Most countries now recommend PEP. The choice of drugs, doses, route of administration, and the length of prophylaxis are somewhat empirical. However, since most studies indicate a time-limited response to PEP, the need for timely and early therapy is vital.

- The starting regime currently recommended in the UK is a combination of nucleoside/nucleotide analogue reverse transcriptase inhibitors plus a combination of protease inhibitors.
- In the United States, guidelines recommend two-drug PEP regimens following lower-risk incidents and three-drug regimens for higher risk incidents.

B. HCV

- No effective PEP exists; recommendations for post-exposure management is aimed at early identification of infection, with appropriate specialist referral.

C. HBV

- HBV immunoglobulin (HBIG) is available for passive protection and is normally used in combination with hepatitis B vaccine to confer passive–active immunity to susceptible individuals after exposure.
- The post-exposure efficacy of combination HBIG and HBV vaccine has not been evaluated in the occupational setting, but increased efficacy (85–95%) has been observed in the perinatally. While HBIG may not completely inhibit virus multiplication, it may prevent severe illness and the development of a chronic carrier state.

The risk of infection depends on the type and severity of the exposure, the infectivity of the source patient, the immune status of the exposed healthcare worker, and the availability of post-exposure treatment.

Prevention is based on minimizing exposure to blood or body fluids, and consists of strict infection control, adherence to universal precautions, immunization against hepatitis B, and prompt management of any occupational exposure.

BBV-infected healthcare workers can potentially transmit infection to their patients, and although the risk is small, guidelines exist in many countries to reduce this risk further (Box 12.7).

Box 12.7 BBV-infected healthcare workers and risk to patients

- Exposure-prone procedures (EPPs) are procedures where there is a risk that injury to the worker may result in the exposure of a patient's open tissues to the blood of the worker. These procedures occur mainly in surgery, obstetrics and gynaecology, dentistry, and some aspects of midwifery.
- In the UK, the UK Advisory Panel for healthcare workers infected with bloodborne viruses (UKAP) is responsible for advising on healthcare workers infected with BBVs. This will include advice regarding restricting the practice of BBV-infected healthcare workers, and on when look-back exercises may be needed as a result of EEPs being undertaken on patients by a BBV-infected healthcare worker.

In the UK the following groups are restricted from performing EPP:

- Those who are HIV positive
- Those who are Hepatitis C RNA positive
- Those who are Hepatitis B e antigen (HBeAg) positive

- Those that are Hepatitis B surface antigen positive but HBeAg negative with a hepatitis B viral load greater than 10^3 genome equivalents/ml – those who are HBeAg negative and have relatively low Hepatitis B viral load may be allowed to perform EPPs, whilst taking continuous antiviral therapy that suppresses their viral load to 10^3 genome equivalents/ml or below, subject to regular monitoring by a specialist occupational health physician

- Worldwide, there have been 3 reports of possible transmissions of HIV from infected healthcare workers performing EPPs: a Florida dentist, a French orthopaedic surgeon, and a Spanish gynaecologist.
- Data available from patient notification exercises support the conclusion that the overall risk of transmission of HIV from infected healthcare workers to patients is very low. From 1988–2003 in the UK, there were 28 patient notification exercises. However, there were no detectable transmissions of HIV from infected healthcare workers to patient despite over 7,000 patients having been tested
- A number of look-back studies involving surgical staff from 1975–1990 have identified HBV transmission risks of 0.9–20%.

In UK, since 1994 there have been 5 reported incidents of HCV transmission to 15 patients from infected healthcare workers during EPPs.

Tuberculosis (TB)

Mycobacterium tuberculosis continues to be the leading cause of adult death from any single infectious agent worldwide. The emergence of multidrug-resistant tuberculosis (MDRTB – tuberculosis resistant to at least isoniazid and rifampicin), with its high case fatality, its prolonged sputum positivity (and consequently, higher transmission risk) and its complex treatment has re-emphasized the importance of TB control.

TB remains a hazard in the healthcare setting, and incidence in healthcare workers parallels (but is higher than) that in the community; a study in the mid-1990s found about a twofold increased risk of TB among healthcare workers in England and Wales. Healthcare workers should therefore be protected against infection, and measures should be taken to detect TB in new or existing staff in order to protect their patients and colleagues (Box 12.8). Protection begins at pre-employment, and continues with strict infection control measures for nursing infected patients.

When a patient or member of staff is found to have TB, infection control and occupational health staff should assess the need for contact tracing (Box 12.9). In the UK, most staff are not considered to be at special risk and should be reassured and advised to report any suspicious symptoms. Those who are immunocompromised, have undertaken mouth-to-mouth resuscitation, prolonged high-dependency care or repeated chest physiotherapy without appropriate protection should be regarded as close contacts and followed up according to national guidelines. Similar precautions should be taken if the index case is highly infectious.

Box 12.8 **In the UK, screening and protection of healthcare workers should follow the guidelines produced by the UK Department of Health and National institute of Health and Clinical Excellence in 2011**

- Those who will be working with patients/clinical specimens should have completed a TB screen or health check, or provide documentary evidence such screening having taken place within the preceding 12 months before starting work
- Health checks should include:
  - assessment of personal or family history of TB
  - symptom and signs enquiry, possibly by questionnaire
  - documentary evidence of tuberculin skin testing (or interferon-gamma testing) and/or BCG scar check by an occupational health professional
  - tuberculin skin test (or interferon-gamma test) result within the last five years, if available
- Those who will have contact with patients/clinical specimens should not start work if they have signs or symptoms of TB
- Those who will have contact with patients/clinical specimens should be offered BCG vaccine (provided there are no contra-indications), whatever their age, if they are tuberculin skin test negative and have not been previously vaccinated
- Those of any age who are from countries of high TB incidence, or who have had contact with patients in settings with a high TB prevalence should have an interferon-gamma test. If negative, BCG vaccine should be offered. If positive the person should be referred for clinical assessment for diagnosis and possible treatment of latent infection or active disease.

Box 12.9 **Hospital infection control and TB**

There are three levels of isolation for infection control in hospital settings:

- Negative-pressure rooms, which have air pressure continuously or automatically measured
- Single rooms that are not negative pressure but are vented to the outside of the building
- Beds on a ward, for which no particular engineering standards are required.

Adults with non-pulmonary TB can usually be nursed on general wards, those with suspected pulmonary without risk factors for MDRTB, should be admitted to a single room vented to the open air until their sputum status is known. In the case of known or suspected MDRTB, particular care must be taken:

- Smear-positive TB patients without risk factors for MDRTB should be cared for in a single room, until they have completed 2 weeks of the standard recommended regimen, or are discharged from hospital.
- Patients with suspected or known infectious MDRTB should be admitted to a negative-pressure room or transferred to a hospital that has these facilities if one is not available. Care should be carried out in the negative-pressure room until the patient is found to be non-infectious or non-resistant.

- Effective control of MDRTB requires a multi-disciplinary approach involving the hospital infection control team, microbiologist, TB physician, consultant in communicable disease control, engineers, and occupational health.

Aerosol-generating procedures such as bronchoscopy, sputum induction or nebulizer treatment should be carried out in an appropriately engineered and ventilated area for:

- all patients on an HIV ward, regardless of whether a diagnosis of TB has been considered
- all patients in whom TB is considered a possible diagnosis, in any setting

Healthcare workers caring for people with TB should not use masks, gowns or barrier nursing techniques unless:

- MDRTB is suspected
- Aerosol-generating procedures are being performed.

Seasonal and pandemic influenza

Influenza is an important cause of morbidity and mortality worldwide, and an important healthcare-associated infection in both acute and long-term healthcare facilities, affecting both patients and staff and disrupting delivery of care. There is evidence that vaccinating health and social care workers reduces mortality among long-term patients and that vaccinating hospital workers decreases the rate of nosocomial influenza in hospitalized patients. Furthermore, immunization of healthcare workers has been shown to be cost-effective and reduces absenteeism.

Pandemic influenza poses a particular challenge as the group of workers most likely to come into contact with the virus are healthcare workers caring for patients with the disease. Limiting transmission of pandemic influenza in the healthcare setting is a major endeavour and requires a range of measures (Box 12.10).

Box 12.10 Control of pandemic influenza in healthcare settings

Infection control requires a range of measures including:

1 administrative controls:

- Early recognition of cases
- Separation of influenza and non influenza patients,
- Occupational health arrangements, including immunization of frontline workers
- Staff, patient, and visitor education regarding infection control
- Implementation of infection control precautions to limit transmission
- Restriction of ill visitors to healthcare facilities
- Instructing staff with symptoms to stay at home
- Planning and implementation of strategies for surge capacity

2 environmental/engineering controls:

- Environmental cleaning
- Adequate ventilation
- Waste disposal

3 use of personal protective equipment (PPE) and hand hygiene:

- Using PPE appropriately
- Consistent and correct hand hygiene.

Despite the evidence that immunization of healthcare workers can have positive benefits, overall rates of influenza immunization among healthcare workers worldwide are disappointingly low, at 40% or less.

Box 12.11 Some infections of significance in a healthcare setting

Measles – Paramyxovirus
Vaccine available (MMR vaccine)
Distribution: Worldwide
Mode of acquisition: Airborne by droplet spread or direct contact with nose and throat secretions. Measles is one of the most highly communicable diseases
Incubation period: 7–18 days. Communicability: Patient is infectious from 4 days before to 4 days after the appearance of rash
Clinical features: Prodromal fever, conjunctivitis, coryza and Koplik's spots on buccal mucosa. Red maculopapular facial rash starts on day 3–4; and then spreads to trunk and limbs. Complications include pneumonia and encephalitis. Subacute sclerosing panencephaltis is a rare late and fatal complication developing several years after initial infection

Non-immune health care workers exposed to a confirmed or likely case should be excluded from work from the 5th day after exposure if there has been any face-to-face contact or exposure for 15 minutes or longer in the same room. Susceptible exposed healthcare workers should receive one dose of MMR (if not contra-indicated) and can return to work 21 days after the final exposure, or earlier if symptom-free and found to be measles IgG positive at least 14 days after MMR vaccine was given.

Human normal immunoglobulin (HNIG) may be considered for those who are non-immune and in high risk groups (immunocompromised, infants, pregnant women).

Meningococcal infection – *Neisseria menigitidis*
Vaccines available against serogroups A, C, W135 and Y
Distribution: Worldwide there are 13 serogroups; in UK following introduction of the meningococcal C conjugate immunization programme (1999), serogroup B strains now account for around 90% of laboratory-confirmed cases. Approximately 10% of the population are asymptomatic carriers.
Mode of acquisition: Person-to-person through respiratory droplets and direct contact with nose and throat secretions. Infectivity is relatively low and transmission requires prolonged close contact.
Incubation period: 3–5 days. Communicability: Patients are generally not infectious within 24 hours of antibiotic treatment.
Clinical features: Presents as meningitis, septicaemia or combination of both. The appearance of a petechial rash signifies septicaemia.

Healthcare personnel are rarely at risk, so routine immunization is not recommended. Only intimate contact with infected patients e.g. mouth-to-mouth resuscitation would warrant antibiotic prophylaxis and if appropriate immunization.

Fifth disease (Erythema infectosum, Slapped Cheek Syndrome) – *Parvovirus B19*

Distribution: Worldwide

Mode of acquisition: Person-to person by droplet spread. Rarely by contaminated blood products. It is highly infectious.

Incubation period: 4–20 days. Communicability: From 7 days before the appearance of rash until onset of rash. In aplastic crises, infectivity may last for up to a week after the rash appears. In the immunosuppressed with severe anaemia, infectivity may last for months or years.

Clinical features: Initially fever which lasts until rash appears. The rash is maculopapular and generally on the limbs. The cheeks often have a 'slapped cheek' appearance. Illness is mild in immuno-competent individuals, although sometimes, persistent joint pain may occur. In those with haemoglobinopathies, transient aplastic crises may occur, and in the immunosuppressed, red cell aplasia and chronic anaemia may occur. Infection in the first 20 weeks of pregnancy can cause hydrops fetalis and fetal loss.

Pregnant women <21/40, immunocompromised individuals or those with heamoglobinopathies who have a significant contact with an infected healthcare worker in the 7 days before onset of rash will need further follow-up. Normal immunoglobulin has been given prophylactically to high-risk patients but its efficacy is not known.

In exceptional circumstances, seronegative healthcare workers who have been exposed may be advised to avoid contact with high-risk patients (e.g. midwives).

German Measles – *Rubella*

Vaccine available

Distribution: Rare in most countries in Western Europe due to immunization programmes.

Mode of acquisition: Direct person-to-person contact by respiratory droplets.

Incubation period: 2–3 weeks. Communicability: 1 week before onset of rash to approximately 4 days later.

Clinical features: Generally mild fever with sore throat and conjunctivitis precedes a macular rash. Persistent joint infection may occur, but complete recovery usual. The main importance is the risk of congenital rubella syndrome.

Methicillin Resistant *Staphylococcus aureus* (MRSA)

Distribution: Worldwide. *S. aureus* is carried as a skin commensal by approximately 30% of the population and a small proportion (1–3% of the total population) are colonized with MRSA; strains resistant to Penicillinase stable beta-lactams are referred to as methicillin resistant *staphylococcus aureus*.

Mode of acquisition: MRSA colonizes the skin, nose, and throat of both patients and healthcare staff. It spreads readily by direct contact, and hence is an important cause of hospital acquired infections. While patients are usually responsible for spread of infection, the introduction of MRSA into unaffected areas by colonized staff is well-documented, and staff hands are an important route of cross-infection.

Incubation period: 4–10 days, but disease may not occur until several months after colonization.

Clinical features: May cause both trivial and deep-seated infections; particular problems include infected bedsores or surgical wounds.

Control of MRSA is essential to patient care, and in the UK mandatory surveillance of MRSA in NHS hospitals has been ongoing since 2001. Since 2009 NHS hospitals have been required to implement screening for MRSA colonization in patients.

Chicken Pox – Varicella zoster

Vaccine available

Distribution: Worldwide

Mode of acquisition: It is highly infectious and transmitted directly by personal contact or droplet spread, and indirectly via fomites.

Incubation period: 10–21 days. Communicability: Most infectious period is from 1 to 2 days before the rash appears until all the lesions have crusted over (about 5 to 6 days after onset of illness).

Clinical features: Initially cold-like symptoms followed by a high temperature and intensely itchy, vesicular rash mostly over the trunk and more sparsely over the limbs. Shingles (Herpes Zoster) is a reactivation of dormant virus in the posterior root ganglion and can be a source of infection generally by contact with the skin lesions, but occasionally by the respiratory route in immunocompromized individuals.

Usually a mild illness; however, severe disease due to fulminating varicella pneumonia is more likely in adults, especially pregnant women and the immunocompromsied. There is also a risk to the fetus and neonate from maternal infection which relates to gestation at time of infection (congenital varicella syndrome in first 20 weeks, Herpes Zoster in otherwise healthy infant in 2nd and 3rd trimesters, and severe or fatal neonatal disease a week before to a week after delivery).

Human Varicella Zoster Immunoglobulin is available for use as post-exposure prophylaxis to high risk groups.

Nosocomial exposure to VZV is a major occupational health problem requiring non-immune healthcare workers to be excluded form patient contact from day 8–21 following a significant exposure.

Other Infections

Other infections worth mentioning include skin infection in engineers associated with the re-use of cutting oils which can lead to oil mists being contaminated with bacteria and fungi, pseudomonal otitis externa in deep-sea divers who use saturation techniques, and legionellosis, which can occasionally be occupationally acquired for example engineering staff working on cooling towers. Finally, travel-associated infections are becoming an important cause of occupationally acquired disease with the increase in international travel and overseas workers (see Chapter 19).

Legionellosis

Legionnaire's disease, Pontiac fever

This is an acute bacterial infection due to a Gram-negative bacillus belonging to the genus *Legionella*. There are two recognized clinical presentations; Legionnaire's disease and Pontiac fever, and the majority of infections are due to *L. pneumophila*. The bacillus is an ubiquitous aquatic organism which thrives in warm environments ($20-45°C$), and is often isolated from natural habitats (e.g. rivers, ponds) and from artificial equipment where the temperature is maintained at levels favouring bacterial proliferation.

Transmission of infection is from inhalation of contaminated aerosols, and both Legionnaire's disease and Pontiac fever present initially with non-specific flu-like symptoms. Pontiac fever occurs

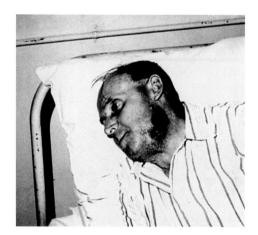

Figure 12.2 A patient with cutaneous anthrax. Recent cases in the UK include two cases of inhalational anthrax associated with manipulation of animal hide drums while drum-making or playing/handling. Since 2009 outbreaks of anthrax among heroin users have also been reported. The likely source is heroin contaminated with anthrax spores, either directly or via a cutting agent.

following an incubation period of 4–66 hours, and is a self-limiting non-pneumonic form of the infection. By contrast, the incubation period for Legionnaire's disease is 2–10 days, and following initial symptoms of fever, malaise, anorexia, and myalgia, there is progression to pneumonia and associated multisystem involvement with diarrhoea, confusion and renal failure. Case fatality can range from 10% to 15%, but may be higher in outbreaks. Treatment is usually with erythromycin (Box 12.12).

Box 12.12 **Legionnaire's disease**

Travel abroad is a major risk factor for Legionnaire's disease in the UK, with nearly 50% of cases being contracted abroad.

Approximately 15% of UK cases are linked to local outbreaks (due to wet cooling systems or hot water systems), and approximately 2% are hospital-acquired. May cases are acquired overseas, or are sporadic, or from an unidentified source. If infection is confirmed, local public health authorities need to be notified as contacts may need to be identified, and the source of infection needs to be established and appropriately controlled.

Hospital outbreaks in particular have high case fatalities.

The highest risk of infection occurs with water systems leading to the aerosolization of water which is stored at temperatures between 25–45°C. This includes:

- Wet cooling systems (e.g. cooling towers and evaporative condensers)
- Hot water systems (especially showers)
- Whirlpool spas
- Indoor and outdoor fountain/sprinkler systems
- Humidifiers
- Respiratory therapy systems
- Industrial grinders

Prevention of infection relies on ensuring that equipment and systems are kept as clean as possible, and regularly disinfected. Where possible, water temperatures should be kept above 50°C or below 20°C. Use of biocides may also need to be considered. In the UK, the Health and Safety Executive provide guidance on the prevention and control of legionellosis.

Conclusion

The extent of occupationally acquired infections is unknown, but it is likely that they are extremely common particularly mild infections in agricultural and healthcare workers. They are an important cause of work-related morbidity and prevention of infection is an important aspect of occupational health practice as it will impact favourably on communicable disease in the general population. Similarly, the control of communicable disease in both the general (and animal population) will decrease the risk to certain occupational groups.

Further reading

Hawker J, Begg N, Blair I, *et al. Communicable disease control handbook*, 2nd edn. Oxford: Blackwell Sciences Ltd, 2005.

Heymann D. *Control of communicable diseases manual*, 19th edn. Washington: American Public Health Association, 2008. *Both these references, while aimed at public health practitioners, provide extensive detail on communicable diseases, their epidemiology, clinical features, prevention and control*

Health and Safety Executive (2008). *Common zoonoses in agriculture.* London: HSE Books 2008. Available at http://www.hse.gov.uk/pubns/ais2.pdf (accessed August 2011) *A useful easy to read overview of agricultural zoonoses in the UK*

Kings Fund Briefing. *Healthcare-associated infections: stemming the rise of the superbug?* London: Kings Fund, 2008. Available at http://www.kingsfund .org.uk/publications/briefings/healthcareassociate.html (accessed August 2011). *This provides some background on HCAIs of most concern and their impact. It also summarizes strategies being used in England to reduce infections, and analysis of their effectiveness*

Department of Health. *Health clearance for tuberculosis, Hepatitis B, hepatitis C and HIV: New healthcare workers.* London: Department of Health, 2007. Available at http://www.dh.gov.uk/prod_consum_dh/groups/dh _digitalassets/@dh/@en/documents/digitalasset/dh_074981.pdf. *UK guidance on screening of new healthcare workers for tuberculosis, hepatitis B, hepatitis C and HIV*

National Institute of Clinical Excellence. *Tuberculosis: Clinical diagnosis and management of tuberculosis, and measures for its prevention and control.* London: NICE, 2011. Available at http://www.nice.org.uk /nicemedia/live/13422/53638/53638.pdf (accessed August 2011). *The principal source of advice on TB management in the UK covering both diagnosis and management and prevention and control*

Department of Health. *Pandemic (H1N1) 2009 Influenza–A summary of guidance for infection control in healthcare settings.* London: Department of Health, 2009. Available at http://www.dh.gov.uk/prod_consum_dh /groups/dh_digitalassets/@dh/@en/@ps/documents/digitalasset/dh _110899.pdf. (accessed August 2011)

Department of Health. *HIV post-exposure prophylaxis: Guidance from the UK Chief Medical Officers' Expert Advisory Group on AIDS.* London: Department of Health, 2008. Available at http://www.dh.gov.uk/prod_consum_dh/groups/dh_digitalassets/@dh/@en/documents/digitalasset/dh_089997.pdf. (accessed August 2011)

http://www.hpa.org.uk

http://www.who.int

http://www.cdc.gov

These websites are excellent resources for infectious disease information (both occupational and non-occupational)

http://www.open.gov.uk/doh/dhhome.htm

The UK department of health website is particularly useful for information on bloodborne viruses, pandemic influenza, healthcare associated infections and UK policy in relation to these

http://www.hse.gov.uk

This site provides practical and clear information on prevention and control of a variety of infectious hazards in the workplace, and is also a source of occupational ill-health statistics

CHAPTER 13

Occupational Cancers

John Hobson

University of Keele and University of Manchester, UK

OVERVIEW

- The overall burden of occupational cancer in Great Britain is currently around 8000 deaths and 14 000 cancer registrations per year. This represents 8% of all cancer deaths in men and about 2% in women
- Asbestos contributes half of the deaths followed by silica, diesel engine exhaust, radon, work as a painter, mineral oils, shift work, environmental tobacco smoke in non-smokers, dioxins, radon and work as a welder
- Work sectors at risk of occupational cancer include construction, painting and decorating, manufacturing, mining, quarrying, utilities and the service industry including personal and household services
- Occupational cancer is a preventable disease and occupational health has an important role in primary prevention

---

Introduction

The first report of cancer caused by occupational exposure was in 1775 by Percival Pott, a British surgeon who described scrotal cancer in boy chimney sweeps. A century later, in 1895, Rehn, a German surgeon working in Frankfurt, treated a cluster of three cases of bladder cancer in workers at a local factory producing aniline dyestuffs from coal tar.

Occupational cancer is any malignancy wholly or partly caused by exposures at the workplace or in occupation. Such exposure may be due to a particular chemical (such as β-naphthylamine), a physical agent (such as ionizing radiation), a fibre like asbestos, a biological agent (such as hepatitis B virus) or an industrial process in which the specific carcinogen may elude precise definition (such as coke production).

The International Agency for Research on Cancer (IARC) was set up to identify carcinogenic hazards to humans. Its role is to conduct and coordinate research into the causes of cancer. It maintains a series of monographs on the carcinogenic risks to humans posed by a variety of agents, mixtures and exposures. Since 1971 over

900 agents have been evaluated and the findings published in over 100 monographs. Over 400 agents have been identified as carcinogenic, probably carcinogenic or possibly carcinogenic to humans (Table 13.1).

Full estimates of the current burden of occupational cancer from a consideration of all 24 cancer sites for which IARC has classified as definite or probable human carcinogens are gradually being published. Emerging findings suggest that the overall burden of occupational cancer in Great Britain is currently around 8000 deaths and 14 000 cancer registrations per year. This represents 8% of all cancer deaths in men and about 2% in women. The World Health Organization estimate that worldwide every year 200 000 die from cancer related to exposures in their workplace (Figure 13.1), and although historically the burden of occupational cancer has fallen mainly in developed industrialized countries, there is increasing concern for the potential growth of occupational cancer elsewhere as industry transfers around the world. This might be the relocation of unsafe processes such as asbestos manufacture or the transfer of old manufacturing equipment. In developing countries industry can be geographically dispersed or fragmented into small workshops where control measures are less likely to be used and less amenable to enforcement agencies or effective legislation, if available. Exposures to silica in small-scale mining,

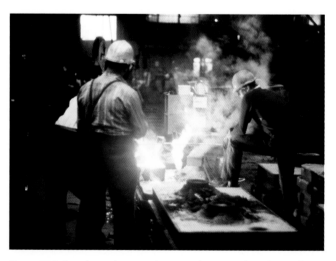

Figure 13.1 Foundry workers may be exposed to a complex mixture of carcinogenic agents in fumes.

ABC of Occupational and Environmental Medicine, Third Edition.
Edited by David Snashall and Dipti Patel.
© 2012 John Wiley & Sons Ltd. Published 2012 by John Wiley & Sons Ltd.

Table 13.1 IARC classification.

Group	Definition	Used when	No	Examples
1	Carcinogenic	Sufficient evidence in humans	107	Asbestos Benzene Wood dust
2A	Probably carcinogenic	Limited evidence in humans and sufficient evidence in experimental animals	58	Engine exhaust, diesel Inorganic lead
2B	Possibly carcinogenic	Limited evidence in humans and absence of sufficient evidence in experimental animals or inadequate evidence in humans or human data non-existent and sufficient evidence in experimental animals	249	Carbon black DDT Nickel Titanium dioxide
3	Unclassifiable as to carcinogenicity in humans	Inadequate or unavailable evidence in humans and inadequate or limited evidence in animals	512	Bitumens Caffeine Volatile anaesthetics
4	Probably not carcinogenic to humans	Evidence suggests a lack of carcinogenicity in humans and in experimental animals	1	Caprolactam

amines in local dye works and asbestos used in construction are good examples of situations where exposures are likely to occur. The concern therefore is that in years to come, the developing world could see a significant increase in the burden of occupational cancer, similar to or even exceeding that seen by the developed world during the twentieth century.

Mechanism

Cancer is a genetic disorder of somatic cells and can be triggered by the genotoxic action of carcinogens. Genetic aberrations can be found in the majority of human cancers. Oncogenes are normally suppressed in mature cells by regulating genes. DNA strand breaks, for instance due to ionizing radiation or chemical carcinogenesis with aberrant repair, can lead to loss of regulation. The activated oncogene uncouples the usual cell loss/gain equilibrium in favour of cell multiplication leading to an increase in cell numbers and ultimately appearance of a clinical tumour. Tumour suppressor genes exist in pairs within the cell and both must be inactivated for a tumour to develop. The p53 gene is the best known tumour suppressor ('the guardian of the genome') and is found to be mutated in the majority of sporadic cancers. Several environmental and occupational carcinogens are linked to p53 mutations such as UV light and skin cancer, tobacco and oral cancer. Other factors linked with p53 include alcohol, vinyl chloride and asbestos.

Tests for genotoxicity such as Ames and fluorescent *in situ* hybridization (FISH) are now well established. The Ames test is the most widely used procedure for assessing the mutagenicity of an agent, indicated by the number of bacterial colonies growing on a plate containing the toxic agent relative to those growing on a plate containing normal medium. FISH is used to assess chromosomal abnormalities.

Epigenetic carcinogens (also known as non-genotoxic or co-carcinogens) act more directly on the cell itself to cause abnormal cell proliferation and chromosomal aberrations that affect gene expression. These carcinogens have a threshold dose for carcinogenicity and it is possible to set exposure levels. For example, all workers involved in distilling β-naphthylamine eventually developed tumours of the urothelial tract, whereas only 4% of rubber mill workers who were exposed to β-naphthylamine contaminating an antioxidant (at 0.25%) used in making tyres and inner tubes developed bladder cancer over a 30-year follow up.

Polymorphisms are different responses to the same factor such as a drug. Slow acetylators who are heavy smokers are 1.5 times more likely to get bladder cancer if exposed to carcinogens. Certain polymorphisms increase the risk of mesothelioma 7.8 times. At the moment there are no readily available tests to determine susceptibility which are appropriate to workplace testing.

Occupationally related cancers are characterized by a long latent period (i.e. the time between first exposure to the causative agent and presentation of the tumour). This latency is not usually less than 10–15 years and can be much longer (40–50 years in the case of some asbestos-related mesotheliomas (Figure 13.2)), and,

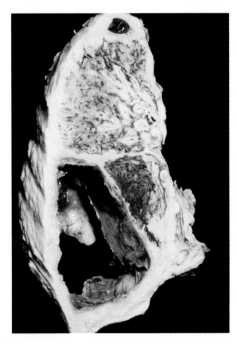

Figure 13.2 Thick-walled mesothelioma of pleura with haemorrhagic cavitation in a former insulation worker.

thus, presentation can be in retirement rather than while still at work. However, susceptibility to occupational carcinogens is greater when the exposure occurs at younger ages. An occupationally related tumour does not differ substantially, either pathologically or clinically, from its 'naturally occurring' counterpart.

Recognition and diagnosis

For a group of workers, occupational cancer is evidenced by a clear excess of cancers over what would normally be expected. Some common malignancies that can be work related also have a well-recognized and predominant aetiology related to other agents, diet or lifestyle (for example, lung cancer from smoking). There are, however, some features which may help to distinguish occupational cancers from those not related to work (Box 13.1, Figure 13.3).

- *History taking* – Taking a patient's occupational history is of paramount importance. It should be defined in detail and sequentially. For example, a holiday job in a factory that lasted only a few months could easily be overlooked, but it may have involved delagging a boiler or handling sacks of asbestos waste.
- *Signal tumours* – Several uncommon cancers are associated with particular occupations. Thus, an angiosarcoma of the liver may indicate past exposure to vinyl chloride monomer in the production of polyvinyl chloride although there have been no cases in workers exposed since 1969. A worldwide registry of all exposed workers exists maintained by the Association of European Plastics Manufacturers.
- *Age* – A younger age at presentation with cancer may suggest an occupational influence. For example, a tumour of the urothelial tract presenting in anyone under the age of 50 years should always arouse suspicion (Figure 13.4).
- *Patients' information* – Patients may speak of a 'cluster' of cancer cases at work or may have worked in an industry or job for which a warning leaflet has been issued.

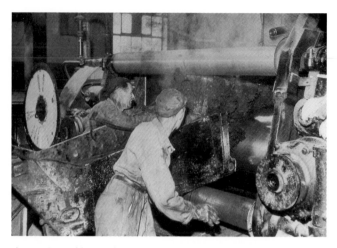

Figure 13.3 Rubber workers in mill room.

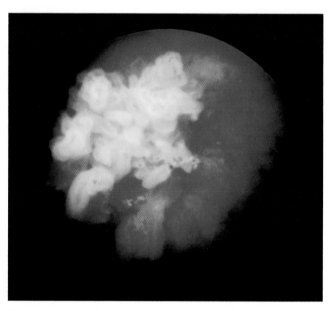

Figure 13.4 Cystoscopic view of papillary carcinoma of the bladder in a 47-year-old rubber worker.

Box 13.1 Diagnosis of work-related cancer is assisted by

- detailed lifelong occupational history
- comparison with a check list of recognized causal associations

Confirmation of requisite exposure

- Search for additional clues: Shift to a younger age; Presence of signal tumours; Other cases and 'clusters'; Long latency; Absence of anticipated aetiologies; Unusual histology or site such as angiosarcoma in vinyl chloride workers and renal pelvic tumours following exposure to amine dyes

---

Prevention and management in the workplace

Primary prevention seeks to actually prevent the onset of a disease. Secondary prevention aims to halt the progression of a disease

once it is established. Tertiary prevention is concerned with the rehabilitation of people with an established disease to minimize residual disabilities and complications or improve the quality of life if the disease itself cannot be cured (Table 13.2).

Primary prevention of occupationally related cancers depends essentially on educating employers and employees; first, about recognizing that there is a risk, and then about the practical steps that can be taken to eliminate or reduce exposure and to protect workers (Box 13.2). Modern risk-based legislation now directs these educational and practical measures.

Secondary prevention

Screening procedures may enable earlier diagnosis but there is little evidence to suggest that screening for most occupational cancer makes a difference to outcomes and in some such as lung cancer screening is not indicated due to the risk of increased x-ray

Table 13.2 Stages and outcome in cancer cycle.

	Stages			Outcomes		
	Health	**Asymptomatic**	*Symptomatic*	*Disability*	*Recovery*	**Death**
Intervention strategies	Health education, immunization, environmental measures and social policy	Presymptomatic screening	Early diagnosis and prompt effective treatment	Rehabilitation		
Levels of prevention	Primary	Secondary		Tertiary		

*Adapted from Donaldson and Donaldson (1999).

Box 13.2 Action for primary prevention of occupational cancers

- Recognizing presence of hazards and risks through process of risk assessment
- Eliminating exposure by substitution and automation
- Reducing exposure by engineering controls (such as local exhaust ventilation and enclosure), changes in handling and altering physical form in processing; limiting access
- Monitoring exposure and maintaining plant
- Educating management and workforce
- Protecting workers by means of personal protective equipment
- Providing adequate facilities for showering, washing, and changing
- Legislative provisions

Table 13.3 Benefits and disadvantages of screening.

Benefits	Disadvantages
Improved prognosis for some cases detected by screening	Longer morbidity for cases whose prognosis is unaltered
Less radical treatment for some early cases	Over treatment of questionable abnormalities
Reassurance for those with negative test results	False reassurance for those with false negative results
	Anxiety and sometimes morbidity for those with false positive results
	Unnecessary medical intervention for those with false positive results
	Hazard of screening test
	Resource costs: diversion of scarce resources to screening programme

exposure. Screening through routine skin inspections is of benefit in cutaneous cancers of occupational origin, mainly because of the excellent prognosis afforded by treatment. Routine urine cytology has been carried out in many industries where there has been previous exposure to known carcinogens. Beta-naphthylamine was withdrawn from use by 1950, but many ex-workers continue to participate in urine cytology screening programmes. Once commenced surveillance should be lifelong. In the UK it is recommended that urinary levels should be checked in those workers exposed to 4,4'-methylene-bis-2-chloroaniline (MbOCA), but periodic urine cytology for those exposed remains controversial (Box 13.3, Box 13.4, Table 13.3).

Box 13.4 Main legislative provisions in United Kingdom

- European Commission Carcinogens Directive (90/934/EEC)
- Chemical Agents Directive (98/24/EC)
- Control of Substances Hazardous to Health (COSHH) Regulations 2002 and associated approved code of practice on the control of carcinogenic substances
- Chemicals (Hazard Information and Packaging) Regulations 2009 (CHIP4)
- Ionizing Radiations Regulations (1999)
- Control of Asbestos at Work Regulations (2006)
- Reporting of Injuries, Diseases and Dangerous Occurrences Regulations (RIDDOR) 1995

Box 13.3 Criteria for screening

- Is the condition an important health problem?
- Is there a recognisable early stage?
- Is treatment at an early stage more beneficial than at a later stage?
- Is there a suitable test?
- Is the test acceptable to the population?
- Are there adequate facilities for diagnosis and treatment?
- What are the costs and benefits?
- Which subgroups should be screened?
- How often should screening take place?

Specific cancers and carcinogens

In men in Great Britain, the top occupational cancer registrations in 2004 were lung, mesothelioma, non-melanotic skin cancer and bladder cancer, and in women breast, lung, non-melanotic skin cancer (NMSC) and mesothelioma (Table 13.4).

In terms of exposures, asbestos contributed half of the deaths followed by silica, diesel engine exhaust, radon, work as a painter, mineral oils, shift work, environmental tobacco smoke in non-smokers, dioxins, radon and work as a welder. In terms of cancer registrations the main exposures were asbestos, shift work, mineral oils and solar radiation. Industries with large numbers of registrations and

Table 13.4 Attribution of work related cancer to occupation.

Established and probable carcinogens IARC group 1 and 2a	Number of registrations attributable to occupation (2004)		Number of deaths attributable to occupation (2005)		Proportion of cancers attributable to occupation (%)	
	Male	Female	Male	Female	Male	Female
Bladder	496	54	215	30	7	2
Larynx	50	6	17	3	3	2
Lung	4632	816	4024	726	21	5
Mesothelioma	1699	238	1699	238	97	83
NMSC	2576	352	21	2	7	1
Sinonasal	101	32	29	10	46	20

deaths included construction including painting and decorating, manufacturing including mining, quarrying and utilities, and the service industry including personal and household services and shift work.

Metals and metalliferous compounds

Arsenic, beryllium, cadmium, chromium (VI), nickel and iron are considered to be proven human carcinogens, either as the metal itself or as a derivative. The risk from iron is related only to mining the base ore and is due to coincidental exposure to radon gas. With all the metallic carcinogens, the lung is the main target organ, but other potential sites include skin (arsenic), prostate (cadmium) and nasal sinuses (nickel).

Aromatic amines

Aromatic amines are among the best known and most studied of chemical carcinogens. The bladder is the main target organ, but any site on the urothelial tract comprising transitional cell epithelium can be affected. The carcinogenic potential of aromatic amines is due to a metabolite formed in the liver and excreted through the urinary system.

The occupations classically associated with risk from these chemicals were in the industries manufacturing chemicals and dyestuffs and to a lesser extent the rubber and cable making industries (Box 13.5). Withdrawal of β-naphthylamine removed the risk for those who started work in the rubber industry after 1950.

Box 13.5 **Occupations causally associated with urothelial tract cancers**

- Dyestuffs and pigment manufacture
- Rubber workers (in tyre, tube, and cable making before 1950)
- Textile dyeing and printing
- Manufacture of some hardener chemicals such as MbOCA (4,4′-methylene-bis-2-chloroaniline)
- Gas workers (in old vertical retort houses)
- Laboratory and testing work (using chromogens)
- Rodent controllers (formally using ANTU ((alpha)-naphthylthiourea))
- Painters
- Leather workers
- Manufacture of patent fuel (such as coke) and firelighters
- Tar and pitch workers (roofing and road maintenance)
- Aluminium refining

Asbestos

Few natural materials used in industry have been the subject of more epidemiological and pathological research than the fibrous mineral, asbestos. Lung cancer due to asbestos was first reported in the 1930s and its association was confirmed in the 1950s. In 1960, Wagner and his colleagues reported 33 cases of the 'rare' tumour mesothelioma in workers exposed to asbestos in South Africa (Box 13.6).

Box 13.6 **Asbestos-related cancers**

- Lung
- Malignant mesothelioma – most commonly of pleura, occasionally peritoneal, and rarely of pericardium
- Larynx
- Possibly gastrointestinal tract

In asbestos workers who have developed asbestosis the risk of lung cancer is increased at least fivefold. For the chrysotile form of asbestos there is a linear relationship between exposure and risk of lung cancer. Each additional fibre exposure (per ml per year) is equivalent to a 1% increase in the standardized mortality ratio.

Smoking with concomitant exposure to asbestos also greatly increases the risk of developing lung cancer; compared with non-smokers not exposed to asbestos, a smoker exposed to asbestos has a 75–100 times greater risk if exposure was sufficient to cause asbestosis, otherwise the risk is about 30–50 times higher. This multiplicative theory on effects of asbestos exposure and smoking, however, has been disputed (Table 13.5).

Over 40% of people with asbestosis die of lung cancer, and 10% die of mesothelioma. Mesotheliomas (Figure 13.5), which are predominantly of the pleura (ratio of 8:1 with peritoneum), have usually been growing for 10–12 years before becoming clinically evident. This latency can be very long; often 30 years and sometimes up to 50 years. However, mean survival from the time of initial diagnosis is 9 months with less than 5% surviving 2 years.

The amphibole fibres in crocidolite (blue asbestos) and amosite (brown asbestos) carry the greatest risk of causing mesothelioma, but the serpentine fibres in chrysotile (white asbestos) can also do so, especially if they contain tremolite. In about 90% of patients with mesothelioma, close questioning will usually reveal some earlier exposure to asbestos. The possible risk to neighbourhoods outside asbestos factories from discharged asbestos dust or contaminated clothing brought home should not be forgotten (Figure 13.6).

The annual number of mesothelioma deaths has increased rapidly from 153 in 1968 to 2249 in 2008 (men and women). The most

Table 13.5 Multiplicative effect of asbestos and smoking on lung cancer.

Asbestos	Tobacco	Lung cancer rate per 100 000
–	–	11
+	–	58
–	+	123
+	+	590

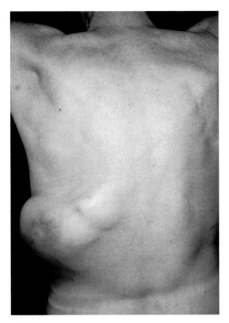

Figure 13.5 Mesothelioma extending through needle biopsy tract.

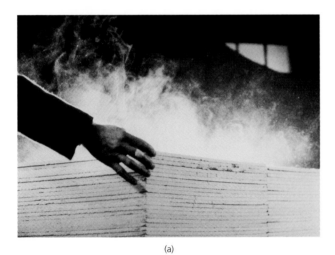

(a)

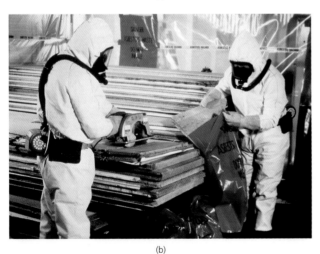

(b)

Figure 13.6 Tyndall beam photography showing asbestos fibres released by mere handling of asbestos boards (a), emphasizing the need for proper protection when dealing with asbestos (b).

frequently recorded occupations on death certificates of men now dying from mesothelioma include carpenters and joiners; plumbers, heating and ventilating engineers; and electricians and electrical fitters (Box 13.7). The expected number of deaths among men is predicted to increase to a peak of 2038 (90% prediction interval: 1929 to 2156) around the year 2016.

Box 13.7 **Occupations involving exposure to asbestos**

- Manufacture of asbestos products
- Thermal and fire insulation (lagging, delagging)
- Construction and demolition work
- Shipbuilding and repair (welders, metal plate workers)
- Building maintenance and repair
- Manufacture of gas masks (in second world war)
- Plumbers and gasfitters
- Vehicle body builders
- Electricians, carpenters, and upholsterers
- Armed forces (historical)

Ultraviolet radiation

Ultraviolet radiation from exposure to sunlight causes both melanotic and non-melanotic skin cancers (basal cell and squamous cell carcinomas) but an excess of skin cancers in outdoor workers is only seen in those with fair skin (Figure 13.7). Initial presentation may be that of solar keratoses or a pre-malignant state. Immunosuppression can increase the risk; other possible additive factors are trauma, heat and chronic irritation or infection.

Mineral oils

The classic epithelioma of the scrotum or groin (Figure 13.8) due to contact with mineral oil is rarely seen today, but these tumours can appear at other sites (such as arms and hands) if contamination with oil persists (Table 13.6).

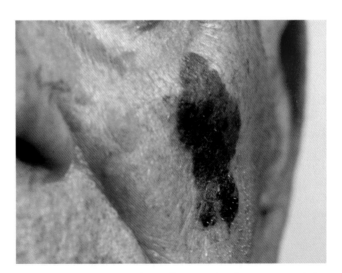

Figure 13.7 Pre-malignant melanosis (lentigo maligna) in a man retired after a lifetime of working outdoors.

Table 13.6 Occupational cancer by exposure and target organ.

Miscellaneous proved human carcinogens by organ	Lung	Bladder	Skin	Haemopoietic	Nasal	Upper GI	Larynx	Scrotum
Aluminium production	✓	✓	✓					
Polycyclic aromatic hydrocarbons and aromatic amines in coal gasification and coke production	✓	✓	✓					
Coal tars and pitch in roofing and road maintenance	✓	✓	✓					
Ethylene oxide as medical sterilizer and chemical intermediary	✓	✓	✓					
Solvents and pigments in painting and decorating	✓	✓				✓		
Soots from chimney sweeping and flue maintenance	✓		✓					
Radon in underground mines	✓							
Benzene in petroleum associated industries	✓							
Bis-(chloromethyl)-ether in production of ion exchange resin	✓							
Antineoplastic agents		✓		✓				
Mineral and shale oils in engineering and metal machining, past exposure to mule spinning in cotton industry and jute processing			✓					✓
Benzene and leather dust in boot and shoe making and repair				✓	✓			
Mists of strong inorganic acid (sulphuric acid) in acid pickling and soap making					✓		✓	
Formaldehyde and hardwood dust in furniture and cabinet making					✓			
Isopropyl alcohol manufacture					✓			

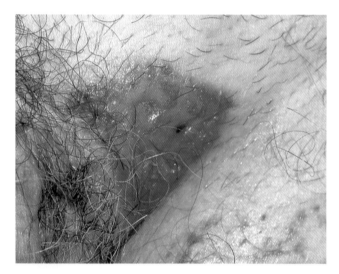

Figure 13.8 Epithelioma of groin due to past exposure to mineral oil.

Other occupational carcinogens

Ionizing radiation is a carcinogen at low dose levels (0.2 Gray or dose rate of 0.05 mSv min). Cancer or hereditary defects are known as stochastic effects and can only be minimized. Cataract, sterility and skin disorders are deterministic effects and can be prevented by keeping exposure below threshold. The recommended effective dose is 20 mSv per year averaged over 5 years for occupational exposures and 1 mSv for the public. Frieben documented the first case of skin cancer on the hand of an X-ray tube factory worker in 1902. Cancer risk estimates on nuclear workers are still not conclusive and the Gardener hypothesis that the children of radiation workers have an increased risk of leukaemia has not been supported. Emergency workers however may have increased incidence and there have been studies concerning airline crew who may receive the equivalent of 100 mSv over a 20-year period from cosmic radiation. No excess cancer has been reported among therapeutic or diagnostic radiologists.

All studies on electromagnetic radiation demonstrate inconsistencies and seldom indicate dose–response trends. This may mean that there is no association between electromagnetic fields and cancer or that there is a risk but studies have not been able to demonstrate it. Particular aspects studied so far have been leukaemia, brain cancer, male breast cancer, electrical workers and welders but a broader research hypothesis is needed.

> **Box 13.8 Shift work**
>
> - Animal studies have demonstrated that disrupting circadian rhythms increases tumour development. Other experimental studies show that reducing melatonin levels at night increases the incidence or growth of tumours
> - Epidemiological studies have found that women who worked shifts for more than 20 years have a statistically higher risk of breast cancer but there is the possibility of bias, chance and confounding in these studies
> - The available evidence does not prove causation or provide a reliable estimation of risk and further studies are needed to clarify if and why shift work may affect breast cancer
> - In the UK the Industrial Injuries Advisory Council have determined that there is insufficient evidence to make breast cancer a compensable disease
> - However IARC have classified overnight shiftwork as a 'probable' human carcinogen (2a)
> - 20% of the European workforce are estimated to undertake shiftwork

Studies of man-made mineral fibres (MMMF) have only looked at small exposures in terms of fibres and years of exposure. An increased risk of lung cancer was found in rock wool workers but it was not possible to conclude that it was caused by MMMF. No risk was found in glass wool/glass filament workers. Five deaths from mesothelioma have been found in various cohorts but at least three of these may have had previous asbestos exposure.

Table 13.7 Cancers covered by Industrial Injuries Disablement Benefit.

	Cancer	Carcinogen
A1	Leukaemia (not CLL) Bone Female breast Testis Thyroid	Electromagnetic radiation or ionizing particles
C7	Acute non-lymphatic leukaemia	Benzene
C21	Skin cancer	Arsenic Arsenic compounds Tar, pitch, bitumen, mineral oil (including paraffin) soot
C22a	Sinonasal cancer	Nickel compounds
C22b	Lung cancer	Nickel compounds (C22b)
D3	Mesothelioma	
D6	Sinonasal cancer	Wood, leather and fibre board dust
D8	Asbestos related lung cancer	Lung cancer with asbestosis or lung cancer and evidence of at least 5 years' asbestos exposure before 1975 in certain jobs
D10	Lung cancer	Due to work as a tin miner, exposure to bis (chloromethyl) ether or to zinc, calcium or strontium chromates
D11	Lung cancer	Silica exposure
C23	Bladder cancer	Exposure to various compounds during chemical manufacturing or processing, including 1-naphthylamine, 2-naphthylamine, benzidine, auramine, magenta, 4-aminobiphenyl, MbOCA, orthotoluidine, 4-chloro-2-methylaniline, and coal tar pitch volatiles produced in aluminium smelting
C24	Angiosarcoma of the Liver	Vinyl chloride monomer

There is sufficient evidence for the carcinogenicity of inhaled crystalline silica in the form of quartz or cristobalite. Studies demonstrate the Bradford–Hill criteria of temporality, consistency, exposure–response gradients, convergence with experimental and clinical evidence. Measures to prevent silicosis are likely to reduce lung cancer risk.

Shift work has recently received attention as a carcinogen (Box 13.8).

Compensation and prescribed disease

The specific forms of occupational cancer which are currently compensable under the UK Department for Work and Pensions Industrial Injuries and Disablement Benefit (IIDB) scheme are listed in Table 13.7. When mesothelioma and asbestos-related lung cancers are excluded there have typically been around 50 or fewer compensated cancers per year during the last 10 years. The figures for asbestos-related lung cancers significantly under-represents the true number. Some cancers are reportable under the The Reporting of Injuries, Diseases and Dangerous Occurrences Regulations 1995 although many occur in those who have retired.

Further reading

IARC monographs on the evaluation of carcinogenic risks to humans. Volumes 1–100. Lyons: International Agency for Research on Cancer, 1972-2010. http://monographs.iarc.fr. *Highly detailed reviews of cancers and cancer causing substances or activities by a committee of international experts*

Rushton L, *et al.* Occupation and cancer in Britain. *Br J Cancer* 2010; 102: 1428–1437. *Groundbreaking research which defines the amount of cancer caused by occupation and the main causative agents*

http://www.hse.gov.uk/statistics/causdis/cancer/ Accessed January 2011. *Contains all the background detail from Rushton's research as well as the impact of control measures on future occupational cancer incidence*

Baxter PJ, Adams PH, Aw, T-C, *et al.* Occupational cancer. In: *Hunter's diseases of occupations*, 10th edn. London: Edward Arnold, 2010. *Authoritative occupational medicine textbook providing in depth detail about occupational cancer*

Wilson JMJ, Jungner G. Principles and practice of screening for disease. WHO Public Health Paper 1968;34.

Donaldson LJ, Donaldson RJ. The Promotion of health in essential public health. 2nd edn. Petroc Press.

Oxford Textbook of Oncology. 2002. *Authoritative oncology textbook providing in depth detail about all aspects of cancer*

CHAPTER 14

Disorders of Uncertain Aetiology

Andy Slovak

University of Manchester, Manchester, UK

OVERVIEW

- The common feature of these conditions is uncertainty
- The commonest uncertainty concerns possible causality
- Uncertainty often extends to both susceptibility and treatment
- Psychosomatic concepts are often relevant but are equally often rejected by those susceptible
- Research is very difficult, arguable and quite often inconclusive

---

Occupational and environmental conditions, by their nature, invite and create contention. This is particularly so where causality is uncertain. Figure 14.1 seeks to explain why this might be. Individual and group beliefs, behaviours, and so on, and their social modulation seem to play as substantial a part in the experience of symptoms as does exposure to the range of putative causal agents.

The issues of causality, attitude and perception that affect approaches to these conditions are discussed first, before describing specific syndromes. From a practical point of view, there is an obvious dichotomy between the support it is proper to give to those affected and the more detached objectivity one would wish to bring to understanding their condition scientifically. This is particularly so when, as is often the case, health professionals are invited to make a commitment to a particular belief system related to the causality of the disorder under discussion. At the same time, those health professionals are all members of the public and as such are susceptible to prevalent, popular, belief systems.

Box 14.1 lists a selection of medical syndromes whose nature and aetiology are at present uncertain. They are an apparently disparate grouping, but as far as broader circumstances are concerned, they tend to reflect some common themes:

- multifactoriality (both symptoms and putative causes)
- lack of control ('involuntary' exposure)
- marked variation in susceptibility
- tendency to ascribe to external causes.

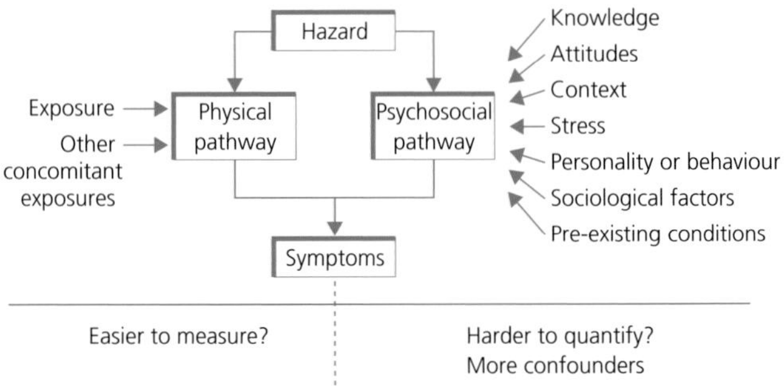

Figure 14.1 Pathways of exposure.

Box 14.1 **Medical syndromes with uncertain nature and aetiology**

- Long-term conditions claimed to be associated with proximity to electromagnetic fields (for example, power lines) and nuclear installations
- Gulf war syndromes
- Multiple chemical sensitivity
- Situational syndromes: the Braer disaster and the Camelford incident
- Sick building syndromes
- Conditions claimed to be associated with proximity to landfill sites
- Long-term conditions claimed to be associated with pesticides used for sheep dipping

---

As such, there are resonances between these conditions and others considered elsewhere in this book or that are beyond its scope. These conditions include non-specific upper limb disorders, regional pain syndromes, fibromyalgia, stress and chronic fatigue syndrome.

To deconstruct the nature of the multifactoriality a little, in the cases of sick building syndromes, multiple chemical sensitivity and war syndromes, the factors implicated are truly extensive and highly varied, whereas in disaster/situational syndromes (for instance oil spills) they are defined by the event, although the nature of the elements of the exposure may still, to some extent, be arguable. The debates about electromagnetic fields and nuclear installations are even more unusual because they are biphasic with more or less distinct occupational and environmental modes.

ABC of Occupational and Environmental Medicine, Third Edition.
Edited by David Snashall and Dipti Patel.
© 2012 John Wiley & Sons Ltd. Published 2012 by John Wiley & Sons Ltd.

Landfill and incinerator sites present another situational pattern. They are numerous, widely distributed and commonly complained of being the source of a range of effects (in time and space) and an even wider range of possible hazards and attendant risks. In contrast to all of the previous examples, the putative causal agents cited for conditions attributed to sheep dipping are highly specific – namely, organophosphate pesticides. Acute effects are well known and well characterized, but the controversy about how they might be implicated in longer term effects, continues.

Electromagnetic fields and nuclear installations

Studies relating to power lines have been pursued for about 40 years and for nuclear installations, about 30 years. Their conclusions, except at the peripheries, are no longer as hotly debated as they were 10 or 20 years ago. Having come to some level of maturation as controversies, they may be taken as 'worked examples' of the assimilation of controversy into common or at least common scientific consensus as explained in the Box 14.2.

> Box 14.2 **Electromagnetic fields**
>
> Electromagnetic field studies by epidemiological methods suggest a weak association for childhood leukaemia. However, biological experimental studies have failed to demonstrate potential mechanisms causally. At the social level, this paradoxical situation has been recognized by labelling electromagnetic fields as a 'possible' carcinogen.'

This consensus, as the relevant WHO monograph (No 238) explains is a 'conceptual framework' where the evidence 'is not strong enough to be considered causal, but sufficiently strong to remain a concern.'

The scientific characteristics of that evidence are educative. They consist of a series of epidemiological studies published since about 1979 which have sparse data and low power. Odds ratios have been in the range 1–1.5 with wide confidence intervals often including unity. Taken together they show some consistency but the doubts noted in the Box 14.2 and other scientific cautionary factors, which include difficulties in precise measurement of exposure and lack of accountability for sources of bias and confounding, have to be recognized.

Numbers are sparse and exposure criteria poorly defined Studies on those occupationally exposed are even weaker. The difficulty in differentiating the 'effect from background noise' is typical of these sorts of long running debates. The rationale for continuing is nevertheless powerful because of the universality of exposure, the likelihood that exposure will increase in the future, the precautionary principle (see Chapter 22) and for reasons of risk perception.

With regard to nuclear installations, concerns have also centred around childhood leukaemia and other childhood cancers (Box 14.3). In the United Kingdom the debate was initiated by a single television programme in 1983. The putative risk factor at

that time was assumed to be installation discharges of radioactive materials. However, such discharges produce doses to the general public that are very small (by several orders of magnitude) when compared with those that might be expected to produce such effects according to robust scientific risk estimations.

> Box 14.3 **Chronology of attributed 'top' cause of childhood acute lymphoblastic leukaemia associated with nuclear installations**
>
> 1983–1990: Local environmental exposure to ionizing radiation
> 1990–2000: Occupational exposure of fathers to ionizing radiation
> 2000–present: Population mixing due to local employment/population movement demographics (viral)

More generally, the risks of ionizing radiation, mainly cancer, have been studied intensively for 60 years. The pivotal cohort, the Hiroshima and Nagasaki survivors (the Life Span Study (LSS)) to which other cohorts are always compared, is now coming to maturation with respect to definitive cancer outcomes. Such outcomes are expressed as a stochastic (statistical) excess of risk attributable to exposure.

From time to time the universal applicability of these stochastic norms are challenged in such a way as to call into question these risk predictions. This has happened recently (2005–2010) with respect to data nested in a very large international, occupational study where the so-called 'all cancer risk' from one participating country was at considerable odds (100–600%) to those of the others and LSS. Eventually this effect was traced to a basic ascertainment error associated with historical transfer of dosimetry data (and thus exposure) from one arrangement to another. However, it took 5 years to work this out. During that time, it permitted those who might have wished more systematically to disbelieve 'conventional' risk estimates to see the events described as grounds to support their views.

Such 'challenge' events are best regarded as a normal part of scientific activity. They are usually a consequence of statistically predictable variations in subsets of data that come to analysis but simple error occurs more frequently than one might expect. Real frameshifts in risk perception are much rarer and are usually less dramatic.

Even though the debate over scientific plausibility has subsided, these matters can still polarize scientific opinion at the extremes of construct belief.

Mobile phones

The explosion in the global use of mobile phones applies to both occupational and public health fields in terms of hazard and risk. Their development has gone forward on the assumption that the well-understood, small, local, heating effects associated with radiofrequencies in mobile phone use are the sole risk and a negligible one.

This view has been challenged in two ways. First, by claims of association with mobile phone use of clusters of a range of illnesses, most prominently cancer. Second, that the universality of use, including by children and young people, demands both experimental reappraisal and epidemiological tracking on a large scale. As with power lines, this latter argument is persuasive as exposure is pretty universal, and so even a small adverse effect would have a significant population impact.

Recent 'toxicological', experimental studies have been unsuccessful in determining any new hazard. The largest cancer study to date, the Interphone Study, addressed head and neck cancers in mobile phone users in 13 countries. The official results were published in 2010 and reported 'no overall risk'. Sub-analyses of the data, especially when adjustments were attempted for sources of possible bias, suggested both small adverse and protective effects and thus, unsurprisingly, the study has become the subject of controversy.

So far the evidence holds that any risk is small or non-existent. The Interphone Study, although large, suffered from the usual problems of case–control studies, which, in the end, means that they are better at raising issues than solving them. Only cohort studies on quite a large scale will give a more definitive answer and these could take decades to deliver.

Gulf war syndromes

The Gulf war conflicts of 1990/91 and 2003 resulted in very low contemporaneous mortality and morbidity for the multinational forces engaged against Iraq. However, subsequent morbidity, usually described as Gulf war syndromes (Box 14.4), has been reported to be high, with quite marked variation between different countries of reporting levels, range of symptoms and persistence. For example, comparatively few French deployed alongside British and American troops developed the disorder. Unsurprisingly, this subject has generated a large amount of sometimes confusing literature.

Box 14.4 **Some of the most popular possible causes of Gulf war syndromes**

- Inoculation programmes
- Prophylaxis against biological warfare agents
- Depleted uranium
- Insecticide spraying
- Pyrolysis due to military action or 'scorched earth' action
- Involuntary dispersal of chemical or biological war agents due to military action

From this research a number of general observations have emerged. Those veterans who have had combat experience or have been in combat theatres have a higher level of protean (tending to change or adapt) symptoms than those not so exposed The excess level of complacency is most strongly associated with 'soft' factors such as unit cohesion and level of prior preparation for war zones. No strong causality or sets of causality have emerged.

It has been extremely difficult to define a syndrome or syndromes let alone agree about this. Not surprisingly, difficulties have been experienced at the strategic level to systematize research methods and objectives.

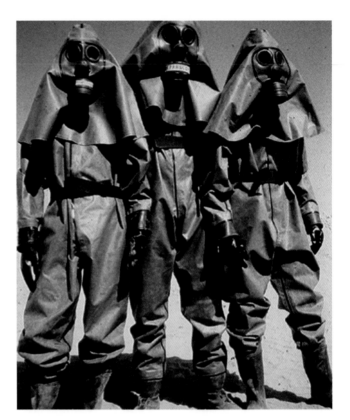

Figure 14.2 Gulf War soldiers in protective clothing.

The strongest inference from all the research activity has been the contextualization of the Gulf war syndromes within the generality of post-conflict psychological and psychosomatic effects (Figure 14.2). These have been reported, more or less consistently, for at least a century. However, this pigeon-holing is likely to be strongly resisted by many veterans as well as those protagonists of particular causal factors or combinations of these.

There is some international consensus that much might be learnt by the more proximate education and monitoring of military personnel prior to and during active deployments as well as systematic follow-up afterwards. The resource implications of such ideas would be very substantial were they to be applied at all comprehensively.

Multiple chemical sensitivity

Multiple chemical sensitivity (MCS) is a difficult entity to position clinically, but over the last decade has tended to be grouped much more emphatically with other hard to define syndromes, as discussed earlier. It is included here because occupational exposures are not infrequently cited as part of the spectrum of precipitating factors.

The range of symptoms observed within the scope of the condition are protean. They include symptoms typical of chronic fatigue, weakness, sleep disturbance, rashes, headache, chest tightness and oppression.

The term multiple chemical sensitivity is used to describe the condition of a group of patients with disabling symptoms whose severity seems to be lessened by restriction of exposure to the everyday environment, particularly by inhalation. It is inferred, therefore, that the aetiology or precipitation of the condition is derived from that environment. Underlying immunological and neurological mechanisms have been proposed but not substantiated.

Diagnostic criteria are hard to define, as are objective investigative methods.

Disaster/situational syndromes

This describes those disasters or events where there has been some unscheduled release or spillage of toxicants. The most common of these are oil spills. Surprisingly the effects of such spillages on human populations potentially exposed have been relatively little studied in comparison with effects on flora and fauna. It may well be that this shortcoming will be remedied following the Gulf of Mexico incident of 2010.

Two situations in the UK have been quite closely observed historically and were sufficiently close together in time to bear meaningful comparison. These were the Braer 'disaster' (1992–3) and the Camelford incident (1988). The Braer, an oil-tanker, ran aground in north Scotland and its cargo of light crude oil was released. At Camelford in Cornwall, an excess of a water treatment agent, aluminium sulphate, was inadvertently introduced into the water supply.

Both incidents resulted in immediate symptoms in local residents. Those associated with Braer were primarily acute, upper respiratory complaints, whereas those in Camelford were more diffuse. The former did not persist; the latter did. The persisting symptoms at Camelford were described as a 'malaise' syndrome (for example fatigue, joint pain, depression, memory loss).

It has been argued that the symptoms associated with the Braer disaster were fleeting because exposures were fleeting as a consequence of vigorous weather dispersion of the pollutants. However, actual exposure to the contaminated water supply at Camelford was also short. Others have argued that the difference lay in the pollutant in question and/or contrasting approaches to the situations by the responsible public authorities. Aspects of societal action that have been perceived as positive in modulating, psychosocial responses to adverse unexpected events are given in the Box 14.5.

> **Box 14.5 Aspects of societal action perceived as positive following situational disasters such as Braer and Camelford**
>
> - Timely communication of an action plan
> - Timely communication of hazard information
> - Effective dialogue with the population at risk
> - Feedback to the population at risk

It is unclear whether recent controversial studies on the long-term effects of Camelford (possible memory loss) have any scientific validity, but it is clear that such situations can cast a long and costly shadow in terms of both human distress and research effort. Curiously, this incident also has a separate existence as a more modern paradigm, that of potential terrorist action on water supplies.

Sick building syndrome

Sick building syndrome (SBS) was originally described in the 1970s and was cast as a mainly respiratory condition associated with newer buildings. It was postulated that there might be a quite wide range of potential causal or contributory factors including ozone, fibres, dust, newbuild volatiles and tobacco smoke. Much official guidance still relates to this model.

A more recent perception of SBS derives from cohort studies of working populations in which the condition might be expected to be found as opposed to earlier studies of symptomatic cases. In the most prominent of these studies, the so-called Whitehall studies of a cohort of British civil servants, the symptoms complained of were much more protean and were most strongly associated with psychosocial aspects of the workplace (e.g. job grade, lack of autonomy) rather than physical elements.

These psychological factors are similar to those associated with work stress and, in such a model, SBS is more easily understood as a predominantly psychosomatic disorder. However, there is no reason why physical and psychosomatic models should not coexist. Also SBS should be differentiated from BRI (building-related illness). BRI is distinguished by the identification of a specific causal agent of which the best known is legionella.

Landfills and incinerators

The figure shows the geographical distribution of UK landfill sites and perhaps also the futility of 'nimbyism.' (NIMBY is an acronym – 'not in my back yard' – denoting resistance to the location of any undesired feature in a particular neighbourhood.) Incinerators are less common although it might be argued that their 'plume shadow' is likely to be greater than any plausible deposition zone around landfills.

In the last 10–15 years, many epidemiologists have taken advantage of the high level of geographic localization available in birth and cancer registries to study their possible associations with landfills and incinerators (Figure 14.3). For cancers, landfill proximity shows the possibility of a small general population excess, but, paradoxically, for landfill workers, who of course are much more likely to have high exposure, no such excess has been seen. For birth defects, the data are still largely driven by a very large UK study in 2001 and its update in 2009 which showed a small proximity association (about 1%). However, 'proximity' encompassed the majority of the UK population.

Data on incinerators (and crematoria) reflect multiple small but inconsistent risks of birth defects. Worker studies suggest a small excess risk of respiratory and gastric cancers but again are not very consistent.

At the technical level, the feasibility of doing the relevant geographical studies has now been demonstrated. There remain serious concerns that, on the one hand, big studies may miss local effects whereas small studies face multiple sources of bias and confounding. In terms of public policy, the scope for using the information to plan the location of landfill sites seems limited but may be greater for incinerator placement.

Landfill and other 'amenity' sites are particularly likely to be the subject of local symptomatic complaint and anecdotal reporting

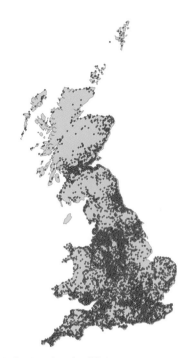

Figure 14.3 Distribution of UK landfill sites.

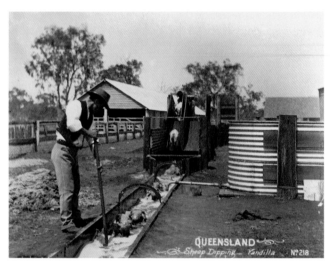

Figure 14.4 Sheep dipping.

of cluster events (for example, cancers). For such investigations, the range of reported conditions and (usually) the lack of easily definable toxic exposures may result in unsatisfactory outcomes for all parties involved.

Organophosphate (OP) sheep dips

Organophosphates are well characterized neurotoxins that exert their effects acutely by inhibiting the widespread neurotransmitter enzyme acetylcholinesterase. This toxic effect has been widely exploited in pesticide applications, as in sheep dips for parasitic infestations. The acute effects have also been widely seen in humans in occupational, domestic, and deliberate overexposures. A typical acute syndrome of stomach cramps, weakness, paralysis, and collapse is directly associated with measurable cholinesterase suppression in a traditional dose–response relation.

Two syndromes of longer duration have been attributed to long-term effects of organophosphate exposure, mainly in sheep dippers who have high and repeated contact with these agents. One, known colloquially as 'dipper's flu', is reported to come on some time after exposure, typically up to a day later. As the name indicates, the illness is described as 'flu-like' in nature and duration. The other syndrome or syndrome set is reported to be truly chronic, and the syndrome range is typical of that described repeatedly in this chapter. Anecdotally, some preponderance of chronic fatigue and cognitive deficits is claimed.

Dipper's flu has been subjected to objective field investigations of exposure and symptoms following dipping. Little difference was observed between symptoms of dippers and unexposed controls when symptoms were grouped (for example, cognitive, visual, flu like). When symptoms were degrouped and analysed separately, some emerged as more common in dippers but these were not those

of flu. Thus, despite quite extensive research, the findings continue to be inconclusive or perverse, and there is no clear dose or dose surrogate relation.

Complaints of neuropathy are more frequent in sheep dippers, especially those handling concentrate, who are also more prone to anxiety and depression (Figure 14.4). Again, no cause and effect relation has been established, and objective signs of damage have not been in evidence.

Puzzlingly, a plausible mechanism of action has not been found for the longer term or chronic effects attributed to organophosphate exposure. The long-term effects are not associated with cholinesterase depletion – the acute toxic mechanism – in any discernible or direct way. It is possible, speculatively, to postulate some 'shadow' effect of cholinesterase inhibition, or some other unknown mechanism of the agent or some contaminant, but the investigations to date have been elusive and discouraging of the existence of such mechanisms.

Little or no progress has been made in the elucidation of these potential long-term OP effects in the last 10–20 years. There continue to be occasional reports of excesses of chronic neurological and psychiatric perturbation in exposed worker groups from time to time. It is to be hoped that more light will be cast on this difficult subject by relatively recently initiated cohort studies such as the US Agricultural Health Study.

Disease hunting and risk attribution

Evidence-based pursuit of these objectives in occupational and environmental subjects has been much advanced by the development of systematically weighted meta analyses (as practised in various Cochrane fields). Practical advisory bodies, such as NICE, also use such techniques. They are not widely understood or practised by the majority of us. In the last few years, well-established instruments for interrogating on-line scientific research data (e.g. PubMed search strategies) have become universally available so it has become open to the interested individual to conduct sophisticatedly modulated searches and analyses. The pursuit of such approaches may be of particular value in teasing out conditions which are currently ill-defined or of unknown aetiology.

Conclusion

The foregoing sections cover a range of occupationally and environmentally ascribed complaints of uncertain origin (Box 14.6).

Box 14.6 **Other environmental ascribed complaints**

- Oestrogenic modulators in water and food chains
- Mercury dental amalgams
- Pesticides residues in foodchains

They bring up scientific problems associated with differentiating between hazard (innate adverse characteristics) and risk (the likelihood of them happening). Ill understood by society, the difference between hazard and risk seems to be marginalized in a society where such issues are now more often subject to perception and the precautionary principle (where ultimately hazard equals risk). However, adoption of the precautionary principle in society at large remains conditional and sometimes perversely inconsistent. Thus the use of mobile phones is universal, even in children, although the risks from their use remain unclear (even if likely to be low). Nevertheless, there is often local resistance to the installation of base stations which the demands of universal usage of mobile phones obviously necessitate. Perverse indeed!

The natural course of issues of the type discussed in this chapter is often a cycle of initial concern, resistance, disturbance, investigation, assimilation and exhaustion. This is shown in the figures, which examine the epidemiological time course of investigations into the nuclear installations issue discussed earlier, and soft tissue sarcoma associated with herbicide application, moving from the sentinel observation towards regression to the mean.

It is not easy to accommodate the uncertainties and paradoxes described in this chapter into rational clinical management strategies to help patients or the 'worried well'. It would be dishonest to set the uncertainties aside as if they did not exist, but these are not grounds for dismissing the distress and anxiety of individuals. Therapeutic handling, regardless of the putative source of the illness, will include acceptance that there is a problem, and painstaking elucidation of symptoms and characterization of the illness behaviour. For the individuals affected the therapeutic journey is also often difficult for it involves acceptance of the uncertainties of causality, at least to some extent, and positive engagement with largely behavioural therapeutic regimens.

References

The reading list below mainly references overviews and other summarizing documents. While usually carried out independently, they cite mainstream, scientific views. In this chapter subject area, such views are often vigorously contested and the interested reader can easily sample the range of alternative views by even the most rapid of internet searches.

Eberlein-Konig B, Przbilla B, Kuhnl P, et al. Multiple chemical sensitivity (MCS) and others: allergological, environmental and psychological investigations in individuals with indoor related complaints. *Int J Hyg Environ Health* 2002; 205: 213–220.

Institute of Occupational Health. *Symptom reporting following occupational exposure to organophosphate pesticides in sheep dip.* HSE Contract Research Report 371/2001. Sudbury: HSE Books, 2001

AGNIR (2001) Electromagnetic fields and the risk of cancer. Docs NRPB,12(1).

Tarn M, Greenberg N, Wessely S. Gulf War syndrome–has it gone away? *Adv Psychiatric Treat* 2008; 14: 414–422.

The Interphone study group. Brain tumour risk in relation to mobile telephone use: results of the Interphone international case-control study. *Int J Epidemiol* 2010: 1–20.

Campbell D, Cox D, Crum J, Foster K, Riley H. Later effects of the grounding of tanker Braer on health in Shetland. *BMJ* 1994; 309: 773–734.

David AS. The legend of Camelford: medical consequences of a water pollution accident. *J Psychosom Res* 1995; 39: 1–9.

Spurgeon A, Gompertz D, Harrington JM. Modifiers of non-specific symptoms of occupational and environmental syndromes. *Occup Environ Med* 1996; 83: 361–366.

Marmot AF, Eley J, Stafford M, et al. Building health: an epidemiological study of 'sick building syndrome' in the Whitehall II study. *OEM* 2006; 63; 283–289.

Impact on health of emissions from landfill sites. RCE 18 2011. www.hpa.org.uk.

CHAPTER 15

Physical Agents

Ron McCaig

Cheshire and Wirral Partnership NHS Foundation Trust, Chester, Cheshire, UK

OVERVIEW

- Physical agents are well characterized and relatively easily measured and knowledge of exposures is important in managing the workplace
- Appropriate control of exposure is essential in preventing harm arising from physical agents
- Administrative controls and the use of personal protective equipment may be necessary in managing workplace exposures
- Administrative controls may include screening of workers to identify any thought to be at particular risk from the exposure
- Health surveillance may be used to monitor the effectiveness of controls, and to identify at an early stage any workers who may have suffered harm

Box 15.1 **Questions to ask about a physical agent**

How is it measured, and what are the units used?
What are the short and long term effects of exposure?
What is the dose response relationship for each health effect?
What are acceptable exposure levels?
Are there groups at higher risk from exposures?
Are there any stochastic effects?
Is there specific legislation relating to this agent?
What are the accepted control measures to prevent harm?

Physical agents

The effects of physical agents have been well studied, and for many of these, exposure criteria are now established at an international level. Fatalities are only likely to occur where established safety procedures are broken

Physical agents impart energy to the body by physical means (for example the effects of noise, vibration, heat, cold or radiations), or through the physical effects of environments which differ from normal ambient conditions (for example those found in diving and compressed air work, at altitude and in flight). The former are much more commonly encountered. In the workplace a healthcare professional may be involved in deciding about an employee's fitness for work that involves exposure to one or more physical agents, in diagnosing health effects thought to have arisen from such exposures or in giving advice to help prevent such harmful effects. GPs may also see ill health from physical exposures at work and need to be alert to this possible aetiology. They may also be consulted by their patients about the health effects of work, particularly where there is a long-term risk of serious effects such as cancer (Box 15.1).

The potential effects of physical agents range from discomfort and interference with work tasks, right through to death, either acutely or many years after exposure. These effects have been well researched and are mostly well understood. Physical agents are amenable to measurement which, when applied in epidemiological studies, allows a dose–response effect to be established and, from this, acceptable exposure standards. These can then be translated into statutory controls. Measurement and exposure standards for physical agents are often published by international agencies. Accessing these standards and national legislation will provide a good introduction to the hazards associated with each of the physical agents. Textbooks of occupational hygiene give details of measurement methods for each of the physical agents.

Stochastic effects differ from direct effects in that there is considered to be no threshold below which there is no risk, and the probability of an effect arising relates to the dose received. The direct effects of physical agents are regarded as having a threshold below which harm does not arise, and a dose–response relationship where the magnitude of the effect is related to the magnitude of the exposure.

Prevention of harm from physical agents relies on controlling exposures. It may be possible to find alternative ways of doing a job that cut down on exposure, for example pulling a bolt through metal, rather than knocking it through–this can cut down on both noise and vibration exposure. If substitution is not possible, then control at source should be considered. Personal protective equipment is often relied on, for example the use of hearing defenders, but is often not perfect in practice, and should be regarded as a last resort. Some exposures cannot be modified such as outdoor work environments or the effects of pressure when

ABC of Occupational and Environmental Medicine, Third Edition.
Edited by David Snashall and Dipti Patel.
© 2012 John Wiley & Sons Ltd. Published 2012 by John Wiley & Sons Ltd.

diving. Administrative controls based on a thorough risk assessment will be necessary and these may include screening the population of workers for individuals at particular risk.

Advice and guidance on controlling exposures to physical agents is well established and a good place to look for such information is on the websites of health and safety organizations such as the Health and Safety Executive (HSE) in Great Britain (Box 15.2) or the National Institute for Occupational Safety and Health (NIOSH) in the USA (Box 15.3). Once there is a good understanding of the principles involved, it may be necessary to involve an occupational hygienist or a health physicist to quantify exposures in a particular workplace of concern.

Box 15.2 **United Kingdom Health and Safety Regulations applying to Physical Agents**

Control of Noise at Work Regulations 2005
Control of Vibration at Work Regulations 2005
Workplace (Health, Safety and Welfare) Regulations 1992
Ionising Radiations Regulations 1999
Work in Compressed Air Regulations 1996
Diving at Work Regulations 1997
The Control of Artificial Optical Radiations at Work Regulations 2010

Box 15.3 **Authorities that provide guidance on exposure to physical agents**

International Organisation for Standardisation (ISO) (www.iso.org)
American Conference of Governmental Industrial Hygienists (ACGIH) (www.acgih.org)
International Commission on Radiological Protection (ICRP) (www.icrp.org)
International Commission on Non-Ionizing Radiation Protection (ICNIRP) (www.icnirp.de)
Other national, transnational, and international authorities

Noise

Occupational noise exposure is one of the most ubiquitous workplace hazards and the harmful effects of noise on hearing have been known since at least the nineteenth century. Progressive deafness beginning with the high frequencies, typically centred on 4 kHz, and gradually spreading to other frequencies, should be a preventable occupational disease. Although hearing loss can be documented by audiometry, tinnitus, which cannot be objectively quantified, can be more distressing for sufferers. Noise also has other effects such as stimulation of the hypothalamic adrenal system and resulting 'stress' and changes in blood pressure as well as effects on performance, which depend on the task duration and type of exposure (Figure 15.1).

The harmful effects of noise depend on both the magnitude and duration of exposure and are dependent on the total noise energy to which the ear is exposed. Sudden massive overexposure to peak noise of 140 dB(A) or more can cause mechanical damage, 'acoustic trauma', resulting in loss of hearing often accompanied by tinnitus.

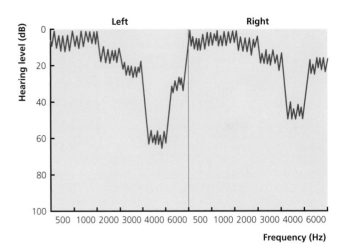

Figure 15.1 Audiogram showing noise-induced hearing loss with classical depression at 4 kHz.

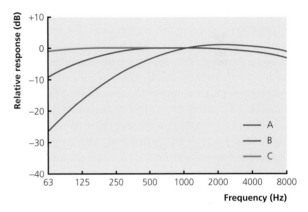

Figure 15.2 A weighting scale.

For continuous noise, exposure criteria for an 8-hour working day have been established and do so using noise measurements which are frequency weighted to take account of the sensitivity of the human ear to noise exposure. This is the 'A' weighting of noise measurements. Sound levels are measured in decibels (dB) where a figure of 0 represents (Figure 15.2) the limit of detection of sound by the human ear and an increase of 3 dB, on a logarithmic scale, represents a doubling of sound intensity. A daily personal noise exposure ($L_{EP,d}$) of 85 dB(A) is a level at which the risk of hearing damage is significant and where employers are usually expected to take action to assess and reduce noise exposures. Within the EU a lower action level is set at a daily personal noise exposure at 80 dB(A), an upper exposure action level at 85 dB(A) and the exposure limit value for continuous sound is set at 87 dB(A). Different actions are required at each of these levels, for example hearing protection must be provided only on request, at or above the lower action value. An area where workers are likely to be exposed at or above the upper action value must be designated as a hearing protection zone. Now, hearing protectors must be provided to employees, who are also required to use them. Details of the many other requirements are to be found in the relevant legislation and associated guidance.

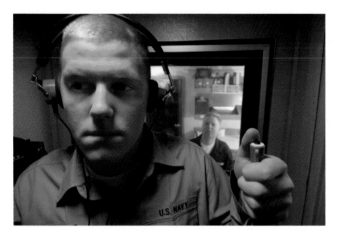

Figure 15.3 Audiometric testing. *Source:* Wikimedia US Navy public domain.

Health surveillance by audiometry will often be required for noise-exposed workers. Testing can be done at the start of a shift to avoid temporary changes in hearing threshold. The results should give a more accurate estimate of hearing function than measurements taken during a shift, although some argue that the latter approach better reflects the overall effects of noise on the individual's hearing at work. If changes are found on a mid-shift audiogram they should be followed up with a pre-shift assessment (Figure 15.3).

The audiogram is not of itself diagnostic of noise induced hearing loss and has to be interpreted along with the occupational and medical history of the individual employee and a clinical examination. A typical high-frequency dip in the audiogram, in the presence of a history of occupational noise exposure, no significant non-occupational noise exposure and no medical factors which could account for the changes would be presumptive of changes of noise induced hearing loss. A full history of occupational and non-occupational noise exposure has to be taken. Leisure noise may occur from shooting, motor sports, attending concerts and night clubs/discos, in-car entertainment systems and from personal music players. Medical factors potentially affecting the audiogram (Box 15.4) include congenital effects, childhood illnesses, trauma to the head, ear disease such as otosclerosis, exposure to drugs such as aminoglycosides and the effects of ageing. Occupational exposure to aromatic solvents such as styrene may act synergistically with noise exposure in the production of sensorineural hearing loss. Clinical examination including Weber's and Rinne's tests will help to classify a hearing loss as conductive or sensorineural. Ageing also results in

---

Box 15.4 Differential diagnosis of noise induced hearing loss

Conductive – Wax, acute otitis media, chronic otitis media, otosclerosis, tympanic membrane injury, barotrauma, ossicular dislocation
Sensorineural – Presbyacusis, congenital (maternal rubella, hereditary, perinatal anoxia), infective (measles, mumps, meningitis), vascular (haemorrhage, spasm or thrombosis of cochlear vessels), traumatic (head injury), toxic (streptomycin, neomycin, carbon monoxide, carbon disulphide), Meniere's disease, late otosclerosis, acoustic nerve tumours (usually unilateral)

---

a high-frequency loss, with the hearing threshold levels falling off at the higher frequencies. Often a pattern suggestive of both noise effects and age is apparent on the audiogram. Other factors with a detrimental effect on hearing thresholds include smoking, high blood pressure and high cholesterol levels.

It will be appropriate to refer the employee to their GP where there is a significant hearing loss that might benefit from the use of a hearing aid, or where undiagnosed medical factors are suspected. One example is where there is a unilateral hearing loss, and particularly where this affects all frequencies. This pattern can be produced by an acoustic neuroma and referral is usually followed by imaging studies which can detect this condition.

Some jurisdictions, for example the United Kingdom, publish guidance based on the audiometric thresholds to help those responsible for advising workers on the significance of their test results. Workers who have developed a mild to moderate hearing loss can usually continue to work in noise exposed environments provided that their future noise exposures are well controlled and they remain under health surveillance.

A clinical assessment following health surveillance is a good opportunity to reinforce messages about the need for meticulous use of hearing protection in all noise exposed workers. For workers with severe hearing loss and limited residual hearing thresholds, the potential risk to that hearing from continuing occupational noise exposure may outweigh the benefits of remaining in the job, even where exposures are thought to be well controlled. Some workers experiencing tinnitus find this exacerbated by noise exposure and may be difficult to place in noisy workplaces (Figure 15.4).

Vibration

Exposure to hand-transmitted vibration (Figure 15.5) is a common experience in a wide range of manufacturing, agricultural and other occupations. Tools are often held with both hands, with one hand being used to operate the controls of the equipment and the other hand used to guide the tool as it is used against the workpiece. The harmful effects of this type of exposure were first noted in the second decade of the twentieth century, as an occupational form of Raynaud's phenomenon. These effects were confirmed in studies during and after the Second World War, and by the latter part of the century three different types of

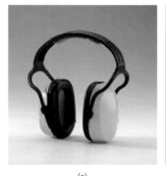

(a)   (b)

Figure 15.4 Hearing protection and warning signs.

Table 15.1 Stockholm workshop classification.

Vascular component

Stage	Grade	Description
0		No attacks
1V	Mild	Occasional attacks affecting only the tips of one or more fingers
2V	Moderate	Occasional attacks affecting distal and middle (rarely also proximal) phalanges of one or more fingers
3V	Severe	Frequent attacks affecting all phalanges of most fingers
4V	Very severe	As in stage 3 with trophic changes in the fingertips

Sensorineural component

Stage	Description
0SN	Vibration-exposed but no symptoms
1SN	Intermittent numbness with or without tingling
2SN	Intermittent or persistent numbness, reduced sensory perception
3SN	Intermittent or persistent numbness, reduced tactile discrimination or manipulative dexterity or both

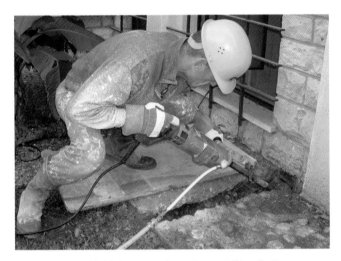

Figure 15.5 Hand-held vibrating tool use. *Source:* Wikimedia Commons public domain.

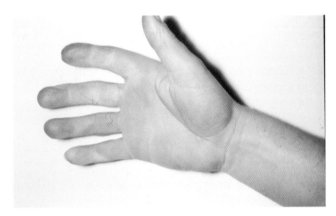

Figure 15.6 Vascular hand arm vibration syndrome, finger blanching. Donated by the late Professor Taylor to HSE.

harm from hand-transmitted vibration were recognized, vascular, sensorineural and musculoskeletal effects, all considered to be components of hand arm vibration syndrome (HAVS). Descriptors for the stages of vascular and sensorineural HAVS were introduced in 1987 following a workshop held in Stockholm (Table 15.1).

The vascular effects of HAVS are similar to naturally occurring Raynaud's phenomenon. Part of one or more fingers experiences intense constriction of superficial blood vessels such that the affected part appears white or dusky yellow in appearance with a clear demarcation between the affected part and the normally perfused skin. Typically the whole circumference of the digit is affected and it is numb and dead to touch during an episode. The finger will rewarm if rubbed or held against a warm body surface but otherwise will stay white or 'blanched' for 15 minutes or more. It is necessary to take a detailed history from patients to establish whether what is being described is an exaggerated but normal response to peripheral cooling or true episodes of finger blanching. Patients can now use a mobile phone to take photographs to show their medical advisers. Primary Raynaud's phenomenon affects about 5% of the normal male population and can occur in vibration-exposed workers. It can be difficult to distinguish between the primary and secondary forms (Figure 15.6).

The sensorineural effects of HAVS are tingling and numbness of the fingers tips associated with reduced tactile sensitivity. These can progress to a level resulting in significant loss of manual dexterity, and so it is important that they are detected early to allow a reduction in, or cessation of vibration exposure. Such symptoms can also occur as a result of other common problems such as nerve entrapment in the neck, and cubital or carpal tunnel syndromes. Carpal tunnel syndrome can also occur in workers exposed to hand-transmitted vibration and may occur more frequently than sensorineural HAVS. A careful clinical assessment has to be made to ascertain the likely cause of sensory symptoms in the fingers of workers exposed to hand-transmitted vibration (Box 15.5).

The musculsoskeletal component of HAVS is poorly defined and derives from reports of radiograph changes and upper limb pain in workers using vibrating tools. As these tools are often heavy and awkward to manipulate upper limb symptoms are more likely to result from the poor ergonomics of tool use.

Workers regularly exposed to significant hand-transmitted vibration should be under health surveillance to detect any early evidence of HAVS. As a diagnosis can have important economic consequences for the worker it is essential to take time to be sure of the findings and it will often be necessary to assess the worker on more than one occasion before reaching a conclusion about the origin of symptoms. Depending on the level of symptoms work

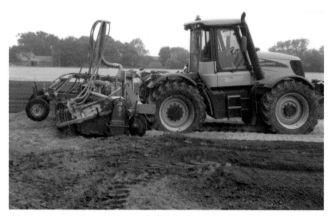

Figure 15.7 Tractor with cultivator. *Source:* Wikimedia; Attribution Nigel Jones.

involving exposure to hand transmitted vibration can be permitted with reduced vibration exposure and ongoing surveillance. This is most easily achieved where there is robust vibration exposure information available to the occupational health professional.

Drivers of mobile machinery and many modes of transport are exposed to vibration principally through their seating, although there may be a small component of hand-transmitted vibration experienced from a steering wheel or other controls. The vibration transmitted through the floor, seat cushion or seat back is whole-body vibration. Some workers who have to stand on vibrating surfaces are also subject to whole-body vibration exposure. Many health effects have been reported from whole-body vibration exposure, but for practical purposes the only one of significance is low back pain. Even here there is some question whether the effect is due to vibration itself or the effects of seated posture, twisting and turning (for example in tractor driving) and associated manual handling tasks. Low back pain arising from vibration exposure cannot be distinguished from that arising from other causes, but workers exposed to whole-body vibration may suffer low back pain at an earlier age that their non-exposed contemporaries. Workers should be aware of this possibility and have a means to report any symptoms. Reduction of exposure can be achieved by the fitting of seating with vibration dampers, by ensuring that the seat is adjusted correctly for the individual driver and by paying close attention to the surfaces that have to be driven over, for example filling in pot holes and removing other rough surfaces on roadways or factory floors (Figure 15.7).

Heat

Exposure to heat can affect comfort, task performance and health. Indoor exposures occur in occupations such as metal manufacturing and processing, kitchen and laundry work. Outdoor exposures include agriculture and construction work in warm climates. Outdoor exposures can be exacerbated by the demands of physical activity and the use of protective clothing, for example if spraying pesticides. Even office workers can be affected by hot conditions in warm summer weather and there can be a demand to specify a maximum acceptable workplace temperature. As many components characterize the thermal environment it is not easy to define a single acceptable temperature value. An International Standard (ISO 7730) gives guidance on assessing moderate thermal environments in relation to comfort. The maintenance of appropriate hydration, wearing loose fitting clothing, ensuring adequate air circulation and providing shielding from sources of radiant heat will mitigate the effects of moderate heat stress.

In more extreme heat the concern is acute heat illness (Figure 15.8, Box 15.6). Regulation of the central (core) body temperature is an essential physiological function – core temperature is normally regulated in a range of about 1°C from a mean of 37°C. The body defends the core temperature by vasodilatation (increasing skin blood flow) and by sweating, both of which facilitate heat loss. If heat gain is greater than heat loss then the body stores heat. As it does so, the temperature of the brain and central organs (such as the liver) – the core temperature–increases and this threatens the survival of the individual. Eventually external cooling must be provided to prevent death. Heat hyperpyrexia (heat stroke) is the most serious effect of exposure to heat. It is generally characterized by a body temperature of 40–41°C, an altered level of consciousness and hot dry skin resulting from failure of the sweating mechanism. These features are not invariable, however, so treatment should not be delayed if heat stroke is suspected (Box 15.7).

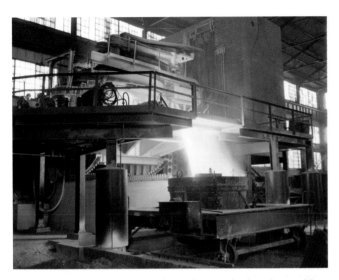

Figure 15.8 Steel furnace. *Source:* Wikimedia US Federal employee public domain.

Box 15.6 **Heat stroke**

Heat stroke is a medical emergency. The body temperature should be lowered by tepid sponging and fanning with cool air. Intravenous fluids may be necessary. The following may predispose to heat exhaustion and heat stroke:

- Obesity
- Lack of fitness
- Age 50 years or more
- Drug or alcohol abuse
- History of heat illness
- Drug treatment (for example, antihistamines, tricyclic antidepressants, or antipsychotics)
- Pre-existing disease of cardiovascular system, skin, gastrointestinal tract, or renal system

Box 15.7 **Groups of people at risk from heat illness**

- Unacclimatized workers in the tropics
- Workers in hot industries who have had a break from exposure
- Workers with an intercurrent illness
- Workers in the emergency services – for example, fire or mines rescue
- People undertaking very heavy physical activity – for example, military recruits
- People working even moderately hard at normal temperatures in all enveloping protective clothing – for example, fire crews dealing with chemical spills
- Older people and the very young when ambient temperatures are raised for prolonged periods

Heat exhaustion results from a combination of thermal and cardiovascular strain. The individual is tired and may stumble, and has a rapid pulse and respiration rate. The condition may develop into heat stroke if not treated by rest, cooling and fluids. Other effects are heat syncope (fainting), heat oedema, (often in the unacclimatized), heat cramps and heat rash (prickly heat). Working in high temperatures can also result in fatigue and an increased risk of accidents.

The prevention of acute heat illness depends on proper selection of workers, training (sometimes including physiological acclimatization to heat) and monitoring of the duration of exposure using appropriate standards (Box 15.8). Personal heat stress monitors are not yet widely available, but their use in some circumstances may confer benefit.

Box 15.8 **The wet bulb globe temperature**

The wet bulb globe temperature (WBGT) index is an index of heat stress. For outdoor use in sunlight it is derived from the natural wet bulb temperature (WB), the dry bulb temperature (DB), and the globe temperature (GT) (a measure of radiant heating) in the ratio:

$$WBGT = 0.7WB + 0.2GT + 0.1DB$$

The WBGT index is measured using a 'Christmas tree' array of thermometers, or purpose built electronic sensors and integrating apparatus.

The index was originally derived to protect troops exercising outdoors by relating environmental conditions to the risk of heat illness. It has since been developed and used extensively in industry and is the basis for International Standard 7243 and guidance by the ACGIH. These documents give upper boundaries of WBGT value for continuous and intermittent work of different intensities. Other standards apply in relation to thermal comfort – for example, ISO 7730.

Cold

In cold conditions the problem is to balance the heat produced by physical activity with the heat lost to the environment. The rate of heat loss depends on the insulation of the clothing and the external climate, including air temperature and wind velocity. The original Wind Chill Index (WCI) (derived in units of kcal/m²/ hour) relates to the risk of freezing of superficial tissues, and gives a value of between approximately 500 and 2500 which has to be interpreted from published charts. Many organizations now use an updated version, the Wind Chill Temperature Index, which has a value expressed in degrees of temperature (C or F). This is easier to understand and use, has a more rational scientific basis and better predicts the risk of frostbite (Figure 15.10).

Large numbers of workers are employed indoors in conditions of moderate to severe cold, mostly in food preparation and storage. Only a few people are exposed to cold in scientific and testing laboratories. Cold stores can operate at temperatures as low as–30°C. Workers in cold stores must be provided with proper insulated clothing and they must have regular breaks in warm conditions. A major problem in severe cold, indoors or outside, is to keep the hands and feet warm. The necessary insulation is bulky, which is less of a problem for footwear than for hand wear. Mitts provide better thermal protection than gloves, but limit dexterity (Figure 15.9).

Indoors, in moderately cold conditions – that is, temperatures below 15°C, it may also be hard to maintain comfort of the

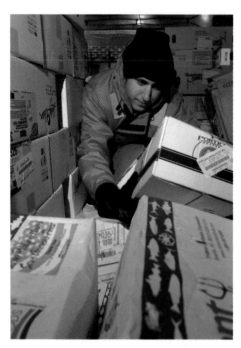

Figure 15.9 Worker in refrigerated store rom. *Source:* Wikimedia US Navy public domain.

Box 15.9 **Conditions that preclude work in moderate to severe cold**

- History of ischaemic heart disease
- Peripheral vascular disease
- Hypertension or Raynaud's phenomenon
- Asthma
- Metabolic disorders
- Sickle cell disease
- Arthritis

---

extremities, and exposure to draughts can be particularly troublesome. Limited evidence indicates that workers regularly exposed to cold conditions such as these may have worse than average general health.

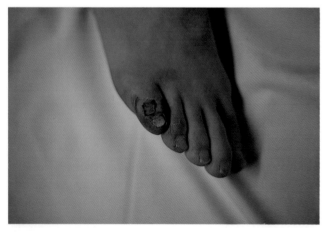

Figure 15.10 Frost bite.

Serious hypothermia should not occur in occupational settings. If there is a risk, people should not work alone, should have good communications with others and should be trained in first aid management of the effects of cold. Hypothermia is initially treated by slow rewarming using the individual's own metabolism, and copious insulation, possibly supplemented by body heat from another person. Active rewarming may be used in medical facilities.

The peripheral effects of cold are freezing cold injury (frost nip and frost bite), chilblains and non-freezing cold injury. Frost nip appears as a white area on the skin that recovers fully within 30 minutes of rewarming. The appearance of frost bite is of marbled white frozen tissue that is anaesthetic to touch. Treatment is by rapid rewarming provided that there is no risk of the tissue refreezing. Non-freezing cold injury usually affects the feet, although the hands can also be affected. It is described as having four stages. During cold exposure sensory changes may result in disturbed gait, although the feet will be cold and numb. On warming the feet may swell and turn pale blue while remaining cold and numb. Then for several weeks the feet will be swollen, hot, red and painful. Finally, limb temperature falls again and there may be long-lasting hypersensitivity to cold and chronic pain. Chilblains are a minor form of cold injury.

Altered ambient pressure

This arises during work in compressed air and diving. Compressed air is used in civil engineering when tunnelling through soft or water permeable strata or when a caisson is used to construct a pier on the surface of a river bed. Commercial diving takes many forms ranging from the use of SCUBA equipment in shallow water for instruction, photography, search and archaeology through to saturation diving at depth in oil exploration and production. The occupational health care of such workers normally requires special training or experience so would be outwith the experience of the newcomer to occupational medicine. Acute symptoms may present to the GP or the hospital emergency department, and long-term effects may be seen in both general practice and occupational medicine (Figure 15.11) (Box 15.10).

Box 15.10 **Working at pressure**

- Atmospheric pressure is 14.7 psi
- 1 atmosphere, 1 bar, 10 m (or 33 feet) of sea water, are broadly equivalent pressures
- Absolute pressure is that of the working environment added to atmospheric pressure
- Decompression illness is very rare at pressures below 1.7 bar absolute. There is no risk from slight elevations of pressure such as in clean rooms
- Typical pressures experienced in civil engineering works are in the range 2–3.5 bar absolute
- Saturation diving techniques become necessary at depths below 50 m, 6 bar absolute

---

The most acute effects arising from hyperbaric exposures are barotraumas to air-filled organs during the increase or decrease

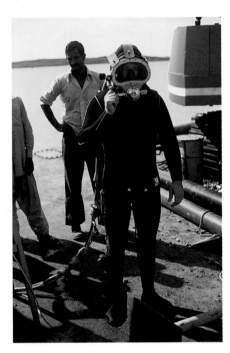

Figure 15.11 Diver.

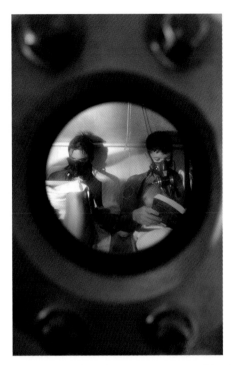

Figure 15.13 Decompression breathing oxygen. *Source:* Wikimedia US Navy public domain.

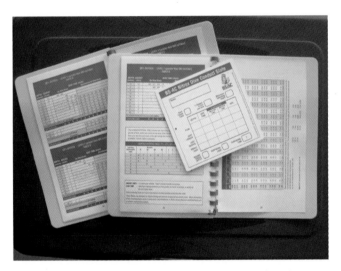

Figure 15.12 BSAC Nitrox decompression tables. *Source:* Wikimedia Commons.

in the ambient pressure. When initially increasing pressure in compressed air work a check is made that no one is suffering from barotrauma before further increasing pressure. The organ most frequently affected is the middle ear, but symptoms can arise from other air-containing structures, principally the respiratory tract. Symptoms arising during decompression may require the chamber pressure to be increased again and then lowered more slowly.

Decompression illness arises as a result of nitrogen gas which is in solution in the body under high pressure coming out of solution and forming gas bubbles in the blood vessels during the

decompression process. Great care is taken with the process of decompression which is staged at defined pressures for specified durations to minimize the risk of symptoms arising from this cause (Figure 15.12). Breathing oxygen during decompression reduces the risk of decompression illness (Figure 15.13). Decompression illness occurs in two types: pain only (previously type 1), in which symptoms occur in the skin (niggles) or around joints (bends), and serious (previously type 2), in which symptoms can occur in the circulation or nervous system. Symptoms can arise from gas bubbles in the pulmonary or coronary circulations (the chokes), or from damage to the brain or spinal cord (the staggers). Serious decompression illness can be life threatening.

The onset of decompression illness can be some hours after the end of a shift working in compressed air, or a dive. Cases can present to GPs or, more likely, to emergency medicine departments. It is important to consider the possibility of serious decompression illness in a worker with previous hyperbaric exposure who presents with central nervous system abnormalities. Compressed air workers are often required to wear a badge stating that they are compressed air workers and giving details of the location of the recompression chamber or a contact number for further advice.

When decompression illness occurs, either pain only or serious, it should always be treated by therapeutic recompression, to manage the worker's symptoms and to reduce the risk of subsequent osteonecrosis. This serious complication of hyperbaric work results from compromise of the blood flow within bone structures. A section of normal bone dies and is replaced by softer material. If this occurs below the surface of a joint, such as the hip joint, there is a real risk of the joint surface collapsing, resulting in permanent disability.

The use of the bisphosphonate alendronate has been shown to significantly reduce the risk of an early collapse of the femoral head in non-traumatic osteonecrosis.

Osteonecrosis will present as pain and loss of function in the affected joint, commonly the hip joint, and can be detected by X-ray or magnetic resonance imaging (MRI) scan. Suspected cases will need referral for specialist orthopaedic assessment.

Risk factors for osteonecrosis are not clearly established. It can occur after one 'bad' decompression, but is normally seen only after higher pressure exposures. Risk factors in compressed air work include the number of hyperbaric exposures and the number of episodes of decompression illness.

Living and working at altitude carries different risks – namely, acute mountain sickness, high-altitude pulmonary oedema (HAPE) and high-altitude cerebral oedema (HACE). Symptoms of acute mountain sickness can occur at altitudes of 2500 metres, with the prevalence reaching 40% at altitudes over 4000 metres. The symptoms include headache, nausea and vomiting, sleep disturbance and muscle weakness. The condition is treated by descent to a lower altitude. Breathing oxygen, and taking acetazolamide and dexamethasone can also help. The main preventive measure is to limit the rate of ascent to altitude. Unlike acute mountain sickness, both HAPE and HCE are life threatening. The former is treated by descent and the use of oxygen. People who live permanently at high altitude show physiological adaptations to their environment, although even these may fail with time. Chronic mountain sickness (Monge's disease) is a loss of tolerance to hypoxia, which occurs particularly in middle-aged men. The condition can only be alleviated by moving to a lower altitude.

Ionizing radiations

Ionizing radiation (Figure 15.14) displaces electrons from their normal orbits around the nucleus of the atom. The resulting ionization alters the nature of biological molecules, especially DNA,

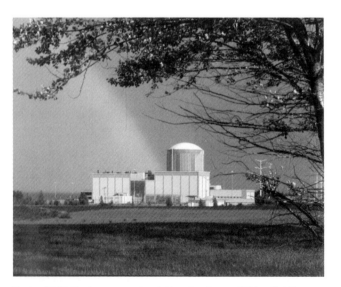

Figure 15.14 Nuclear power plant in America. *Source:* Wikimedia US Federal Government public domain.

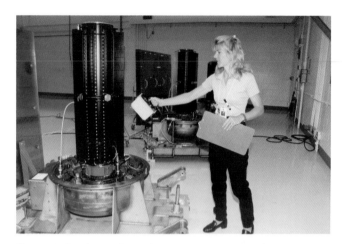

Figure 15.15 Using a radiation dose rate meter. *Source:* Wikimedia NASA public domain.

resulting in gene mutation or cell death. *Alpha* particles are relatively large and easily stopped. *Beta* particles are small and can penetrate up to a centimetre in tissue. *Neutrons* are smaller than *alpha* particles but are much more penetrating. *Gamma* radiation and *X-rays* are packets of energy transmitted as electromagnetic radiation, and are highly penetrating.

External irradiation is that arising from a source – either a radiation generator, such as an X-ray machine, or a radioactive substance – that is external to the body. The irradiation ceases when the generator is switched off or the source is moved away or shielded (Figure 15.15). The body can be *contaminated* by particles of radioactive material that lie on the skin externally or are incorporated into the tissues, resulting in *internal* irradiation. This will persist as long as the radioactive material is in the body. Alpha emitters such as plutonium are particularly harmful sources of internal irradiation (Box 15.11).

Typical occupations in which there is the potential for significant exposure to ionizing radiations are work in the nuclear energy sector, for example in power generation or fuel processing and recycling and in the use of X-ray generators in industrial radiography to check the integrity of metallic components. Ionizing radiations are used widely in healthcare settings, in medical and dental radiography, and in the investigation and treatment of disease.

Box 15.11 **Doses and units of radiation**

- Absorbed dose – the energy of ionizing radiation a body absorbs, measured in Gray
- Dose equivalent – an adjustment of the absorbed dose, using a quality factor for the type of radiation involved, to take account of the effectiveness of the different types of radiations in harming biological systems; measured in Sieverts
- Effective dose – an integrated index of the risk of harm, derived by multiplying the dose equivalent for each of the major tissues by a weighting factor based on the tissue's sensitivity to harm by radiation. The weighted values are summed. The unit is the Sievert

Table 15.2 The probabilities of harm from exposure to ionizing radiation derived by the ICRP (2007). Values are expressed as percentage risk per Sievert dose received (the values in the table are multiplied by 10-2 Sv-1 to give the actual risk).

	Whole population	Adult population
Fatal cancers	5.5	4.1
Hereditary disorders	0.2	0.1
Total risk	5.7	4.2

The ICRP recommends an effective dose limit of 20 mSv (averaged over a defined 5-year period) for workers, and 1 mSv per year for the public. Limits are also set for exposure of the eye lens, the skin, and the hands and feet. The dose limit for the fetus is the same as the public dose limit of 1 mSv a year.

The ICRP also publishers 'reference levels' for radiation exposure to guide planning of work emergency situations.

In the Fukushima nuclear accident in march 2011 a number of workers received exposures in excess of the ICRP reference level of 100 mSv.

Large doses of ionizing radiation cause death by damage to the brain, gut and haemopoietic system. Such exposures only occur in the event of accidents, which can often be traced to a failure to operate established controls in a proper way. Lower doses can damage the skin or the lens of the eye. This may occur if sources are mishandled or exposures are prolonged: for example, in industrial radiography or interventional radiography.

Ionizing radiations are recognized to have stochastic effects, including the induction of cancer, and hereditary effects. These do not have a threshold, and the likelihood of the effect is related to the dose. Risk estimates for the stochastic effects of radiation have been derived from epidemiological studies (cancer) and animal studies (hereditary effects) (Table 15.2). The most important epidemiological data are from the Life Span Study of survivors of the atom bombs used in 1945. The risk estimates are published by a number of bodies of which the International Commission on Radiological Protection (ICRP) is the most influential. The ICRP also publishes dose limits derived from the risk estimates, and these are the basis of the statutory dose limits applied in many countries.

Workers who are substantially exposed to ionizing radiation are subject to regular medical surveillance. This is to ensure that they are fit for their proposed work with radiation: for example, the need to work with unsealed sources or to use respiratory protective equipment. They are also subject to dose monitoring. Doctors involved in this area of work may need to undergo specialist training, and must be familiar with the terminology relating to the measurement of radiation exposures as well as the legislation governing work with ionizing radiations. Exposure to ionizing radiation should be as low as reasonably practicable (ALARP) by the provision of appropriate controls, including shielding and reduction of exposure time. As legislative controls have been tightened, so workers' typical exposures to ionizing radiations have fallen. In the United Kingdom, average annual occupational doses are 1–2 mSv per year (about the same as background radiation).

Studies of large cohorts of workers occupationally exposed to radiation consistently show a healthy worker effect. Nevertheless, cases of cancer of types known to be produced by ionizing radiation do occur in these populations. Individuals may be compensated for

such disease on the basis of 'presumption of origin' or 'probability of causation', depending on national arrangements.

Electromagnetic fields

Electromagnetic fields with wavelengths shorter than 0.1 mm, that is ultraviolet and below, contain insufficient energy to break molecular bonds and so do not cause ionization. This 'non-ionizing radiation' does, however, have other frequency-dependent effects on biological tissues. Broad divisions of this radiation include microwave and radiofrequency radiation, as well as extremely low frequency, which includes the frequencies of power distribution (Figure 15.16).

At high frequencies – for example, microwaves used in communication systems – the main effect is tissue heating, a phenomenon made use of in the microwave oven. This effect is quantified by the specific absorption rate (SAR) of energy into the body, and in most situations there are unlikely to be ill effects. This might not be the case where the individual is also working physically hard, or is exposed to a hot environment. At lower frequencies the effects of electric and magnetic fields are considered separately. Exposure to magnetic fields can set up circulating currents within the body, which have the potential to interfere with physiological processes if sufficiently great. For example, muscle activation could potentially occur during magnetic resonance imaging. Low-frequency electric fields do not penetrate the body, but can generate charges on the body surface.

Other recognized but rarer effects include the phenomenon of microwave hearing. Some people hear repeated clicks when exposed to pulsed sources of electromagnetic fields, usually radars. A visual illusion of flickering lights (magnetophosphenes) can be produced when the retina is exposed to intense magnetic fields. Exposure standards which reflect the frequency dependence of these effects have been derived to protect against the established effects of electromagnetic fields (Box 15.12).

Increasingly, active implantable medical devices which operate electrically are being used in the treatment of medical conditions;

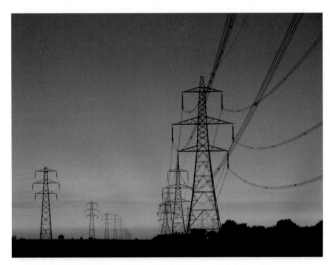

Figure 15.16 Power lines. *Source:* Wikimedia Commons.

examples include implanted cardiac pacemakers and defibrillators. If a worker with an implanted medical device may be exposed to strong electric or magnetic fields at work they should initially seek advice about possible interference with its function from the medical team which fitted the device or its manufacturer. Any interference which may occur is usually temporary and alleviated by moving away from the source of the interference (Boxes 15.13 and 15.14).

Since the late 1970s there has been increasing public concern about exposure to electromagnetic fields. This was prompted by epidemiological studies of the association between childhood cancer and residential exposure to magnetic fields. Although some individual studies have not demonstrated an effect, a pooled analysis did show a statistical association between an average exposure greater than 0.4 microtesla, which is relatively large, and a twofold increased risk of childhood leukaemia. In 2001 the International Agency for Research on Cancer concluded that there was limited evidence that residential magnetic fields increase the risk of childhood leukaemia, resulting in a classification of '2B"possibly carcinogenic' for extremely low frequency magnetic fields. The position has not changed since then and it remains only a possibility that high magnetic field exposures may be implicated in some way in the origin of some cases of childhood leukaemia.

Public concern also extends to the possible effects of exposure to electromagnetic fields from mobile phone handsets and base stations. In the United Kingdom an independent expert group was commissioned to study the evidence in relation to mobile phone technology. This group, which reported in 2000, concluded that exposure to radiofrequency radiation below the International Commission on Non-Ionizing Radiation Protection guidelines did not adversely affect population health, but in view of other biological evidence it concluded that it was not possible to say that exposures below current guidelines were totally without potential adverse health effects. The group therefore advocated a precautionary approach in the use of this technology – for example, suggesting that the use of mobile phones by children for non-essential calls should be discouraged. INTERPHONE, a major multinational epidemiological study collected data on brain cancer and mobile phone use between 2000 and 2004 and reported key findings in 2010. In May 2011 the International Agency for Research on Cancer classified radiofrequency electromagnetic fields as possibly carcinogenic to humans (2B) based on an increased risk of glioma associated with wireless phone use, a result found in one group of cases in the INTERPHONE study. However, the data were interpreted differently by the Standing Committee on Epidemiology of the International Commission on Non-Ionizing Radiation Protection. They noted methodological difficulties with the INTERPHONE study and concluded that the evidence is increasingly against there being a link between mobile phone use and brain tumours in adults.

There is no evidence that exposure to electromagnetic fields from the use of display screen equipment has any harmful effects.

Optical radiations

Optical radiations comprise ultraviolet, visible and infrared radiation, which have wavelengths between 100 nm and 1 mm (Box 15.15). Their harmful effects are largely restricted to the skin and the eye. Ultraviolet radiation is implicated in non-melanoma and melanoma cancers. Outdoor workers, for example farmers and the deck crews of ships, have an increased risk of non-melanoma cancer. Fortunately, this is usually curable. As a sensible precaution, all those who work outdoors should avoid overexposure of the bare skin to sunlight, and sunburn, in order to reduce their risk of melanoma cancer. Some evidence suggests that exposure to ultraviolet radiation can impair the function of the immune system.

Ultraviolet radiation is responsible for the painful symptoms of arc eye (photokeratoconjunctivitis), which occurs some hours after unprotected exposure to a bright source of ultraviolet radiation such as a welding arc. Often, bystanders who are adventitiously exposed get this condition (Figure 15.17, Box 15.16).

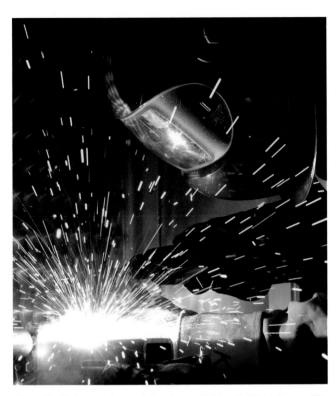

Figure 15.17 Gas metal arc welding. *Source:* Wikimedia US Air Force public domain.

Box 15.15 **Wavelengths of optical radiation**

- Ultraviolet C (UVC) – 100–280 nm
- Ultraviolet B (UVB) – 280–315 nm
- Ultraviolet A (UVA) – 315–400 nm
- Visible – 400–760 nm
- Infrared – 760 nm–1 mm

Box 15.16 **Possible effects of optical radiation on the eye**

- Ultraviolet C/B – arc eye
- Ultraviolet B – pigmentation of lens
- Ultraviolet A – retinal damage in aphakia
- Visible – accelerated ageing (high power sources), burns of retina (lasers)
- Infrared – corneal burns, usually prevented by blink reflex, cataract, retinal burns, from infrared A sources including lasers

---

Infrared radiation can cause thermal damage to the skin and eyes, both of which are easily protected, the latter with appropriate goggles. In developed countries occupational cataract from exposure to infrared radiation is largely of historical interest, given proper protection. In developing countries, however, cataracts may occur as a result of overexposure to infrared radiation, for example from molten metal in steel mills, possibly exacerbated by episodes of dehydration (Box 15.17).

Sources of optical radiation where the light waves are in phase (for example from lasers) can cause serious thermal damage to the retina and skin burns. Lasers are classified according to their potential to cause harm to the eye and skin. Engineering and administrative controls and personal protection are needed to prevent damage where high-powered lasers are in use. Routine eye examination is not appropriate for laser workers, although a baseline assessment of visual acuity is useful to identify the functionally monocular individual, for whom a greater duty of care exists.

For control of harm arising from optical radiations, as for that arising from the other physical agents, controlling exposure is the key. Fortunately there is good guidance available (Box 15.17).

Box 15.17 **Guidance on exposures, and international standards**

ICNIRP. Guidelines for limiting exposure to time-varying electric, magnetic, and electromagnetic fields (up to 300 GHz). *Health Phys* 1998;74:494–522

ICNIRP. Statement on the 'Guidelines for limiting time-varying electric, magnetic and electromagnetic fields (up to 300 GHz). *Health Phys* 2009;97:257–259

ICNIRP. Guidelines for Limiting Exposure to Time-Varying Electric and Magnetic Fields (1 Hz–100 kHz). *Health Phys* 2010;99:818–836

ICNIRP. Guidelines on Limits of Exposure to Ultraviolet Radiation of Wavelengths Between 180 nm and 400 nm (Incoherent Optical Radiation) *Health Phys* 2004;87:171–186

ICRP, 2007. The Recommendations of the International Commission on Radiological Protection. ICRP Publication 103. Ann ICRP 37 (2–4)

International Organisation for Standardisation. *Hot environments– estimation of the heat stress on working man, based on the WBGT index (wet bulb globe temperature).* Geneva: ISO, 1989 (ISO 7243)

International Organisation for Standardisation. *Moderate thermal environments – determination of the PMV and PPD indices and specification of the conditions for thermal comfort.* Geneva: ISO, 1993 (ISO 7730)

International Organisation for Standardisation. *Ergonomics of the thermal environment – Medical supervision of individuals exposed to extreme hot or cold thermal environments.* Geneva: ISO, 2001 (ISO 12894)

Further reading

Cherrie J, Howie, R, Semple S. *Monitoring for health hazards at work,* 4th edn. Chichester: Wiley-Blackwell, 2010. *A practically oriented handbook covering all aspects of occupational hygiene. It has separate chapters on the measurement and assessment of noise, vibration, heat and cold, ionizing radiation and non-ionizing radiation*

Maltby M. *Occupational Audiometry, Monitoring and Protecting hearing at work,* Oxford: Butterworth-Heinemann, 2005. *A practical guide to setting up an audiometric surveillance programme with advice on interpretation of the audiogram as well as background material on the wider aspects of hearing conservation and the science of hearing and hearing loss*

Mason H, Poole K. *Evidence review on the clinical testing and management of individuals exposed to hand transmitted vibration.* London: Faculty of Occupational Medicine, 2004. *An evidence based review on issues surrounding the diagnosis and management of Hand Arm Vibration Syndrome. The results* are presented as answers to practical questions such as 'How is the diagnosis made?' and 'What is the optimum management of an individual case?'

Youle A, Collins K J, Crockford G, et al. *TG12 The thermal environment*, 2nd edn. British Occupational Hygiene Society, 1996. *This is a guide for all those who may need to investigate or assess the thermal environment in the workplace. It provides an overview of the science, but is not a step by step guide. It is available at www.bohs.org/library/technical-publications*

Youle A, Parsons K C, TG12 *The thermal Environment addendum to the second edition*. British Occupational Hygiene Society, 2009. *A technical update to TG12 The Thermal Environment (second edition) also available at www.bohs.org/library/technical-publications/*

Parsons K. *Human thermal environments*, 2nd edn. London: Taylor and Francis, 2002. *A reference work for those wishing to get to grips with the detailed science of human heat transfer in hot, cold and moderate environments. It also covers the effects of dehydration, psychological responses and interference with tasks and performance*

Edmonds C, Lowry C, Pennefather J, Walker R. *Diving and sub aquatic medicine*, 4th edn. London: Hodder Arnold, 2005. *A comprehensive textbook covering all aspects of diving medicine*

Mettler FA, Upton AC. *Medical effects of ionising radiation*, 3rd edn. Philadelphia: WB Saunders, 2008. *A comprehensive reference on all aspects of the health effects of exposure to ionizing radiations; hereditary effects, carcinogenesis and direct effects. It does not cover radiation protection issues however*

http://www.hse.gov.uk. *The Health and Safety Executive website has pages covering all of the physical agents covered in this chapter and from which it is possible to access both the relevant United Kingdom legislation and the comprehensive guidance documents published to support employers in complying with that legislation. There is a lot of other useful supporting material also for employees, employers and health professionals*

http://www.icrp.org. *The International Commission on Radiological Protection website has a listing of their publications with access to summaries or journal articles but not the full original documents, which may be purchased*

http://www.icnirp.de. *The International Commission on Non-Ionizing Radiation Protection website lists their publications and also gives direct access to the full documents*

CHAPTER 16

Ergonomics and Human Factors

Joanne O. Crawford

Institute of Occupational Medicine, Edinburgh, UK

OVERVIEW

- Humans are diverse – one size does not fit all
- Ergonomics and human factors aim to design both work and the workplace to fit the user
- Taking an ergonomic approach involves understanding the user from the commissioning of a work system through design, building and testing
- Work elements that affect humans such as posture or mental workload can be modified by job design
- Human performance including safe behaviour is influenced by time pressure, experience and fatigue

---

Basic concepts

The terms human factors and ergonomics are synonymous, ergonomics being used in the United Kingdom and human factors in the United States. According to the International Ergonomics Association, Ergonomics (or human factors) is the scientific discipline concerned with the understanding of interactions among humans and other elements of a system, and the profession that applies theory, principles, data and methods to design in order to optimize human well-being and overall system performance.

Ergonomists seek to understand the work system, the human-system interactions both physical and psychological and develop work systems or solutions with allied professions such as engineering, psychology and occupational medicine.

Within ergonomics there are three broad areas of specialism: physical ergonomics (anatomy, anthropometry, workplace design and layout, manual handling, upper limb disorders and environmental ergonomics); cognitive ergonomics (mental workload, decision making, human computer interaction, human reliability, human error and stress); and organizational ergonomics (sociotechnical systems, safety culture, job design and cooperative work). Ergonomists often work across domains or in specific areas, such as patient safety, where a multifaceted approach is required.

ABC of Occupational and Environmental Medicine, Third Edition.
Edited by David Snashall and Dipti Patel.
© 2012 John Wiley & Sons Ltd. Published 2012 by John Wiley & Sons Ltd.

Epidemiology

Internationally, the majority of self-reported sickness absence is due to backache and muscular pain. This is closely followed by issues of fatigue and stress. The role of the ergonomist in analysing issues within the workplace is in examining the work system; identifying potential hazards (which can be physical and/or psychological); and developing risk reduction measures either through workplace redesign, job redesign or organizational change. This often involves working in conjunction with other professionals in occupational health, psychology or engineering.

Many sources of problems can be removed from a work system through effective design of the physical environment, particularly the workplace size and layout and consideration of the end user and their role in the system. Unfortunately, ergonomic considerations at the outset are often omitted, leaving problems to be addressed either by changing the workplace dimensions or adding warnings to the system after commissioning. The physical environment also has an impact on the postures adopted when working so can have either a positive or negative effect.

Consideration of ergonomics is an important aspect of the design of workplaces and equipment used therein. Poorly designed equipment can directly influence the chance of human errors occurring. For example, the layout of controls and displays can influence safety if switches are placed so that they can inadvertently be knocked on or off, or if controls are poorly identified and can be selected by mistake, or when critical displays are not in the user's normal field of view. The controls on different pieces of equipment may not be compatible; for example, a switch in the up position may be 'on' in one case but 'off' in another. An analysis of the Kegworth (UK) air crash in 1989, identified that the aircraft had undergone a change in design and the pilots were not aware of all the changes; thus they mistakenly switched off the right-hand engine when it was the left-hand engine that was on fire. The vibration indicators would have highlighted this but they were known to be unreliable in previous aircraft so were effectively ignored and their new design (small with a needle going around the outside) did not help comprehension.

Alarm systems are sometimes designed so that high-priority alarms are not clearly differentiated and are thus easily missed. Figure 16.1 shows the dimensions an individual should possess in order to use the layout of controls presented.

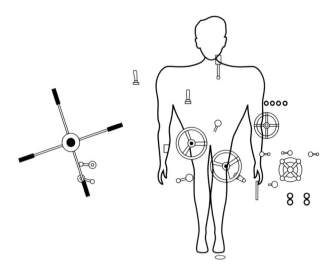

Figure 16.1 Arrangement of the controls on a lathe and 'ideal' operator who should be 1.3 metres tall, 61 cm across the shoulders with a 2.4-metre arm span.

Many sources of human error can be removed through effective design of equipment and procedures. Such 'error-tolerant' designs consider the tasks that the equipment is intended for and the errors the user may make. For example, accidental administration of vincristine intrathecally rather than intravenously has been recognized as a major risk to patients. The appreciation of this risk resulted in changes to the process of prescribing and administering the drug, the labelling of the drug, the use of a minibag system and recommendations on equipment design. This redesign process examined the whole work system, the people involved and the processes and equipment they used.

Designing tasks, equipment and workplaces to suit the users can prevent or reduce human errors and thus accidents and ill health. A key message is that effective use of ergonomics will make work safer and more productive.

At-risk occupations

Ergonomic problems can exist in all workplaces but problems are more prevalent in certain industries. Musculoskeletal problems are more prevalent in construction and agriculture as are physical hazards such as exposure to extreme thermal environments – heat and cold, wind and humidity or lack of it. A high mental workload is characteristic of certain jobs such as air-traffic control, offshore working and other safety critical work and high emotional demand characteristics of healthcare, social work and teaching where the research base is now informing better practice.

Management in the workplace

When managing ergonomic risks there are a number of approaches that can be taken depending on the risk factor and whether there is relevant legislation that has to be complied with. Box 16.1 lists some initial considerations to be made when procuring equipment for the workplace. For example, in preventing back injuries in the UK, there is a requirement to carry out a risk assessment for all

work tasks where there is a risk of injury to the person carrying out the task (Manual Handling Operations Regulations 1992 as amended 2004). The risk assessment should also be followed up by risk reduction measures such as redesigning the workplace, the work organization and the task. Although training in lifting and handling is one risk reduction measure, this should be seen as a last resort in relation to manual handling tasks and not just because its effectiveness has been called into question – primary prevention is almost always more effective. Research on the prevention of work-related upper limb disorders has been published to identify the source of problems (not always ergonomic ones) and again risk reduction measures may be feasible. The relevant ergonomic input is to evaluate the workplace, the work organization and the tools in use. To reduce the risk of work-related upper limb disorders occurring, it is necessary to assess the postures adopted by the individual, the level of repetitiveness of the work tasks, the vibration from tools and the force requirements of the job. Risk reduction measures may include workplace redesign to ensure

---

Box 16.1 Examples of ergonomic criteria for procuring equipment

- Does the equipment suit the body size of all users?
- Can users see and hear all they need to easily?
- Is it easy to understand the information displayed?
- Would the equipment cause discomfort if used for any length of time?
- Is it easy to learn how to use the equipment? Are instructions and any warning signs clear? Is the language used appropriate for the users?
- What errors may occur? Can these be detected easily and corrected?
- Is the equipment compatible with other systems in use?
- Can users reach controls easily?
- Can users move safely between operating positions?
- Is the equipment too noisy, does it vibrate too much, is it paced too fast?

the workplace fits the user, the use of different tools to reduce postural strain and reorganization of the work to reduce the level of repetitiveness of the task. Some factors to consider when assessing workplaces are listed in Box 16.2. Notwithstanding this ergonomic approach to prevention as with heavy lifting tasks, training may have a place. A participatory approach to workplace changes and involving managers, supervisors and employees in change is key to the success of any risk reduction approaches.

> ### Box 16.2 **Factors to consider in workplace assessment**
>
> - Can the users fit, reach and see all they need to?
> - Do users have to adopt awkward postures?
> - Do users have to handle heavy loads?
> - Is the work repetitive?
> - Are the rest breaks adequate between tasks?
> - Have the tools been designed to avoid static loading?
> - Are the tools designed for use by either hand?
> - Is seating designed to fit all users?
> - Does the seat support the worker in a good posture?
> - Do hazards need to be identified and risks assessed in order to comply with legislation?

In understanding the work tasks to be assessed, task analysis may be used to break down the individual work components. The aim of task analysis is to give the assessor tools to be able to understand the roles that people play in complex work situations. What task analysis allows is a description of the work tasks that people carry out and from this the ergonomist can identify tasks where individuals are overloaded or under loaded by either physical or mental demands. When carrying out task analysis, information about the work tasks is collected via interviews, surveys, walkthroughs or verbal protocols from supervisors or employees within the work group. The information collected is then presented in a format such as a hierarchical task analysis to show the individual work tasks that an employee has to complete. Linking this to risk identification measures allows a better understanding of where in the work system an individual is at risk and provides for a focused intervention. An example of a hierarchical task analysis is presented in Figure 16.2.

Although it is often feasible to prevent accidents and incidents by the effective design of workplaces and equipment, problems may arise due to human factors such as fatigue or working practices such as the institution of non-standard shifts. Examples are drivers falling asleep at the wheel or other workers (such as healthcare staff) in high-risk environments unable to remain awake on night shifts. Many people do work shift systems including night work or extended hours on overtime. Shift work has been associated with a number of health problems, including fatigue, sleeplessness, gastrointestinal symptoms, cardiovascular disease and, most recently, breast cancer in nurses working nights. A number of strategies

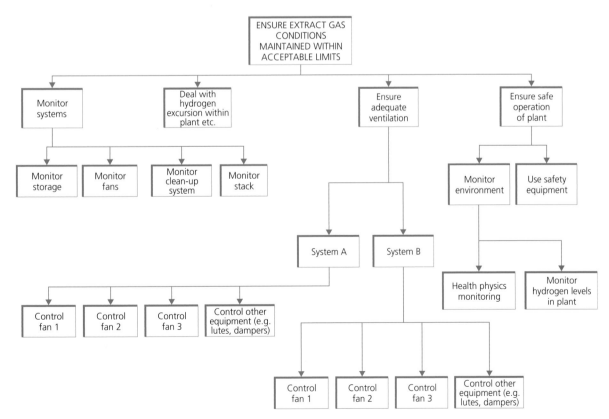

Figure 16.2 Example of a hierarchical task analysis. From Kirwan, B. and Ainsworth, L.K (1992). Reproduced with permission of Taylor and Francis.

can be used to reduce the impact of shift work (Box 16.3). Major incidents that have identified shiftwork and fatigue as a factor in their occurrence include the Exxon Valdez oil spill, the Chernobyl nuclear reactor explosion and the sinking of the Herald of Free Enterprise ferry. Studies of driver fatigue and accidents have identified shift work as a major risk factor.

Box 16.3 **Factors to consider in planning shift work**

- Reduce night work so far as is practically possible
- Set limits for maximum hours of duty and time needed for recovery. In Europe this is prescribed in legislation
- Ensure that the shift system in place rotates forward, has a quick rotation and early shifts do not start before 06:00
- Consider reducing the duration of night shifts longer than 8 hours
- Plan safety critical tasks to avoid night shifts.
- Allow so far as is practically possible employee control over shift allocation
- Advise employees on the maintenance of health and fitness and to take advantage of health assessments
- Improve social support among supervisors and colleagues
- Recognize that people can have sleep disorders such as narcoplepsy or sleep apnoea and refer for further help

---

A large body of research on shift work and its effects on health and performance exists, but the findings are rarely put into practice. Working patterns are usually seen as matters to be negotiated between employees and the employer. Overtime is perceived more as a financial advantage than a potential health and safety issue. However, in high-hazard industries awareness of the relation between sleepiness and accidents is growing.

'Human error' is often invoked as an explanation for an accident, whether a minor incident in the workplace or a major disaster

---

Box 16.4 **Typical causes of human failures in accidents**

Job factors

- Illogical design of equipment and instruments
- Constant disturbances and interruptions
- Missing or unclear instructions
- High workload
- Noisy and unpleasant working conditions

Individual attributes

- Low skill and competence levels
- Tired staff
- Bored or disheartened staff
- Individual medical or fitness problems

Organizational aspects

- High work pressure because of poor work planning
- Poor health and safety culture
- One-way communications (messages sent but no checks to ensure they are received or are appropriate)
- Lack of safety systems and barriers
- Inadequate responses to previous incidents

---

entailing significant loss of life. When the term is used by the media it is seen as being the fault of the human in the work system. Research in high-risk industries has shown that understanding the role of the individual and where human failure occurs is crucial to reducing the numbers of incidents and accidents. Human errors in the work system can be intentional, unintentional or violations. These categories of errors are also influenced by factors such as distraction, time pressure, workload, communication systems, employee morale and physical agents such as noise. Box 16.4 lists some of the typical causes of human failures in accidents. Our understanding of the human in the system has been greatly enhanced by research in high-risk industries. The post-accident investigation of events such as the Piper Alpha oil rig and the Challenger Space Shuttle explosions are examples (Figures 16.3 and 16.4).

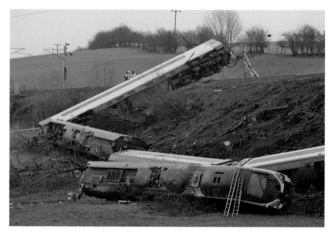

Figure 16.3 Human failures are often caused by poor system design. *Source:* Wikimedia Commons.

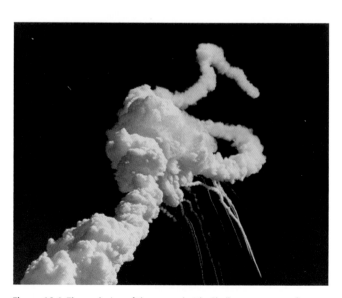

Figure 16.4 The explosion of the space shuttle Challenger – poor safety culture and communication was seen as a contributor to this. *Source:* Wikimedia Commons.

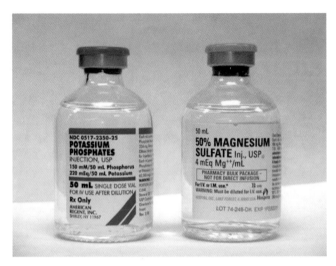

Figure 16.5 Poor drug packaging design can increase the likelihood of errors.

> ## Box 16.6 **Common errors relating to drugs**
>
> - Unavailable drug information (for example, lack of up-to-date warnings)
> - Miscommunication of drug orders (for example, through poor handwriting, confusion between drugs with similar names, misuse of zeros and decimal points, confusion between milligrams and micrograms)
> - Incomplete patient information (such as not knowing about other medicines they are taking)
> - Poorly designed packaging with different drugs similarly packed
> - Lack of suitable labelling when a drug is repackaged into smaller units
> - Workplace factors that distract medical staff from their immediate tasks (such as poor lighting, heat, noise and interruptions)

Modern healthcare is also a complex and, at times, high-risk activity where adverse events regularly occur. However, a substantial proportion of adverse events results from preventable human failure by healthcare staff. Boxes 16.5 and 16.6 present some examples of human failures in medicine and Figure 16.5 demonstrates the issue of drug packaging design. They occur in about 10% of admissions to hospital in the United Kingdom – a rate of 850 000 adverse events a year and 400 people die or are seriously injured every year in adverse events associated with faulty or improperly used medical devices. Hospital-acquired infections are estimated to cost the NHS nearly £1 billion every year, but about 15% of such infections may be avoidable. In the United States it is estimated that between 44 000 and 98 000 people die annually because of medical errors. Yet healthcare is not unique: there are many parallels with other high-risk sectors such as the nuclear and aviation industries, which have been examining the need to reduce human failures in complex systems for over three decades. The response to these data in the United Kingdom has been to develop tools for healthcare staff to build a safer culture, enable openness for reporting of incidents and use root cause analysis to investigate incidents and report on the findings and through this improve safety in patient care. Box 16.5 lists the typical causes of human failures in accidents.

At an organizational level, a number of factors influence safety performance. These concern not only human factors issues but also the 'safety culture' of the organization. A 'culture' means shared attitudes, beliefs and ways of behaving. An effective safety culture establishes good ways of informing and consulting with all staff, recognizes that everyone has a role to play in safety, provides a visible commitment by managers to involving all staff, and promotes cooperation between members of the workforce, open two-way communications and high-quality of training. An organization that continually improves its own methods, and learns from mistakes (including accidents and 'near misses') will tend to have a better safety performance than one that blames individuals for 'being careless' when accidents happen.

Websites

International Ergonomics Association http://www.iea.cc.
Institute of Ergonomics and Human Factors http://www.ergonomics.org.uk.

Further reading

HSE, Managing Shiftwork: health and safety guidance, HSG256 2006. *Guidance on the health effects of shiftwork and designing shift systems*

HSE. *Reducing error and influencing behaviour.* Sudbury: HSE Books, 1999. *Guidance to industry on understanding and control of human factors in health and safety management. Covers understanding human failures, designing for people, and control measures for human errors*

HSE Upper limb disorders in the workplace HSG60, HSE Books 2002. *Guidance on ULDs, identification assessment and risk reduction methods*

Kirwan, B. and Ainsworth, L.K., *A guide to task analysis.* Taylor and Francis, London 1992. *A key influence on those involved in carrying out task analysis*

National Patient Safety Agency, *Seven steps to patient safety: an overview guide for NHS staff NPSA,* London 2004. *A guide to concepts and methods to improve patient safety*

> ## Box 16.5 **Examples of human failures in medicine**
>
> - A patient is inadvertently given a drug to which they are known to be allergic
> - A clinician misreads the results of a test
> - A child receives an adult dose of a toxic drug
> - A patient is given medicine that has a similar sounding name to that prescribed
> - A patient is given medicine
> - A toxic drug is administered by the wrong route, for example intrathecally
> - A heart attack is not diagnosed by emergency department staff in an older patient with ambiguous symptoms

NHS. *An organisation with a memory*. London: NHS Publications, 2000.

Reason J. *Human Error*. Cambridge: Cambridge University Press, 1990. *An influential work on human error that has impacted on all future research*

Reason J. *Managing the risks of organisational accidents*. Ashgate Publishing, 1997. *Seminal work on the causes of major accidents. A key influence for those looking at medical errors*

Moore-Ede M. The 24-hour society: the risks, costs and challenges of a world that never stops.

Wilson JR., Corlett EN. (eds) *Evaluation of human work: A practical ergonomics methodology*, 3rd edn. London: Taylor & Francis, 2005. *Covers the main methodologies and tools available in ergonomics*

CHAPTER 17

Genetics and Reproduction

Nicola Cherry

University of Alberta, Edmonton, Canada

OVERVIEW

- Genetic differences may make some workers more susceptible to the impact of occupational and environmental exposures
- Such exposures might also be passed to future generations through changes to the DNA of the germ cell or through epigenetic changes, although there is at present little evidence to support this
- Exposures at work can affect male fertility and, where the mother is exposed during pregnancy, the viability of the pregnancy and the health of the infant
- Given our current state of knowledge, selection for employment using the results of genetic screening cannot be well justified on either ethical or practical grounds
- The duty of the employer is to provide a workplace that is safe for all workers, including those with genetic susceptibilities and those contemplating pregnancy

---

All healthcare professionals concerned with the health of patients who have reached working age need to consider whether a specific pathology or set of symptoms is related to exposures at work. Given our new knowledge of the human genome it is reasonable to ask also whether genetic susceptibility might help to explain why one worker develops the disease while many others with the same exposure do not. The question of interest here is whether some workers are genetically less able than others to respond to chemical or other challenge at work. Such gene–environment interactions are particularly difficult to study as the effect will be seen only where exposure has occurred and will only be correctly attributed if pains are taken to explore and document the exposure history. Such knowledge of the environment – in addition to the genome – is essential if we are to fully understand the impact on workers' health: the genome is not readily manipulated, but exposures can in principle be controlled and health effects prevented. With our current knowledge such genetic susceptibility to a specific exposure would very rarely be a reason for excluding a worker, but may lead to greater understanding of the mechanisms by which disease occurs, and suggest approaches to prevention or treatment.

ABC of Occupational and Environmental Medicine, Third Edition.
Edited by David Snashall and Dipti Patel.
© 2012 John Wiley & Sons Ltd. Published 2012 by John Wiley & Sons Ltd.

There is also concern that occupational or environmental exposures may affect subsequent generations through changes to stem cells. By this means an infant born to such a parent may be at greater risk of disease even if exposure of the parent has ceased long before the child is conceived. Recently the picture has become even more complex with the emergence of environmental epigenetics – examining the effects that the environment can have on gene expression while leaving unchanged the structure of the DNA. There is troubling (though not conclusive) evidence that some epigenetic changes resulting from occupational or environmental exposures (for example methylation of the germ cell) may be heritable by future generations, thus linking the three topics of this chapter (work, genetics and reproduction).

In all these areas, genetic susceptibility, genetic alteration and reproductive health, exposures in the working population may be of particular concern as these tend to be higher than exposures in the general population – they occur in a sub-population in which a large proportion is of reproductive age and where exposures are preventable. Exposure standards designed to protect workers do not currently take account of genetic differences in susceptibility. Environmental exposures to the general public (including the very young and pregnant or nursing mothers), through contaminants in food, water and in the air we breathe, may also be suspected of affecting reproductive health. Pressing questions remain about whether such exposures may cause infertility, affect the outcome of pregnancy or influence the development of the infant in later life.

Work and genetics

Why should those professionally involved in occupational health be concerned with the genetic make-up of people in the workforce or who seek to join it? First, there are those whose genetic inheritance, even in the absence of a specific occupational exposure, will lead to disease that will put at risk themselves, their fellow workers or the general public. For example, a worker genetically programmed to develop Huntington's disease may, if employed as a driver of a high-speed train, put the public at risk in the early stages of the disease before a diagnosis can be made that permits redeployment or retirement on medical grounds. Second, there may be genetic conditions, for example sickle cell disease, where work environments (such as in deep sea diving) that can be tolerated by other workers may induce a crisis in a worker carrying this gene and, as a result, the worker and others put at peril. Third, it may be that a particular genetic variant (or polymorphism) or a combination of variants, carries a risk of ill health if a worker is exposed to a chemical that is detoxified by the enzyme produced by the gene. Where such a disease is a serious threat to quality of life or life itself, it may be tempting to consider introducing screening to monitor such workers and exclude them from exposure.

The arguments for and against such genetic screening are summarized in Box 17.1. It should be noted that other reasoning may apply in different societies. Where there is no universal healthcare, for example screening for genetic disease might reduce the employer's overall healthcare bill although the temptation to do this, for example in the United States, may be tempered by ethical and legal considerations. In the United Kingdom there is currently little or no genetic screening for employment. Following the 1995 Statement of the Human Genetics Advisory Committee (Box 17.2), which suggested consensual evidence-based genetic screening, the Human Genetics Commission recommended in 2002 that any employer considering offering testing should inform the Commission and employers are now required to do so. The balance of opinion is that, with our current state of knowledge, such screening for genetic susceptibility is seldom, if ever, justified either from an ethical or practical standpoint.

Box 17.1 Genetic testing in employment

Arguments for	Arguments against:
1 May identify predispositions to disease that would put others at risk in certain jobs (e.g. Huntington's disease)	1 Potential for unethical and illegal discrimination
2 May identify those at increased risk from specific job demands or exposures (e.g. sickle cell and diving: PON1 polymorphisms and organophosphates)	2 Risk of invasion of privacy if not confidential and consensual
3 Allows individuals to make informed choices about where to work	3 Failure of employers in their duty to provide a workplace safe for all
4 May reduce healthcare costs of society as a whole	4 Poor predictive value with current level of Knowledge

---

A further issue is whether the potential for a substance to cause mutation and ultimately cancer can be monitored through genetic biomarkers such as the formation of 'adducts' when a chemical binds to DNA following exposure (for example to polycyclic aromatic hydrocarbons) and can be measured in lymphocytes or red blood cells obtained from a routine blood sample. Those with the highest number of adducts may be thought to be at the greatest risk of developing cancer, either because their exposures have indeed been higher (perhaps because of poor environmental controls) or because a finding of a particularly high level of adducts may, in itself, be an indication of an inherent inability to detoxify a particular mutagen (or to repair damage when it occurs). Given the wide

---

Box 17.2 Statement of the Human Genetics Advisory Committee 1995

i An individual should not be required to take a genetic test for employment purposes – an individual's "right not to know" their genetic constitution should be upheld.

ii An individual should not be required to disclose the results of a previous genetic test unless there is clear evidence that the information it provides is needed to assess either current ability to perform a job safely or susceptibility to harm from doing a certain job.

iii Employers should offer a genetic test (where available) if it is known that a specific working environment or practice, while meeting health and safety requirements, might pose specific risks to individuals with particular genetic variations. For certain jobs where issues of public safety arise, an employer should be able to refuse to employ a person who refuses to take a relevant genetic test.

iv Any genetic test used for employment purposes must be subject to assured levels of accuracy and reliability, reflecting best practice. We recommend that any use of genetic testing should be evidence-based and consensual. Results of any tests undertaken should always be communicated to the person tested and professional advice should be available. Information about and resulting from the taking of any test should be treated in accordance with Data Protection principles.
Furthermore, test results should be carefully interpreted, taking account of how they might be affected by working conditions.

v If multiple genetic tests were to be performed simultaneously, then each test should meet the standards set out in (ii), (iii) and (iv).

---

variation in adducts in the same individual measured on two occasions, and the uncertainty in interpreting the importance of such measures in assessing the risk of cancer in later years, the routine use of DNA adducts as exposure effect markers for individual workers may not be defensible. However occupational health professionals need to understand the potential importance of such measures as evidence of a relevant mechanism. Such evidence in humans is already being used by the International Agency for Research on Cancer in the designation of chemicals such as ethylene oxide as carcinogens.

Genetic analysis may also have a place in the attribution of causality after disease has occurred. Mutations in p53, a suppressor gene, have been found in most types of cancer and, in individual cases, it may be helpful to consider whether the mutation observed is one that occurs more frequently in tumours associated with one type of exposure than another, increasing the *post facto* probability that this is the exposure that was responsible. In epidemiological studies, where an excess of ill health is observed but the importance of exposure is uncertain, demonstrating that those with a genetic susceptibility to the exposure are more likely to develop the disease may again shift the balance towards acceptance of causality.

Genetics and reproduction

The time window for genetic damage in reproductive stem cells differs markedly between men and women. In females, ova that will be available for fertilization in adulthood go through most phases of development while the fetus is *in utero*. The implication is that exposure of a pregnant woman may bring about genetic changes not only in the female infant she is carrying but also children born to her daughter, as the ova that will produce those grandchildren are already forming in the fetus. In practice, there is little evidence that this does occur (at least for occupational exposures). In the male, in contrast, damage to stem cells that may affect the genetic complement of the resulting child may happen at any time, from the *in utero* exposure important in the female to the point at which production of the sperm occurs. There is then a further 3-month window for adverse environmental effects as the sperm that will eventually fertilize the ovum moves through its final stages of development. Although the time period of opportunity for damage is much greater for the male, and the protection from external influences less stringent than *in utero*, the evidence of such effects, from occupational exposure in humans is sparse. Despite the belief that epigenetic changes resulting from environmental exposures are erased from sperm cells there remains unexplained 'inheritance' of some traits in some species that have led to the hypothesis of some epigenetic changes being transmitted. Of particular interest to occupational and environmental health is the suggestion of effects transmitted after exposure of rats to viclozolin, an endocrine-disrupting fungicide.

Finally there is the suspicion that environmental exposures *in utero* may lead to childhood cancers, although the best evidence for this again comes from pharmaceutical products (with mothers' use of diethylstilboestrol (DES), for example, responsible for vaginal cancers in female offspring as they reach adolescence and beyond). It is likely that mutations to stem cells, which would perpetuate genetically mediated disorders through the generations, are much less common than such somatic mutations.

Work and reproductive health

Although the fertility of both men and women can be adversely affected by exposure to chemical compounds (Boxes 17.3 and 17.4) (particularly certain pesticides and solvents), metals, the physical environment (heat, radiation) and other factors at work, evidence suggests that only a limited number of exposures have such effects (although when they do the outcome can be dramatic, as seen some 35 years ago with azoospermia following exposure to the nematocidal soil fumigant dibromochloropropane (DBCP) in many workers). Once the fertilized ovum is implanted, and begins to develop, the risk appears much greater, with exposure – to chemicals, infective agents, radiation – having the capacity to interrupt fetal development during the period of organogenesis (as happened with thalidomide), to interfere with the development of the nervous system (with effects on hearing or eyesight, for example, and possibly on rates of spina bifida) or to result in retardation – not evident at birth – in the infant as it develops. Importantly, there is good epidemiological evidence that heavy physical demands at work are related to fetal death and prematurity. Few occupational cohort studies have been able to follow the offspring of workers into childhood to determine subtle effects on development that may result from exposure *in utero*, but if community studies of

environmental exposures are correct in their interpretation, similar effects of occupational exposure would be anticipated.

Box 17.3 **Agents associated with risk to male fertility***

Chemical
- Cabaryl – abnormal sperm morphology
- Carbon disulphide – oligospermia, abnormal morphology
- Chlordecone – oligospermia, reduced sperm motility, abnormal sperm morphology
- Dibromochloropropane – oligospermia/azoospermia
- Glycol ethers – oligospermia, reduced sperm motility
- Lead – oligospermia, reduced sperm motility, abnormal sperm morphology

Physical
- Heat – oligospermia
- Ionising radiation – oligospermia/azoospermia

Biological
- Mumps – oligospermia/azoospermia

*For some of these hazards, there is conflicting epidemiological evidence.

Box 17.4 **Some hazards associated with adverse pregnancy outcome***

Chemical
- Anaesthetic gases – spontaneous abortion, growth retardation, intrauterine death
- Organic solvents – spontaneous abortion
- Lead – spontaneous abortion, intrauterine death, prematurity
- Polychlorinated biphenyls (PCBs) – congenital PCB syndrome

Physical
- Ionising radiation – spontaneous abortion, growth retardation, central nervous system malformation, childhood cancer
- Heavy physical demands, shift work, extremes of temperature – spontaneous abortion, prematurity, growth retardation, intrauterine death

Biological
- Rubella – spontaneous abortion, intrauterine death, congenital rubella syndrome
- Varicella zoster infection – neonatal infection, congenital varicella syndrome
- Parvovirus B19 – hydrops fetalis and fetal loss

*For some of these hazards, there is conflicting epidemiological evidence.

Environment and reproductive health

Many of the concerns about effects on the developing infant come from the interpretation of community studies of the relation between exposure to lead (from flaking paint or gasoline), household pesticides (used repeatedly in poor quality housing in hot climates) and neurotoxic substances (for example organic mercury), from diet (fish, game) or water. Of particular interest in recent years has been the suggestion that endocrine modulators, from water, diet (phytoestrogens such as soya) or exposures to, for example, plasticizers such as phthalates, have effects *in utero* on the male fetus leading to congenital malformations (hypospadias), low sperm count and testicular cancer. Results of research into such effects in humans are not wholly supportive of this overarching hypothesis, but the impetus arising from this elegant synthesis has pushed environmental (and occupational) reproductive health into the focus of regulators throughout the Western world.

Further reading

Bonde JP. Workplace exposures and reproductive health. In Baxter PJ *et al.* (eds) *Hunter's Diseases of Occupations*, 10th edn London: Hodder Arnold, 2010. *Useful overview of reproductive issue in occupational health, particularly good on male fertility*

Bonzini M, Coggon D, Palmer KT. Risk of prematurity, low birth weight and pre-eclampsia in relation to working hours and physical activities: a systematic review. *Occup Environ Med* 2007; 64: 228–243. *Review of the effects of ergonomic factors at work on the health of the fetus*

Daxinger L, Whitrlaw E Transgenerational epigenetic inheritance: more questions than answers. *Genome Res* 2010; 20: 1623–1628. *Thought provoking discussion of the evidence for environmental effects being passed through the generations*

Palmer KT, Poole J, Rawbone RG, Coggon D. Quantifying the advantages and disadvantages of pre-placement genetic screening. *Occ Environ Med* 2004; 61: 448–453. *Consideration of pre-employment screening and the information needed to make a rational judgment about the circumstances under which it might be justified*

Pullman D, Lemmens T. Keeping the GINA in the bottle: assessing the current need for genetic non-discrimination legislation in Canada. *Open Med* 2010;4E95. *Discussion of the US Genetic Information Nondiscrimination Act (GINA) and whether similar legislation might be desirable (or not) in other jurisdictions*

Vineis P, Ahsan H, Parker M. Genetic screening and occupational and environmental exposures. *Occ Environ Med* 2005; 62: 657–662. *Good discussion of the arguments for and against screening, with an interesting discussion of susceptibility to arsenic in drinking water in rural Bangladesh.*

Information on genetic testing is on www.hgc.gov.uk

CHAPTER 18

The Ageing Workforce

Sarah Harper

Oxford Institute of Ageing, University of Oxford, Oxford, UK

OVERVIEW

- Nearly one-fifth of all workers in the industrialized world are over 50 and the number of younger workers entering the labour force each year is declining
- Increasing the economic contribution of older workers could ameliorate the looming pensions deficits and promote better health
- Many countries have now enacted legislation to ban age discrimination in employment
- There is a degree of physical and mental decline with age, but this is highly variable and a degree of compensation can occur
- Initiatives to encourage employers to engage older workers are in place in many countries; adaptation of workplaces and working practices is the key

Introduction

All industrialized nations are currently experiencing dynamic changes to both their population structures and their workforces. Already nearly one-fifth of all workers in the industrialized world are over 50. By 2030, half the UK population will be aged over 50, and one-third over 60. At the same time the ageing of the population structure will have significantly reduced the number of younger workers entering the labour force each year. This alongside growing age discrimination legislation in European countries will require employers to address the needs of retaining its older workers in suitable occupations.

Demographics and policy initiatives

The next decade will thus see a rapid shift towards increased elderly dependency ratios in most industrialized countries. The EU-25 Elderly Dependency Ratio is set to double as the working-age population (15–64 years) decreases by 48 million between now and 2050, and the EU-25 will change from having four to only two persons of working age for each citizen aged 65 and above

(European Commission, 2006). In 2010 the working age population comprised 70% of Europe's population, with older and younger dependents equal in size, and representing a total dependency ratio of 46:100 workers. From 2010 to 2050, the total dependency will increase to 73:100 workers (Table 18.1). There is thus a widespread assumption that the structural ageing of the European population will lead to a *demographic deficit*, whereby the population of working age is insufficient to support the increasing proportion of older dependents.

It is now accepted by most OECD governments that some remedial measures will be needed. These measures may be approached by altering the age composition of the population through encouraging changes in fertility and migration rates to increase the proportion of young people, and by increasing the productivity of the population by encouraging higher labour force participation rates and extending working lives by altering entry and exit ages. Increasing the economic contribution of older workers is an important measure for industrialized countries to consider. This is particularly the case in those European countries where early retirement rates are high.

Encouraging longer working lives:

- reduces pension longevity for the individual and societies
- has the potential to tackle issues emerging from the demographic deficit, through the retention of experience and skills held by older workers
- should in the longer term reduce national public health bills by increasing the wellbeing of its older population through continued usefulness and mental and physical activity in later years.

There is now general acceptance that future cohorts of older men and women, with higher levels of education, skills and training, will be able to maintain high levels of productivity given supportive and conducive working environments (Harper, 2010).

Lengthening working lives

Although there is a general acceptance that, faced with population ageing, longer working lives must be encouraged (OECD 2006) there are also concerns. These include:

- the relationship of life expectancy to healthy life expectancy
- the changing physical and mental capacity of individuals as they age

ABC of Occupational and Environmental Medicine, Third Edition.
Edited by David Snashall and Dipti Patel.
© 2012 John Wiley & Sons Ltd. Published 2012 by John Wiley & Sons Ltd.

- the need to adapt working practices and environments for older workers
- the need to provide specialist training for older workers.

The relationship of life expectancy to healthy life expectancy

There is considerable debate over whether healthy or disability-free life expectancy has kept pace with life expectancy. Whereas some predictions for Europe and the United States forecast that both men and women in their early 70s can expect to live well into their 80s, enjoying most of those years disability free (Manton *et al.* 2006), historical data for the UK suggests that for both men and women the increases in 'healthy life expectancy' (HLE), and 'disability-free life expectancy' (DFLE) in particular, have not kept pace with total gains in life expectancy. This is important, as both of these measures provide an indication of the length of time an individual remains 'healthy' and are thus more closely aligned with an individual's ability to work later in life, and in turn the ability to defer reliance on the state pension to an older age (Figure 18.1 and Table 18.2).

Table 18.1 Distribution of the population of major areas by broad age groups, 2010, 2030 and 2050 (medium variant).

Major Area	Population by age group (%)											
	2010				2030				2050			
	0–14	15–59	60+	80+	0–14	15–59	60+	80+	0–14	15–59	60+	80+
UK	17.4	60	22.7	4.7	17.2	55.7	27.2	6.2	16.4	54.7	28.8	8.6
EU 27	15.4	62.6	22	4.2	14.7	56.0	29.3	6.1	15.0	50.8	34.2	9.6
More developed regions	16.5	61.7	21.8	4.3	15.4	55.8	28.8	6.4	15.4	52.0	32.6	9.5
Less developed regions	29.2	62.1	8.6	0.9	24.0	61.7	14.2	1.6	20.3	59.5	20.2	3.5
Least developed regions	39.9	54.9	5.2	0.4	33.3	59.3	7.0	0.6	27	61.9	11.1	1.1

Source: UN 2008.

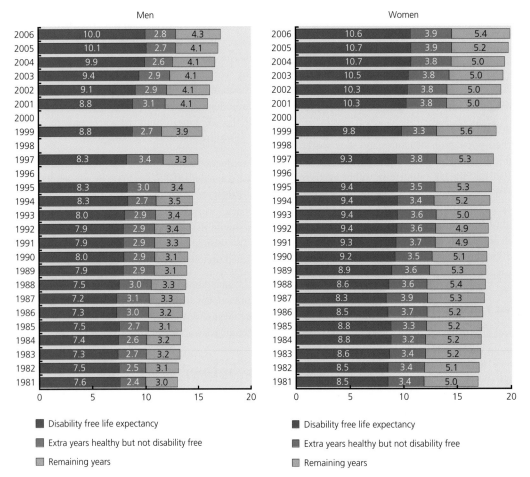

Figure 18.1 Disability free, healthy and total life expectancy in Great Britain (1981–2006). *Source:* ONS Club Vita calculations Harper *et al.* 2011.

Table 18.2 Healthy life expectancy (HLE) at birth and age 65: by country and sex, 2006–2008.

	At birth		At age 65	
	Males	Females	Males	Females
United Kingdom	62.5	64.3	10.1	11.3
Great Britain	62.7	64.4	10.1	11.3
England	63.0	64.5	10.2	11.4
Wales	60.2	62.7	10.1	10.5
Scotland	60.9	64.2	9.6	11.1
Northern Ireland	60.8	62.9	9.5	10.9

Source: ONS (2010) Health expectancies at birth and at age 65, United Kingdom, 2006–08. Statistical Bulletin.

Changing capacity

Despite stereotypes to the contrary, there appears to be no direct relationship between ageing and decline in occupational capacity among those under age 70. As research, especially in Finland, has long revealed, muscle strength, heart and lung function and some mental capacity do decline with age, but these can be compensated for by changing working conditions (Illmarinen 2001) (Figure 18.3, Table 18.3 and 18.4).

In general, the average health level tends to decrease markedly with age. However, the extent of the decline depends to a significant degree on individual factors such as the levels of environmental exposures, variable lifestyle, previous working habits and genetics (Harper and Marcus 2006).

Age-related changes that are most likely to be important to job exposures and job experience among older workers occur in the following organ systems: skeletal muscle, bone, vision, hearing, pulmonary function, skin, metabolism and immunity (Wegman and McGee 2004).

Many authors point out that functional capacities appear to decrease after the age of 30, with the declines in physical work abilities occurring at a younger age and exceeding those of either mental or social abilities (Illmarinen 2001). These declines are primarily associated with reductions in cardiovascular, respiratory,

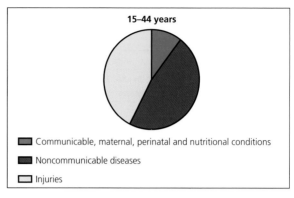
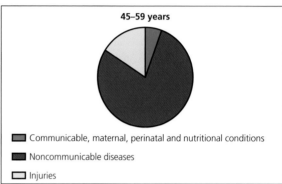
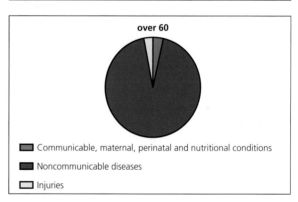

Figure 18.3 Leading causes of death, 2009, Europe by age. *Source:* WHO 2009 Database.

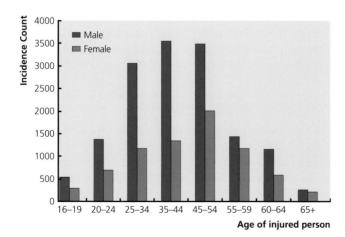

Figure 18.2 Injuries to employees by age and sex of injured person reported to all enforcing authorities in the UK, 2009/2010. *Source:* Health and Safety Executive, UK.

metabolic and muscular functions. An average decline of 20% in physical work capacity has been reported between the ages of 40 and 60 years, due to decreases in aerobic and musculoskeletal capacity (Illmarinen 2002; Glen *et al.* 2008).

Average muscle strength decreases by roughly 10% per decade for ages 20–60, by approximately 15% each decade for ages 60–80, and 30% each decade after age 80. Age-related muscle loss may have an important effect on other functions, such as respiration, joint mobility, and speech.

Hearing ability declines with age. Workers after age 50 typically begin to lose higher frequency hearing.

Eyesight is affected by age through several mechanisms. Older individuals need objects to be 50–70% lighter and with a stronger contrast to have the same visual ability as younger individuals.

Many workers above the age of 50 begin to have problems with balance, risking injuries from trips and falls. Figure 18.2 shows

Table 18.3 Work-related musculoskeletal disorders: percentage age distribution (a) of estimated cases by age and diagnostic category, for 2007–2009, UK.

Diagnostic category	Age distribution (%)					
	16–24 years	25–34 years	35–44 years	45–54 years	55–64 years	65+ years
Upper Limb disorders	4	15	28	34	19	1
Raynaud's/HAV/VWF	1	7	29	36	27	–
Other hand/wrist/arm	6	21	25	31	16	1
Elbow	3	6	39	38	14	–
Shoulder	4	11	20	44	21	1
Spine/back disorders	4	22	28	31	13	1
Neck/thoracic spine	3	19	29	31	17	1
Lumbar spine/trunk	5	23	28	32	11	1
Lower Limbs	6	16	25	33	16	3
Hip/knee/leg	7	20	21	30	19	3
Ankle/foot	4	8	37	38	13	–
Others	5	24	23	33	11	3
Total number of diagnoses	4	17	27	34	17	1
Total number of individuals (b)	4	17	28	33	17	1

Age is not recorded for some cases: percentage breakdown is calculated for all those cases for whom age is known.
Individuals can have more than one diagnosis.
Source: HSE – http://www.hse.gov.uk/statistics/tables/thorm02.xls

Table 18.4 Work-related respiratory disease: percentage age distribution (a) of estimated cases by diagnostic category, 2007–2009, UK.

Diagnostic category	Age distribution (%)					
	16–24 years	25–34 years	35–44 years	45–54 years	55–64 years	65+ years
Allergic alveolitis	–	3	28	20	50	–
Asthma	2	17	34	28	19	1
Bronchitis/emphysema	–	2	1	7	43	48
Infectious diseases	9	26	28	26	9	1
Inhalation accidents	25	2	42	30	1	–
Lung cancer	–	–	–	5	16	79
Malignant mesothelioma	–	–	–	4	23	73
Benign pleural disease	–	–	–	2	26	72
Pneumoconiosis	–	–	1	8	5	85
Other	4	23	18	22	22	10
Total diagnoses (b)	1	4	7	9	22	56
Total individuals	1	4	7	9	23	56

A small proportion of cases within each diagnostic category are of unknown age: percentages are calculated from those cases for which age was known, and may not sum to 100% due to rounding.
Individuals can have more than one diagnosis.
Source: HSE http://www.hse.gov.uk/statistics/tables/thorr02.xls.

injuries to employees by age and sex of injured person reported to all enforcing authorities in the UK in 2009/2010.

Older workers may become less tolerant of extended hours and shiftwork.

The impacts of age on cognitive function are more complex, because cognitive abilities decline with age whereas others tend to be relatively robust over the life cycle. A number of aspects of cognition are detrimentally affected by ageing, including processing speed, memory and reasoning; the negative age trends are often large; and the decline often begins before age 50. At the same time, ageing is related to an increase in the control of language

and the ability to process complex problems (Ilmarinen 2001). Furthermore, in some occupations, the cognitive abilities that remain stable are the ones most closely correlated to job success. Senior employees can remain highly productive within a field that they know well and where relatively long experience is beneficial.

Screening and indexes

There exist a variety of work indexes and assessment kits which enable testing of workers for both capacity and health and safety. With a few exceptions (Finnish Workability Index;) these have not included capacity changes with age. Indeed both Scandinavia and Australia in particular are far more advanced than the United Kingdom in the development of such capacity testing. Yet new screening measures mean that such assessments may become more sophisticated and relevant for employers coping with ageing work-forces. Indeed, there is now growing recognition by human resource departments in particular of the lack of such evidence, and the need to develop it.

Legislation

Since 1999, the UK government has introduced an array of measures and programmes to promote best practices and age diversity in employment. Among others, the government, in cooperation with the social partners, launched the Age Positive campaign and a Code of Practice on Age Diversity in Employment in June 1999. Legislation making age discrimination unlawful was introduced in 2006 in the Employment Equality (Age) Regulations 2006. These Regulations are now incorporated in the Equality Act 2010.

Some key points are:

- The Regulations protect people of all ages in employment regarding recruitment, promotion, reward and recognition, redundancy and vocational training.
- The Regulations apply to all employers, providers of vocational training, trade unions, professional associations, employer organizations and trustees and managers of occupational pension schemes.
- Occupational pensions are covered by the Regulations, as are employer contributions to personal pensions although, generally, the way in which pension schemes work is not affected.
- The Regulations do not affect state pensions (CIPD, 2010).

International perspectives

The Age Discrimination in Employment Act (ADEA) has existed in the United States since 1967 and protects individuals who are 40 years of age or older from employment discrimination based on age. Its 1986 amendments prohibited mandatory retirement in most occupations by eliminating the upper age limit altogether (OECD 2006).

In Australia, the Age Discrimination Act is the most recent of the federal antidiscrimination laws. Australian federal antidiscrimination laws are related to the international human rights system because each of its Acts is based in part on international human

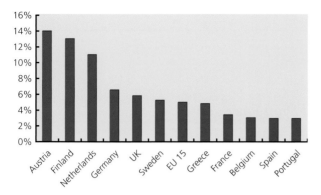

Figure 18.4 Age discrimination at work (percentages). *Source:* OECD 2006.

rights conventions or agreements (Australian Human Rights Commission, 2010).

In 1985, Canada passed legislation proscribing age discrimination within a comprehensive human rights act. The Canadian legislation is on several counts more universal than the British equivalent, but both the United Kingdom and (some provinces of) Canada tolerate compulsory retirement within the purview of their statutes.

Figure 18.4 represents the results of the 2000 European Survey on Working Conditions, where workers aged 50 and over in the EU-15 countries were asked whether during the previous 12 months they had either personally experienced age discrimination or witnessed it occurring at their workplace.

European initiatives to retain older workers

French companies hiring unemployed people age 50 or above can take advantage of the *Contrat Initiative Emploi* (contract to promote employment), a subsidy which reduces the employers social security contribution.

Germany has an integration subsidy *Eingliederungszusschusse* equivalent to 50% of their wages for hiring unemployed older people.

Sweden's *Special Employment Subsidies* programme encourages employers to recruit unemployed people over 57.

Norway has a tripartite agreement (government, employers, trade unions) under which the employer must establish systems to address the problem of ill health and declining functions among older workers, and provide training.

Conclusion

The past 20 years have seen a growing recognition, especially in OECD countries, of the need to facilitate an integrated workplace, one which adapts the working environment by ergonomic improvements, work rotation, reorganization of working tasks, flexibility in working time, part-time work, skills enhancement and training.

References

Australian Human Rights Commission. *Age discrimination* – exposing the hidden barrier for mature age workers. AHRC, 2010. *A clear expansive example of the barriers to older employment*

CIPD. *Age and Employment.* CIPD, 2010. *Factsheet. Key facts*

European Commission *The demographic future of Europe – from challenge to opportunity.* Luxembourg: EC, 2006. *The European view on the demographic challenges*

Harper S, Marcus S. Age-related capacity decline: a review of some workplace implications. *Ageing Horizons.* 2006; 5: 20–30. *An overview of some of the mental and physical changes which occur in later life*

Ilmarinen J. Aging workers. *Occup Environ Med* 2001; 58: 546–552. *The classic paper raising key issues around older workers*

Kenny GP, Yardley JE, Martineau L, Jay O. Physical work capacity in older adults: implications for the aging worker. *American Journal of Industrial Medicine* 2008; 51: 610–625. *An overview of some of the mental and physical changes which occur in later life*

Manton KG, Gu X, Lamb VL. Change in chronic disability 1982 to 2004/2005 as measured by long-term changes in function and health in the US elderly population. *PNAS USA* 2006; 103: 18374–18379. *An exposition of the morbidity/mortality debate*

OECD. *Live Longer, Work Longer* Paris: OECD, 2006. *The OECD view of the challenges ahead*

Wegman DH, McGee JP (eds). *Health and safety needs of older workers.* Washington, DC: National Academies Press, 2004. *Addressing health and safety issues*

Further reading

Skirbekk, V. (2008) Age and Productivity Capacity: Descriptions, Causes and Policy Options. *Ageing Horizons*, 8: 4–12. *How policy can address ageing and productive capacity*

Silverstein, M. (2008), Meeting the challenges of an aging workforce. *Am J Industrial Med* 51: 269–280. *The US view of the challenges ahead*

CHAPTER 19

Travel

Derek R. Smith[1,2], Peter A. Leggat[2,1] and Dipti Patel[3]

[1] School of Health Sciences, University of Newcastle, Ourimbah, New South Wales, Australia
[2] School of Public Health, Tropical Medicine and Rehabilitation Sciences, James Cook University, Townsville, Australia
[3] Foreign and Commonwealth Office, London; National Travel Health Network and Centre, London, UK

OVERVIEW

- Travelling abroad has now become a common feature of many types of employment
- Hazards faced by occupational travellers may appear similar to those of the general tourist but various interrelated factors can combine to make travelling for work a less favourable experience
- The majority of problems experienced by overseas travellers are minor, self-limiting conditions; but a small proportion will result in hospital admission, repatriation and death
- Employers retain a duty of care for staff while they are abroad
- Preparation of the occupational traveller should include consideration of individual, occupational and destination related risks

---

Box 19.1 **Why occupational travellers differ from tourists**

- Locations, times and dates are not chosen for enjoyment, interest or potential adaptability to the traveller
- Country, language, people and culture are not usually chosen for their potential compatibility with the traveller
- There is usually no chance for rest upon reaching the overseas destination, although some companies insist on rest on arrival at destination and advise against scheduling important meetings in the first 24 hours
- The occupational traveller is often very busy when away, usually travelling for the sole purpose of working
- The nature of the work may render occupational travellers targets for violence, kidnapping, etc.
- There is usually limited opportunity to recover after returning home as schedules often require a prompt return to work

---

Introduction

In recent years as the world embraces a global economy, travelling abroad, has now become a common feature of many types of employment. Advances in air travel and accessibility have led to the acceptance of this scenario as a typical job task, and many companies often assume that their employees are now 'transnationally competent'.

Those who travel overseas for work (from hereon referred to as occupational travellers) represent an important group of international travellers, and include both short- and long-term travellers (including expatriates), across a range of occupations. They are exposed to a variety of hazards, including those that may not be present in their home country, and while the hazards faced by occupational travellers may appear similar to those of the general tourist; various interrelated factors can combine to make travelling for work a less favourable experience (Box 19.1). Therefore, protecting the health and safety of those who travel overseas for work has become an increasingly important aspect of occupational and environmental medicine.

Travel-related health problems

Various studies have made it possible to obtain some consensus regarding the type of illness and the degree of risk experienced by travellers. Diarrhoea, upper respiratory infections and skin disorders are the most common travel-related illnesses. Although the majority are minor, self-limiting conditions, of those travellers who become unwell up to 30% may be confined to bed, 19% will need to consult a doctor and 2% are admitted to hospital. Deaths are fortunately rare; with cardiovascular disease followed by accidents and injuries being the most frequently recorded cause of death. Accidental death being highest in men in the 20–29 year age group.

Research on occupational travellers reveals similar findings, although illness rates tend to be higher and psychological problems more prominent. For expatriates in particular, as a result of their longer stay overseas, illnesses (including unusual infections), hospital admission, injury, violence and psychological problems are more frequently reported, while accidents and injury account for most deaths. Key findings from some studies on the health of occupational travellers are summarized in Box 19.2.

Air travel

Air travel itself may pose a risk to health and wellbeing, and although illness directly due to air travel is uncommon, exacerbation of

---

ABC of Occupational and Environmental Medicine, Third Edition.
Edited by David Snashall and Dipti Patel.
© 2012 John Wiley & Sons Ltd. Published 2012 by John Wiley & Sons Ltd.

pre-existing conditions due to changes in air pressure, humidity and oxygen concentration, relative immobility during flights and close proximity to passengers with communicable diseases are all potential risks (Box 19.3).

Jet lag

Jet lag is a syndrome associated with rapid long-haul flights across several time zones. It is characterized by sleep disturbances, day-time fatigue, reduced performance, gastrointestinal problems and generalized malaise. The incidence and severity of jet lag increase with the number of time zones crossed, with eastward travel being worse than westward travel. The adjustment of circadian rhythms to a new sleep–wake schedule can be protracted, although jet lag is generally worst immediately after travel and gradually resolves over 4–6 days as the person adjusts to the new local time. The more time zones crossed, the longer the effects take to wear off. For the short-term occupational traveller, in particular, recovery can be impeded by time and other practical constraints due to inflexible work and/or flight schedules (Box 19.4).

Box 19.4 **Jet lag**

Symptoms

- Poor sleep during the new night-time, including delayed sleep onset (after eastward flights), early awakening (after westward flights), and fractionated sleep (after flights in either direction)
- Poor performance (both physical and mental tasks) during the new daytime
- Negative subjective changes (fatigue, headaches, irritability, decreased concentration)
- Gastrointestinal disturbances (indigestion, frequency of defecation, changed consistency of the stools) and decreased interest in, and enjoyment of, meals

Combating jet lag

- Be as well rested as possible before departure
- Eat light meals and limit consumption of alcohol
- Limit caffeine to normal amounts and avoid within 4–6 hours of an expected sleep

A. If the journey crosses fewer than three time zones, then jet lag is unlikely to be a major difficulty for most people

B. If the stay is too short for adjustment of the body clock (for most less than 3 days), remain on home time, and attempt to arrange sleep and engagements to coincide with this

C. If the journey is across more than three time zones and the stay is more than 3 days, then:

  ○ a minimum block of 4 hours sleep during the local night (anchor sleep) is thought to be necessary to allow adaptation to the new time zone so, at destination, it helps to get as much sleep as possible in the 24 hours after arrival
  ○ total sleep time should be made up by taking naps during the day in response to feelings of sleepiness
  ○ exercise during the day may help, but should be avoided within 2 hours of trying to sleep
  ○ as the cycle of light and dark is one of the most important factors in setting the body's internal clock, a well-timed exposure to daylight (preferably bright sunlight) will usually help
  ○ when flying west, exposure to daylight in the evening and avoidance in the morning (e.g. by using dark glasses) may be helpful
  ○ when flying east, exposure to light in the morning and avoidance in the evening is recommended
  ○ short-acting sleeping pills may be helpful
  ○ melatonin is available in some countries, and is effective in preventing or reducing jet lag. Occasional short-term use appears to be safe, and should be considered for adult

---

  travellers flying across five or more time zones, particularly in an easterly direction
  ○ individuals react in different ways to time zone changes. Frequent flyers should learn how their own bodies respond and adopt habits accordingly

---

Infectious diseases and the occupational traveller

Travellers are exposed to a variety of infectious diseases (Box 19.5). Traveller's diarrhoea is the most common travel-related infectious disease, although malaria remains the most significant. With the exception of influenza and hepatitis A, travellers are generally believed to exhibit a relatively low risk of vaccine-preventable diseases. On the other hand, sexually transmitted infections (STIs) continue to be problematic due to a generally increased opportunity for casual sex when travelling abroad. Vector-borne diseases, such as dengue fever and chikungunya, are becoming more prominent in travellers.

Box 19.5 **Some important travel-related infections and predominant mode of transmission**

The changing pattern of travel, climate change, the emergence of new or previously unrecognized organisms, the re-emergence of infections (particularly in areas where they had not previously existed or had been eradicated), and microbial drug resistance pose an increasing challenge

- **Food and water borne** – cholera,* hepatitis A,* hepatitis E, paratyphoid, polio,* travellers' diarrhoea, typhoid*
- **Insect or animal bites** – African trypanosomiasis, American trypanosomiasis, chikungunya, Crimean-Congo haemorrhagic fever, dengue fever, Japanese encephalitis,* leishmaniasis, Lyme disease, lymphatic filariasis, malaria, onchocerciasis, plague, rabies,* Rift Valley fever, Rocky Mountain spotted fever, tick-borne encephalitis,* tick typhus, West Nile virus, yellow fever*
- **Close contact and other** – diphtheria,* ebola, hantaviirus hepatitis B,* hepatitis C, HIV, influenza,* Lassa fever, legionellosis, leptospirosis, Marburg virus, measles,* meningitis ACWY,* tuberculosis*

*Vaccine preventable.

Malaria

Malaria represents one of the most important disease hazards for the tropical traveller. Five types of malaria parasites cause disease in humans, although *Plasmodium falciparum* malaria is responsible for almost all fatalities. In humans, malaria is transmitted by the bite of an infected female anopheles mosquito, and risk of infection is influenced by destination, infected vector density, infected population density, infrastructure, seasonality, duration of exposure, compliance with preventive measures, style of travel and individual factors such as semi-immunity or pregnancy.

Prevention is based on the ABCD of malaria (Box 19.6). Failure to take antimalarial drugs or not taking the appropriate drugs remain key reasons for contracting malaria. Those at particular risk are individuals visiting friends and relatives in their country of origin. Apart from the military, who often spend extended periods of time in areas with endemic malaria, occupational travellers account for a minority of cases.

Box 19.6 Malaria Prevention of malaria depends on the ABCD of malaria prevention

A – Be aware of risk, the incubation period and the main symptoms

Worldwide, malaria risk is generally greatest in sub-Saharan Africa (particularly West Africa), to a lesser extent in South Asia (such as India), and lowest in Central and South America and South East Asia. Risk can however vary widely within countries depending on location

B – Avoid being bitten by mosquitoes, especially between dusk and dawn

Measures to reduce contact with mosquitoes include:

- Staying in well-screened areas or air conditioned rooms
- Sleeping under mosquito bed nets (preferably insecticide-treated)
- Wearing appropriate clothes that cover most of the body.
- Using insect repellents for use on exposed skin (DEET is the most effective).
- Using a pyrethroid-containing insect spray in living and sleeping areas during evening and nighttime hours

C – Take antimalarial drugs (chemoprophylaxis) to suppress infection when appropriate

D – Immediately seek diagnosis and treatment if symptoms develop 1 week or more after entering an area where there is a malaria risk

Malaria symptoms may develop from as early as 5–6 days following an infected bite. Most *P. falciparum* infections will have presented within 1 month, although this time window may be extended, especially among those taking chemoprophylaxis. *P. vivax*, *P. malariae* and *P. ovale* infections commonly have slightly longer incubation periods, with durations of 6 to 12 months having been reported with *P. vivax*.

Adapted from WHO ABCD of malaria protection http://www.who.int/malaria/travellers/en.

Traveller's diarrhoea

Traveller's diarrhoea (TD) represents one of the most common travel-related illnesses and depending on destination affects 20–60% of travellers (Box 19.7). Symptoms are generally mild and self-limiting, although in about 10% symptoms persist for more than a week, and in about 2% for more than a month. Up to 40% of travellers alter their plans because of diarrhoea, and up to 5% seek medical care. Most TD is due to infective enteropathogens, and while the innate risk initially appears similar to that faced by tourists, destinations visited by the occupational traveller are not usually chosen for their cuisine or suitability to the individual. Furthermore, the occupational traveller may have little or no choice in this regard. Even though the evidence for its effectiveness is contradictory, prevention of TD is usually based on careful attention

---

Box 19.7 Travellers' diarrhoea (TD)

- Classic TD is defined as three or more loose stools in 24 hours with or without at least one symptom of cramps, nausea, fever, or vomiting
- Bacterial pathogens (most commonly enterotoxigenic Escherichia coli) account for approxiamtely 80–90% of TD. Intestinal viruses (such as norovirus and rotavirus) usually account for 5–8% of illnesses, and protozoal pathogens (e.g. giardia) account for approximately 10% of diagnoses in longer-term travellers
- In special circumstances (short-term travelers who are high-risk hosts such as those who are immunosuppressed or who are taking critical trips during which even a short bout of diarrhoea could affect the trip), prophylactic antibiotics can be used. More commonly, treatment is supportive, with occasional self-treatment with antibiotics. For the latter, flouroquinolones are typically the drug of choice, and the combination of loperamide with an antibiotic in moderate TD may lead to more rapid clinical improvement

---

to food and water hygiene, and while the risks of unhygienic conditions are usually well known; occupational travellers (who often have to 'eat on the go') may not have the luxury to abide by the cardinal rule to 'boil it, cook it, peel it or forget it'.

Sexually transmitted infections

STIs are a major consideration for any traveller, as there is a well-established association between travel and these diseases. Up to 50% of short-term travellers report having had sex with a new partner, with up to two-thirds of this group reporting variable condom use. In occupational travellers, high rates of sexual contact with overseas nationals have been reported amongst seafarers, military personnel and expatriates.

Occupation and infectious diseases

Infectious disease poses a significant risk for healthcare workers, researchers, disaster relief workers and other aid workers who travel to developing countries and disease-endemic areas as part of their employment (see Chapter 12). This group will be exposed to some of the sickest and most infectious people, and exposure to endemic diseases in the country being visited may therefore be significant and should not be overlooked, particularly as 'traditional' tropical diseases such as dengue fever, for example, are now on a continuous rise. Furthermore, exposure to microorganisms which are genetically unfamiliar to the traveller will tend to increase their risk of contracting a particular disease.

Travellers can also contribute to the global spread of disease – outbreaks of severe acute respiratory syndrome (or SARS) during 2002 and pandemic (H1N1) influenza in 2009, clearly demonstrated how air travel can have an important role in the spread of newly emerging infections. Healthcare workers in particular can be implicated in the spread of healthcare associated infection – for example, the transatlantic spread of methicillin-resistant *Staphylococcus aureus* (MRSA) in 2003.

Psychological issues

Occupational travellers (particularly expatriates) and their families are believed to be particularly prone to a range of additional psychological pressures while overseas, and, indeed, expatriates have been shown to have a consistently high incidence of affective and adjustment disorders, with mental health problems being one of the principal causes of repatriation and premature departure from overseas assignments. This concept is not new: as early as a century ago, attrition rates among workers sent to tropical environments had been shown to reach 40%, with the majority of ailments relating to 'nervous conditions'.

More recently, a study of international business travellers working for the World Bank showed that over one-third of respondents reported experiencing high to very high levels of travel-related stress. The traveller's spouse may also suffer, with one study revealing that around half of all spouses in this situation experienced high to very high levels of stress. Travel-related stress may also manifest as *culture shock* – a term coined in the 1960s as an occupational disorder suffered by individuals who had been suddenly translocated abroad. Culture shock is now recognized as a condition that can occur whenever a person enters a new culture or returns to their original environment. The latter situation, reverse culture shock, is a particularly important though often overlooked issue for occupational travellers returning after long periods abroad.

Potential impact on the employer

Organizations sending their employees overseas have a duty of care to their staff, both in their home country and while they are abroad. This responsibility includes ensuring that individuals are prepared for their assignment and that adequate procedures are in place to take care of them if they become ill or are injured while overseas. Issues employers need to consider are summarized in Box 19.8. Aside from potential compensation costs, given that the occupational traveller is usually being paid a salary, falling ill when travelling for work will usually incur a financial loss for the employer. While these costs may often go unrecognized, they can easily become substantial – a study from Switzerland, for example, showed the average period of time lost due to illness was 3 days, which corresponded to 2% of the entire time abroad. Costs are also incurred by occupational travellers compared with equivalent non travelling employees. When travelling staff have been compared to non-travelling staff, for example, there have been 80% higher medical insurance claims across all ICD-9 categories, especially infectious diseases and psychological disorders, with 16% higher claims for mental health problems.

For these reasons, travel-related illness can amount to a significant burden. Aside from lost time, direct financial expenditure and lost productivity, dispatching employees overseas also incurs a duty of care because employers may inadvertently be exposing their staff to hazards not present at home, and occupational health and safety standards may be less stringent. To a large extent, this will depend on where employees are sent, how long they go for, and what their activities comprise at the overseas destination (both work and leisure). For example, issues of expatriate health

> **Box 19.8 Potential Issues for employers regarding occupational travel**
>
> - Travel-related illness may incur lost work-time and lost productivity
> - Employees can be seriously injured or killed when travelling overseas
> - Employers may be inadvertently exposing their staff to unknown hazards
> - Occupational health and safety standards may be lower in other countries
> - General health and hygiene facilities may be lower in other countries
> - Occupational travellers who frequently fall ill may be unwilling to travel any more
> - Illness or injury incurred overseas may require, medical care overseas or in extreme cases, medical repatriation
> - Illnesses and injuries incurred overseas or which remain or become problematic on return may attract claims for compensation
> - Travel-related infectious diseases confirmed or diagnosed on return may require notification to public health authorities
> - Employee or work activities may have an adverse impact on local environmental and public health

are generally perceived to be more significant when moving from a developed to a less developed country. Long-term travellers are generally exposed to greater risk than short-term travellers, and certain occupations are more inherently hazardous. Given the complexity of these issues, combined hopefully with aspirations to corporate social responsibility the legal, ethical, and moral issues brought up by imposing work-related travel on employees should always be seriously considered by management.

Clinical assessment of the occupational traveller

The clinical assessment of the occupational traveller need not be a daunting process, and will generally be no different to the strategies used in the assessment of tourists. Risk assessment is a fundamental part of any assessment prior to travel and determines the advice given and interventions proposed. The focus should be the employee's fitness to travel and work overseas (see Chapter 7), the provision of preventive advice, immunizations and malaria prophylaxis, and a process for the management of problems while overseas. The degree of detail should be informed by the risk assessment, and relevant employment legislation should always be considered. It is important to note however that health and safety concerns or country-imposed entry restrictions (e.g. legality of medication overseas, or restrictions on those with certain conditions such as HIV) may affect fitness decisions which would not be relevant in their home base.

Where pre-existing health issues are identified, the stability of the condition and any impact it has on functional ability should be considered in conjunction with the efficacy of preventive measures, the effect of travel and the overseas environment, the availability of adequate local medical facilities including the accessibility of medication/medical equipment. (Table 19.1).

Table 19.1 Preparation of traveller.

Traveller details	Basic demographic details Medical history Immunization history Drug and allergy history (including adverse reactions) General attitudes to risks Experience
Itinerary and activity related information	Dates of travel Duration of trip Type and style of travel Destination (season, climate, environment) Accommodation Purpose and planned activities Occupational risks
Immunization	Routine, required, recommended, contraindications
Advice and other preventive measures	Air travel Malaria prevention Food and water precautions Insect bite avoidance Accident prevention Sun safety Destination specific disease advice Sexual activity Environmental issues (for example, heat/cold/altitude/air pollution/natural disaster), cultural issues Medical arrangements (including repatriation) Personal safety and security Reporting Illness on return Other issues identified during assessment Specific occupational advice (long working hours, infection control for health care workers, etc.)

Assessment of psychological risk is one of the most difficult tasks, particularly for long-term or expatriate assignments, and while in depth psychological assessment if often advised for long-term assignments, evidence in relation to its utility appears to be sparse.

Assessment of the returned occupational traveller can often follow the protocols of assessment of returned travellers. Specific clinical manifestations of individual diseases to which occupational travellers may have been exposed vary, and are described in detail in Chapter 12 and the Further reading section. When assessing returned travellers, clinicians are advised to consult the latest evidence-based guidelines, although some factors to consider are displayed in Box 19.9.

Treatment and recovery

Occupational travellers generally have little or no time to recover from the innate pressures of long distance travel when they arrive at their final destination, particularly if it entails structured events with schedules that cannot be altered. Owing to their tight schedules and relatively short durations of stay (often a result of tight travel policies that do not permit the inclusion of 'down time'), occupational travellers may experience reduced opportunity for access to medical services in the host country. This is in addition to the intrinsic differences in healthcare delivery between the area being visited and one's home country. One result may be that illnesses progress to more advanced clinical states, a problem which could have been avoided had they been effectively treated at an earlier stage (for

example poorly managed/controlled diabetes mellitus). It is also important for returning occupational travellers, who are seeking medical advice for conditions potentially contracted abroad, to tell their treating health professional that they have been travelling (and where), as this alters the differential diagnoses (Box 19.9).

Box 19.9 Effective treatment and recovery

- Seek medical advice early post-travel, especially for fever
- Understand that many conditions, such as travellers' diarrhoea and jet lag, are self-limiting
- Liaise early with travel insurers and employers regarding accidents and injuries
- Appreciate that animal bites abroad need to be evaluated as soon as possible for rabies prophylaxis

Factors to consider in assessing ill returning travellers

- Travel itinerary
- Duration of travel
- Type of accommodation
- Association with mass gathering (Hajj, for example)
- Pre-travel immunization history
- Adherence to preventive advice (e.g. food and water hygiene, bite prevention, malaria prophylaxis etc)
- Activities and exposures during travel (e.g. source of water, consumption of contaminated food, insect and arthropod bites, activities in fresh water, leisure/adventure activities, animal bites and scratches, sexual contacts, tattoos, body piercing, and shared razors, hospitalizations and other medical/dental care while overseas, including injections, transfusions and surgery)

NB: Occupational health professionals will not generally be involved in the management of a newly returned ill occupational traveller, but may often be the first point of contact. They should ensure that the traveller accesses appropriate medical care (often the individual's GP, but in some situations a hospital with experience in infectious/tropical disease).

Conclusion

Although the clinical needs of the occupational traveller may appear similar to that of the general tourist, various interrelated factors may combine to make travelling for work a less pleasant experience. While we have emphasized the various problems likely to be experienced by the occupational traveller, and why their needs differ from those of regular tourists, it is equally important to remember that occupational travellers are often a self-selected group, and one that might generally be expected to be in reasonable health due to the 'healthy worker effect'. They may also have the additional benefits of more structured preparation, support from colleagues, corporate medical schemes, better access and more reliable communications, and networks.

Further reading

Bhatta P, Simkhada P, van Teijlingen, Maybin S. A Questionnaire study of voluntary service overseas (VSO) volunteers: health risk and problems encountered. *J Travel Med* 2009; 16: 332–337.

Chen LH, Wilson ME, Davis X, *et al.* Illness in long-term travelers visiting GeoSentinel clinics. *Emerg Infect Dis* 2009; 15: 1773–1782.

Cossar JH, Reid D, Fallon RJ, *et al.* A cumulative review of studies on travellers, their experience of illness and the implications of these findings. *J Infection* 1990; 21: 27–42.

Dahlgren AL, Deroo L, Avril J, *et al.* Health risks and risk-taking behaviors among International Committee of the Red Cross (ICRC) expatriates returning from humanitarian missions. *J Travel Med* 2009; 16: 382–390.

Herxheimer A, Petrie KJ. Melatonin for the prevention and treatment of jet lag. *Cochrane Database of Systematic Reviews* 2002; 2:CD001520.

Kemmerer T, Cetron M, Harper L, Kozarsky P. Health problems in corporate travellers: risk factors and management. *J Travel Med* 1998; 5: 184–187.

Leggat PA. Risk assessment in travel medicine. *Travel Med Infect Dis* 2006; 4: 127–134.

Liese B, Mundt K, Dell L, Nagy L, Demure B. Medical insurance claims associated with international travel. *Occup Environ Med* 1997; 54: 499–503.

Patel D. Occupational travel. *Occup Med* 2011; 61; 6–18.

Patel D, Easmon C, Seed P, Dow C, Snashall D. Morbidity in expatriates–a prospective cohort study. *Occup Med* 2006; 56: 345–352.

Silverman D, Gendreau M. Medical issues associated with commercial flights. *Lancet* 2009; 373: 2067–2077.

Smith DR, Leggat PA. Occupational travel medicine: Protecting the health and safety of those who regularly travel overseas for work. *Ann Australas Coll Trop Med* 2010; 11; 8–11.

Steffen R, Rickenbach M, Willhelm U, Helminger A, Schär M. Health problems after travel to developing countries. *J Infect Dis* 1987; 156: 84–91.

Waterhouse J, Reilly T, Atkinson G, Edwards B. Jet lag: trends and coping strategies. *Lancet* 2007; 369: 1117–29.

Additional reading

Keystone JS, Kozarsky PE, Freedman DO, Nothdurft HD, Connor BA (eds). *Travel medicine*, 2nd edn. Philadelphia: Mosby; 2008.

DuPont H, Steffen R (eds). *Textbook of travel medicine and health*, 2nd edn. Hamilton: BC Decker Inc, 2001.

Zuckerman J (ed). *Principles and practice of travel medicine*, 1st edn. Chichester: John Wiley & Sons, 2001.

Three useful reference books with comprehensive information on all aspects of travel medicine

Useful websites

http://wwwnc.cdc.gov/travel/
http://www.hpa.org.uk/
http://www.nathnac.org/pro/
http://www.who.int/ith/en/

Websites with a comprehensive collection of information on travel medicine providing a US, UK, and international perspective. Excellent resources for important travel related publications and epidemiological data

CHAPTER 20

Emerging Issues

Judy Sng[1] and David Koh[1,2]

[1] Saw Swee Hock School of Public Health, National University of Singapore, Singapore
[2] PAPRSB Institute of Health Sciences, Universiti Brunei Darussalam, Brunei Darussalam

OVERVIEW

- Emerging occupational and environmental health issues can broadly be categorized as either due to environmental changes, to the changing nature of work, or to the composition of the workforce. They provide new challenges to occupational health professionals.
- Environmental: Climate change–exposure of outdoor workers to heat stress, emergency workers to flooding, or exposure of agricultural workers to different infectious disease due to changes in distribution (e.g. West Nile fever and dengue fever)
- Work-related: New technologies, changing patterns of work, psychosocial hazards.
- Worker-related: Migrant workers, ageing workforce, chronic diseases and work

A rapidly changing physical and social environment has a profound impact on health and healthcare, and provides new challenges in the practice of occupational and environmental medicine. Technological advances and social and organizational change lead to the emergence of new risks, and the impact of pre-existing issues may be altered. For example, new technologies may be implemented in industry before potential health risks are adequately understood, and at times of organizational change and economic crisis psychological stress may become more prevalent. Global and country-level economic changes can also lead to an increase in the number of migrant and informal sector workers; and both groups often experience hazardous working conditions. Work arrangements that are gaining in popularity such as self-employment, outsourcing and time-limited contracts give rise to new occupational health (OH) concerns, and rapid globalization has also resulted in a number of new challenges for OH practitioners to consider. With easy access to a wealth of information on the internet, not to mention the increasingly popular social networking sites, workers are now more connected and informed than ever before. This has led to workers having higher expectations of their employers and also their OH practitioners, and has possibly resulted in greater litigiousness.

Forces that drive emerging issues

Technological and scientific advances

When technology advances, job processes change and new materials are introduced. This changes the profile of the work as well as the resultant risks to health and to the environment. OH professionals are faced with the challenge of workers who present with conditions that could have resulted from new and poorly understood workplace risks.

With improved scientific understanding and increasing recognition, a better appreciation of certain occupational and environmental risks can occur: the effects of shift work on health, for example. Changing perceptions of the importance of certain risk factors may also influence which of them comes to prominence. An example is the effect of psychosocial factors on work-related stress (ILO 2010).

One important step is to recognize the work-relatedness of many health issues. For example, high work stress may manifest with vague symptoms such as headaches or dizziness. These may easily be misclassified as malingering or non-compliance with medication if work-relatedness is not considered (Figure 20.1).

An example of a work-related disease that was initially ill defined, but subsequently officially recognized is 'karoshi' (Box 20.1).

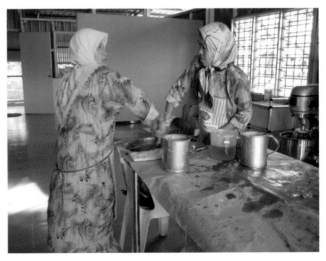

Figure 20.1 For women, juggling work with caring for their families can put them at higher risk of work-related stress which may present with vague, non-specific symptoms.

ABC of Occupational and Environmental Medicine, Third Edition.
Edited by David Snashall and Dipti Patel.
© 2012 John Wiley & Sons Ltd. Published 2012 by John Wiley & Sons Ltd.

Box 20.1 **Karoshi: death from overwork**

Karoshi

- First reported in Japan in 1969, legally recognized in the 1980s, now recognized in Japan, Korea, Taiwan
- Sudden death of any employee who works an average of 65 hours per week for more than 4 weeks or an average of 60 hours a week for more than 8 weeks may be karoshi
- Major medical causes are acute myocardial infarction and cerebrovascular accidents
- Likely to gain prominence as more people worldwide are working longer hours
- Higher risk if long working hours are combined with high job demand, low control and poor social support
- *Karojisatsu*, the term given to suicide due to overwork, is an issue in the Far East
- Over the past decade there has been an increase in *karojisatsu* in Europe

Box 20.3 **The triple burden of traditional occupational diseases, work-related disorders and emerging occupational risks**

Traditional occupational diseases:

- Pneumoconiosis, e.g. silicosis
- Pesticide poisoning
- Heavy metal poisoning

Work-related disorders:

- Musculoskeletal pain from workplace ergonomic issues
- Stress-related conditions, e.g. hypertension
- Chronic non-specific respiratory disorders

Emerging occupational risks:

- Infections, e.g. SARS (severe acute respiratory syndrome)
- New materials/processes, e.g. nanotechnology
- Psychosocial hazards, e.g. karoshi

Changing demographic and employment patterns

With an ageing workforce and an increasing prevalence of lifestyle-related illnesses, there is a growing need for health promotion and preventive services in the workplace. This century will see the world's population ageing at an unprecedented rate, with profound effects on many facets of life, including work (www.un.org/esa/population/publications/worldageing19502050/) (see Chapter 18)

The global financial meltdown in 2008 led to record unemployment levels and a global crisis of 'discouraged jobseekers, involuntary temporary and part-time workers, informal employment, pay cuts and benefit reductions' (ILO 2010). Although some types of work can be hazardous to health, lack of work (or worklessness) is also known to be associated with increased adverse health effects (Box 20.2) (Chapter 2). This in itself should be considered to be a type of work-related health hazard. (Dorling 2009).

Box 20.2 **Health effects of unemployment/worklessness***

Unemployment has been associated with increased overall mortality and greater risk of morbidity from:

- cardiovascular disease
- cerebrovascular disease
- lung cancer
- depression
- suicide and parasuicide

*Covered in greater detail in Chapter 2.

Development and globalization

Newly industrializing countries (NICs) are less developed nations that experience rapid economic growth. The potential effects of such rapid growth are the amplification of pre-existing risks and the introduction of new risks. As such, many of these countries grapple with a 'triple burden' of occupational and work-related diseases. Box 20.3 presents some examples for each category.

Over the past few decades, regional economies, societies and cultures have become increasingly integrated and acculturated. To some degree, the same integration occurs in the workplace and has resulted in practices such as outsourcing and supply chaining. This has given rise to some new and emerging issues in occupational and environmental health such as working non-standard hours, home working, increasing measurement of work rate and quality, competitiveness within workforces, presenteeism and the uncertainty of continuous employment

Emerging work issues

New technologies

The application of new technological discoveries in industry has often run ahead of adequate health and safety research. One example is nanotechnology, defined by The Royal Society and The Royal Academy of Engineering as the 'design, characterization, production and application of structures, devices and systems by controlling shape and size at the nanometre scale'. Given the diversity of nanomaterials and nanotechnology research, the potential applications for nanomaterials in industry are boundless. Consumer products containing nanomaterials began to appear at the turn of the 21st century, and by 2011 there were over a thousand such products on the market (Box 20.4). However, the potential health and environmental risks are still poorly understood and cannot be ignored, as nano-sized (Figures 20.1 and 20.2) materials exhibit properties that are different from those of bulk materials. (Table 20.1).

Another application of technology in the workplace is that work processes become automated and enclosed. Although this reduces the risk of accidents and high level chemical exposures, there is still a potential for long-term exposure to low doses of mixtures of chemicals. An example is afforded by the semiconductor industry, where many different chemicals such as arsenic, beryllium and hydrofluoric acid are used in automated processes. Such changes may also transfer risks to workers performing cleaning, maintenance or repair work.

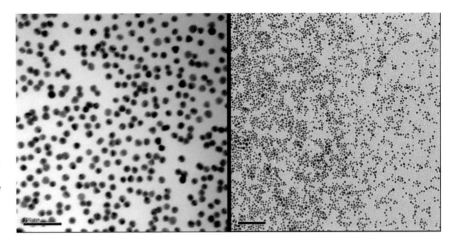

Figure 20.2 Gold nanoparticles with diameter of 20 (left frame) and 7 (right frame) nanometers. This is about a hundred thousandth the diameter of an average human hair. Although bulk gold is relatively inert, gold nanoparticles have been documented to cause oxidative damage to human lung fibroblasts (Li J, *et al*. 2008).

Box 20.4 **Examples of nanomaterial-containing consumer products currently on the market**

Category	Examples of products
Appliances	Refrigerators coated with silver nanoparticles to keep food fresher for longer
Automotive	Automotive parts such as fenders made from nanotubes for greater strength and paint retention
Coatings	Tableware coated with silver nanoparticles for antibacterial effect
Electronics	High-capacity memory chips produced using nanotechnology-centred semiconductor manufacturing methods
Food and beverages	Shatter-proof beer bottles that keep beer fresher for longer (exact material not specified)
Health and fitness	Sunscreens with nanoparticles of zinc oxide and titanium dioxide for greater transparency
Home and garden	Air purifiers incorporating nanofilters

Source: Project on Emerging Nanotechnologies: Inventories (http://www.nanotechproject.org/inventories/consumer/browse/categories/)

Table 20.1 Example of a widely used nanomaterial and the toxicity of its bulk and nano form.

	Carbon black (bulk form)	Carbon nanotubes
Distribution (following inhalation)	Deposition in lungs and via phagocytes to lymph nodes	Potential for translocation via nerve axons
Effects in animal models	Intratracheal instillation – mild pulmonary inflammation	Intratracheal instillation – inflammatory, granulomatous, fibrogenic response. Impaired bacterial clearance (Shvedova *et al*, 2005)
Fire and explosion risk	Small fire potential, when exposed to heat or flame	Main safety hazard. May unexpectedly become chemical catalysts, causing unanticipated reactions

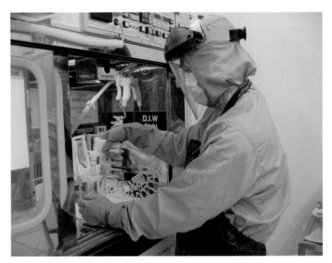

Figure 20.3 A silicon nano-device research facility. It has been estimated that nanotechnology industries worldwide will require 2 million workers by 2015.

Moreover, new technologies are increasingly present in developing countries and NICs, where occupational and environmental health practice, standards and enforcement may be less rigorous. In China, for instance, there were over 1000 enterprises involved in nanotechnology-related business and an estimated 3000 people employed in nanotechnology industries in Shanghai alone as of June 2010.

Impacts of globalization

With our increasingly interconnected world, many people perform work that spans different time zones (the 24/7 world). A common scenario is of an employee working in Asia who needs to coordinate with enterprises in the United States and Europe via email and teleconferencing. Irregular work hours and remote working are now commonplace and have blurred the boundary between home and the workplace, making the achievement of a healthy work–home balance an even greater challenge.

Another aspect of globalization is increasing air travel. At present, there are approximately 4.8 billion airport passengers per year, with aircraft movements highest in North America, Europe and the Asia-Pacific.

As a result, contagious diseases that previously took many weeks to traverse international borders can now spread across the globe within hours. Emerging biological hazards have been a major OH issue in the healthcare, aviation and other service-related industries in the past decade. This was especially seen during the outbreak of severe acute respiratory syndrome (SARS) in 2003 which originated in China and affected over 8000 persons in 29 countries, resulting in 916 reported deaths. In all affected countries, healthcare workers were the worst hit occupational group – accounting for one-fifth of all cases worldwide and over 40% of cases in Canada and Singapore.

Migrant workers and the informal economy

Every year, approximately 100 million people migrate to seek work. These individuals are often inadequately protected by prevailing labour laws and are subject to exploitation, particularly those who are undocumented migrants. Many high-income countries depend on migrant workers to perform 'dirty, dangerous and degrading (the 3-D)' jobs that indigenous workers are unwilling to take up (Benach J *et al.* 2010). For instance, over 90% of construction site workers in Singapore are from other Asian countries, whereas nearly 40% of construction workers in London are migrants from countries such as Poland, Romania and India. Large numbers of migrants work in the construction industries of the Middle East.

In developing countries the informal sector (defined by the World Bank as 'performing activities and earning income partially or fully outside government regulation, taxation and observation') is estimated to account for one- to four-fifths of non-agricultural employment. Workers in the informal sector are often vulnerable and exposed to poor working conditions and a lack of basic OH provision. For example, in a 2009 study, 90% of workers in Bangkok over the age of 60 were in the informal sector. Many of these were working in agriculture, manufacturing, hotels, restaurants, construction and transportation (Figure 20.4).

Psychosocial hazards

Psychosocial hazards in the workplace have been identified as significant emerging risks. Related issues such as work stress and workplace violence are increasingly recognized to be major challenges for occupational health and safety. The topic of mental health and stress is covered in greater detail in Chapter 9.

Healthcare for a workforce with lifestyle-related illnesses

With changes in work and work patterns over the years, there has been a concomitant change in the workforce. Many populations, especially in developed nations, are ageing (see Chapter 18). There are more women in the workforce, even in roles that were previously reserved for men, such as heavy manual work. Also, more women over the age of 50 are continuing to work or return to work after their children have grown up. For example, in the United States, labour force participation rates for women over 55 years of age increased to 30.5% in 2004 from 24.0% in 1994 and 25.6% in 1999.

Those with disabilities or chronic diseases such as diabetes and renal failure are now living longer and also have a better quality of life. The integration of such individuals into the workforce is

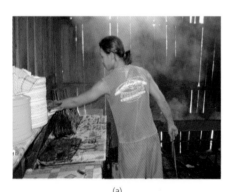
(a)

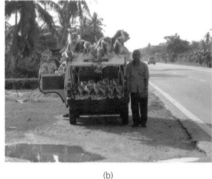
(b)

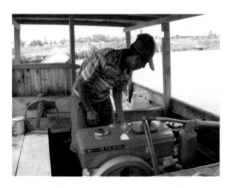
(c)

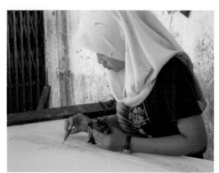
(d)

Figure 20.4 (a–d) Workers in the informal sector are often vulnerable and need access to basic occupational healthcare services.

therefore important, and OH professionals need to be aware of possible interactions between workers' diseases/conditions, their treatment, and exposures in the workplace.

For example a diabetic employee on shift work may have problems with glycaemic control due to disruption of their circadian rhythm (Box 20.5). Treatment would have to be tailored accordingly, and if not possible the person might have to avoid shifts. In such situations the OH professional may need to provide advice to their employer on necessary workplace adjustments (see Chapter 7).

Box 20.5 Managing a diabetic shift worker

Mr X works on a rapid rotating shift system (where he switches from morning to afternoon to night shifts every 2 or 3 days. He is a diabetic who has been treated with oral hypoglycaemics for the past 10 years. However, his glucose control has been problematic with a glycated haemoglobin (HbA1c) ranging from 9.5% to 10% (target <6.5%) in the last 2 years. His oral medication is already at the maximum dose and any increase unlikely to improve his glycaemic status. However, insulin injection in the face of a changing wake–sleep time pattern poses a problem.

Mr X is insulinopenic and would benefit from insulin injections at this stage. Concerns about hypoglycaemia are valid. A reasonable insulin initiation strategy would be to start him on once daily basal insulin. Insulins such as glargine and detemir are relatively peakless. They can be given once daily and are therefore generally more acceptable to patients. Being peakless, they avoid the actions of some other insulins which give rise to hypoglycaemia if peaks are not appropriately matched with food intake.

After starting on insulin, Mr X is comfortable with the injections, and his HbA1c declines to 8.5%. However, his post-meal sugars are not controlled, although his fasting sugars have improved considerably.

Mr X may have to be persuaded to improve his control by the addition of pre-meal insulins. Various options can be considered. The human analogue insulins (e.g. aspart, lispro and glulisine) have a rapid onset of action, allowing meals to be taken soon after the injections. This is an added convenience for shift workers whose meal times are not fixed. In all such cases, efforts should be directed to making use of modern therapy to enable rehabilitation and the restitution of workers to normal fitness as far as possible. In the case of workers with diabetes, this will include self blood glucose monitoring, diabetes education, avoidance of hypoglycaemia and regular screening for complications.

Obesity

Obesity is a global public health challenge, with a rising worldwide prevalence. There are few jobs for which a person is unfit purely on the grounds of being obese and the health consequences thereof. Examples are professional diving and the military. Generally, the risks such employees pose to others are not as significant as those to themselves.

There has been concern about the rising per capita medical expenditure on obese workers. One estimate suggests that between 1987 and 2001, obesity was responsible for 27% of the rise in inflation-adjusted health care expenditure among workers. Besides the medical costs, overweight and obese workers have been reported as being more likely to be less productive and to have higher absenteeism and presenteeism rates (Finkelstein et al. 2010).

There has also been much debate about the ethical aspects of obesity prevention and issues of stigma and interference with autonomy are raised repeatedly. However, there should be no disagreement with the assertion that, however well intended, health promotion programmes have to be sensitively planned. Programmes that create conditions conducive to a healthy lifestyle are more acceptable than programmes that target specified groups.

Challenges in the provision of occupational health services

Challenges for the provision of OH services include the need for more research and more evidence of effectiveness. The Cochrane reviews of Occupational Health, the NHS Plus Evidence Based Guidelines, and the NHS National Institute for Health and Clinical Excellence (NICE) provide an evidence base for the effectiveness of some interventions but more work in this area is needed.

In this age of information people have more access to knowledge and this raises their expectations for better healthcare and an optimal work–home balance, especially among employees in developed countries. At the same time, OH services have to sift through a lot more data and meet employer expectations of reducing healthcare expenditure costs while helping to keep workers healthy and productive.

At the other end of the spectrum, is the lack of provision for the 80% of workers worldwide who do not have access to OH services (Sim 2010). In many developing countries, there is still a need for adequate training and equipping of personnel to provide even basic OH services.

References

Benach J, Muntaner C, Chung H, Benavides FG. Immigration, Employment relations, and health: developing a research agenda. *Am J Industrial Med* 2010; 53: 338–343. *Summary and critical examination of data from various sources on immigration employment relations and health.*

Finkelstein EA, DiBonaventura Md, Burgess SM, Hale BC. The costs of obesity in the workplace. *JOEM* 2010; 52: 971–976. *Quantification of medical expenditures and productivity loss from obesity among employees in the United States, using data from the 2006 Medical Expenditure Panel Survey and the 2008 National Health and Wellness Survey*

ILO. Emerging risks and new patterns of prevention in a changing world of work. Geneva: International Labour Organisation, 2010. http://www.ilo.org/wcmsp5/groups/public/ – ed_protect/ – protrav/ – safework/documents/publication/wcms_123653.pdf *Concise overview of new and emerging occupational health issues around the world*

Li J, Zou L, Hartono D, Ong CN, et al. Gold nanoparticles induce oxidative damage in lung fibroblasts in vitro. *Adv Mater* 2008; 20: 138–142. *Experimental study exposing human fetal lung fibroblasts (commercial cell line) to gold nanoparticles*

Sim M. Occupational health services–standards need to be underpinned by better research on effectiveness. *Occup Environ Med* 2010; 67: 289–290. *Editorial on the need for more stringent evaluation of occupational health services*

Shvedova AA, Kisin ER, Mercer R, *et al*. Unusual inflammatory and fibrogenic pulmonary responses to single-walled carbon nanotubes in mice. *AmJ Physiol–Lung Cell Mol Physiol* 2005; 289:L698–L708. *Experimental study showing that mice exposed to carbon nanotubes experienced much greater inflammation than those exposed to equivalent doses of ultrafine carbon black*

Further reading

European Agency for Safety and Health at Work, 2009. *Outlook 1 – New and emerging risks in Occupational safety and health. European Risk Observatory*. Luxembourg: Office for Official Publications of the European Communities. *Overview of ERO's (European Risk Observatory) main projects*

Dorling D. Unemployment and health. *BMJ* 2009; 338:b829*Editorial outlining the relationship between unemployment and poor health*

Occupational Health: Regional Issues and Challenges, World Health Organization Regional Office for South-East Asia. http://www.searo.who .int/EN/Section23/Section1214/Section1730.htm *Covers occupational issues unique to South-East Asia, as well as initiatives by the WHO to improve occupational health in the region*

Health and Safety Executive: Working in Great Britain from overseas. http://www.hse.gov.uk/migrantworkers/index.htm *Covers health and safety laws, workers' rights for migrant workers in Great Britain*

United Nations Department of Economic and Social Affairs, Population Division. World Population Ageing: 1950-2050. www.un.org/esa/population /publications/worldageing19502050/ *Description of global trends in population ageing*

Fujioka R, Thangpet S Decent work for older persons in Thailand. ILO Asia-Pacific Working Paper Series, February 2009. *Comprehensive review of current and emerging issues surrounding older workers in Thailand*

Finnish Institute of Occupational Health: Occupational Safety and Health Review Group. http://osh.cochrane.org *Collation of systematic reviews on the effects of specific worker protection measures*

National Institute for Health and Clinical Excellence : NICE Guidance. http://www.nice.org.uk/guidance/index.jsp?action=bypublichealth& PUBLICHEALTH=Occupational+health#/ *Comprehensive evidence-based guidance on occupational health and wellness issues developed by multi-disciplinary expert committees*

National Health Services Plus Evidence Based Guidelines. http://www.nhsplus .nhs.uk/providers/clinicaleffectiveness-guidelines-evidencebased.asp *Downloadable guidelines on commonly encountered occupational health issues*

Scott A, Zhou E. The Increased Use Of Nanotechnology In China's Biotech Industry. Life Science Leader, June 2010. http://www.lifescienceleader.com /index.php?option=com_jambozine&layout=article&view=page&aid= 4059. *Account of the growth of China's nanotechnology industry by experts in the life sciences industry*

National Institute for Health and Clinical Excellence: NICE Guidance. http://guidance.nice.org.uk/

CHAPTER 21

Pollution

Robert Maynard

University of Birmingham, Birmingham, UK

> **OVERVIEW**
>
> - Air pollution continues to be a major threat to health in both developed and developing countries
> - Long-term exposure to fine particles shortens life expectancy: the effect is a result of an increased risk of death from cardiovascular disease
> - Indoor air pollution in developing countries is now recognised as a very serious public health problem
> - Some of the effects on health of the ambient aerosol might be explained by very small particles but this is, as yet, uncertain

Pollution of the air, soil and water is a major problem in many parts of the world. In developed countries the worst excesses of industrial pollution are coming under control but have been replaced by pollutants generated by motor vehicles. In developing countries the rapid increase in industrialization combined with the increased use of motor vehicles is producing conditions as bad, if not worse, than those seen in developed countries a century ago. Dense chemical smog is common in megacities such as Mexico City and São Paulo and is an increasing problem in many of the cities of China and India.

Photochemical air pollution is a problem in the Mediterranean area; in fact, only the dense and damp smogs so characteristic of London until the late 1950s seem to have disappeared (Figure 21.1). The combination of a damp, foggy climate and intensive use of soft coal in inefficient household fireplaces does not seem to have been repeated on such a scale elsewhere, although similar conditions may have occurred in Eastern European countries and in Istanbul. High concentrations of coal smoke and sulphur dioxide do occur in some Chinese cities, and forest fires have, over recent years, caused significant 'haze' conditions in South East Asia.

Air pollution is not solely an outdoor problem: in many countries indoor pollution produced by the use of biomass as a fuel damages health, especially that of women and young children who may be exposed for much of a 24-hour day. The seemingly inevitable link between poverty and poor environmental conditions persists, and

Figure 21.1 Classic London 'smog'.

efforts to resolve this and instil a sense of environmental justice are only now beginning. (see also Chapter 22).

Air pollution is a major problem, but so is pollution of water. Attention has been drawn to the contamination of drinking water with arsenic leached from soil in West Bengal. High levels of lead, nitrates and pesticides have also been detected in drinking water in various countries. A problem in California has been the seepage of methyl *tert* butyl ether (MTBE) into drinking water: an ironic problem as MTBE was added to petrol as an oxygenating agent designed to reduce the production of air pollutants. In October 2010, the collapse of a storage reservoir for waste produced by an aluminium refinery in Hungary led to widespread contamination of the Danube. Local residents were exposed to deep red slurry: iron oxide accounted for the colour. Concerns about heavy metals reaching the food chain were expressed widely.

Air pollution

Air pollution is a worldwide problem. Concentrations in cities in developing countries often exceed the WHO Air Quality Guidelines by a wide margin (WHO 2005). The impact of air pollution on health is large: some 3 million deaths each year are attributed by the WHO

ABC of Occupational and Environmental Medicine, Third Edition.
Edited by David Snashall and Dipti Patel.
© 2012 John Wiley & Sons Ltd. Published 2012 by John Wiley & Sons Ltd.

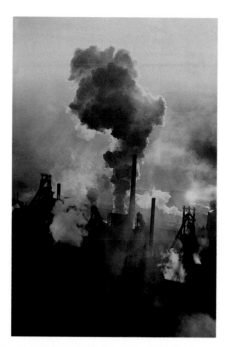

Figure 21.2 Mixture of water vapour and smoke being emitted from an industrial site.

to air pollution. Of these, 2.8 million result from indoor exposure (1.9 million occurring in developing countries) and only 0.2 million occur as a result of outdoor exposure. It is salutary to consider how much effort is put into controlling outdoor concentrations of air pollutants compared with indoor concentrations (Figure 21.2).

Particulate air pollution

Until about 1990 it was believed that ambient concentrations of particles in countries like the United Kingdom had fallen to such levels that effects on health had essentially disappeared. This is now known to be untrue.

An increase in the daily average concentration of particles monitored as PM_{10} (the mass of particles of, generally, less than 10 μm diameter per cubic metre of air) of 10 μg/m^3 is associated with about a 0.7% increase in non-accidental, daily deaths. The effect on hospital admissions is of the same order. Even in a small country like the United Kingdom, this leads to a large impact on health: 8100 deaths brought forward (all causes) and 10 500 hospital admissions (respiratory) either advanced in time (i.e. the admissions would have occurred but occur earlier as a result of exposure to pollution) or caused *de novo*.

It has been argued that the extra deaths calculated in this way are merely deaths advanced by just a few days in those who are already seriously ill: an example of a so-called 'harvesting effect'. This does not seem to be true: recent work by Schwartz has suggested that at least some of the deaths may be advanced by months. Studies in the United States have shown that living in a city with a comparatively high level of particles leads to a reduction in life expectancy. The effect is significantly larger than that of daily variations in concentrations of particles: an increment of 10 μg/m^3 in the long-term average concentration of particles

monitored as $PM_{2.5}$ (the mass of particles of, generally, less than 2.5 μm diameter per cubic metre of air) is associated with a 6% increase in non-accidental all-cause mortality at all adult ages. The effect seems to be mainly on deaths from cardiovascular disease.

Calculating the extent of the impact at an individual level is impossible because we do not know how many in a population are affected. If all people were affected equally, then at levels of particles found in the United Kingdom, the individual impact would be of the order of a 6-month loss of life expectancy. This effect can be represented by the number of premature deaths occurring each year due to long-term exposure to current levels of fine particles. The effect, expressed in this way, is large: more than 30 000 premature deaths per year in the UK. Whether expressing the effect in these terms is informative, though arithmetically accurate, is open to debate. It is very unlikely that all these deaths can be attributed *solely* to the effects of exposure to particles; it is more likely that exposure increases the risk of death in a large number of people in whom other contributing causes play a large, and perhaps more important, role.

If this is the case in the relatively unpolluted United Kingdom then the effect in much more polluted developing countries must be large indeed. Predicting the size of the effect in developing countries is not easy as it will, in part, depend on the background prevalence of disease. If the effect of exposure is to increase the rate of development of disease, then as the background level of cardiovascular disease rises so will the impact of particles.

These calculations of the impact of particles on health have produced a revolution in thinking in inhalation toxicology.

Some, being unable to understand the mechanism of effect of ambient particles, have argued that the reported associations are not causal. Others, rather more usefully, have set out to find the mechanisms of action of ambient particles and research has flourished.

Ultrafine particles (less than 100 nm in diameter) have been suggested to play an important role (Figure 21.3). These particles contribute little to the mass concentration of the ambient aerosol but a great deal to its number concentration. The idea that the number of particles in every cubic metre of air may be more important than the mass per cubic metre has gained ground since it was suggested in 1995. More recently, the idea that total particle surface area per unit volume of air may be important has been suggested. If this is true then air quality standards, currently defined in terms of mass concentrations, will need revision (Box 21.1).

Box 21.1 New trends in research on particulate air pollution

- Effects are not limited to the respiratory system; effects on the cardiovascular system are likely to be more important
- Small particles (less than 2.5 μm in diameter) are likely to play an important role
- The production of free radicals, perhaps as a result of metals acting as catalysts, is likely to be important
- Changes in the control of the heart's beat to beat interval and in the production of clotting factors may be important

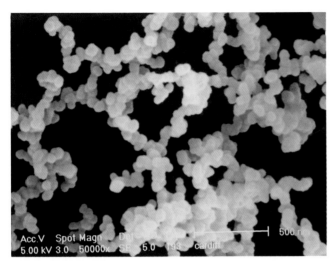

Figure 21.3 Electron micrograph of diesel particles. Individual particles are about 25 nm in diameter. Photograph kindly provided by Professor RJ Richards, Cardiff University.

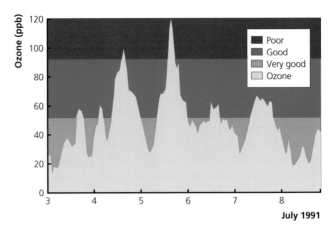

Figure 21.4 Daily variations in ozone concentrations.

Table 21.1 Numbers of deaths and hospital admissions for respiratory diseases per year caused by ozone in both urban and rural areas of Great Britain during summer only.

GB, threshold (in parts per billion)	50	0
Deaths (all causes)	700	12 500
Hospital admissions for respiratory disease	500	9900

Photochemical air pollution

Concern about secondary pollutants generated from primary (emitted) pollutants by photochemical reactions began in Los Angeles in the late 1940s. Ozone is the best-known photochemical air pollutant produced from nitrogen dioxide (Box 21.2) particles; other chemical species, including peroxy radicals derived from volatile organic compounds, are also important. Ozone is the classic example of a secondary air pollutant: essentially no ozone is emitted by sources of outdoor air pollution (Figure 21.4)

Box 21.2 **Ozone production reactions**

$$NO_2 + h\nu_- \rightarrow NO + O^\bullet$$

$$O^\bullet + O_2 \rightarrow O_3$$

$$RO_2 + NO \rightarrow NO_2 + RO$$

It will be appreciated that as long as sunlight (represented by $h\nu_-$), oxygen, nitrogen dioxide and peroxy radicals (RO_2, produced from volatile organic compounds emitted by motor vehicles) are present, ozone production will continue. The reactions stop at night and levels of ozone fall, to build up again the next day. Ozone is thus a problem in cities with heavy traffic and bright sunlight: Athens, Los Angeles and Mexico City are examples. In the United Kingdom ozone is a greater problem in rural than in urban areas, the formative reactions taking place in polluted air masses drifting from the city to the countryside.

Ozone is a strong oxidizing agent and at concentrations above 100 parts per billion ($200 \mu g/m^3$) produces inflammation of the respiratory tract. This is reflected in a reduction in the forced expiratory volume in 1 second (FEV_1) and peak expiratory flow rate (PEFR). Pain on deep inspiration occurs and these effects lead, unsurprisingly, to a reduction in athletic performance. Interestingly, the effect is short lived, and daily exposure studies have shown that the effect is much reduced by about the fourth or fifth day. Epidemiological studies show that daily deaths and hospital admissions for asthma and other respiratory diseases are related to daily ozone concentrations. Discussion of a possible threshold of effect remains unresolved. If no threshold is assumed then a much larger impact on health can be calculated (Table 21.1). Further research to resolve this question of a threshold of effect is urgently needed.

Combinations of air pollutants

Chemical air pollutants never occur alone: there is always a mixture, and it is likely that effects on health are caused by the mixture and might vary with the composition of the mixture. Separating out the more important pollutants has proved to be difficult, and recent studies have shown that the effects of one pollutant may be modified by co-pollutants. This seems to be the case in co-exposures to particles and nitrogen dioxide. The effects of nitrogen dioxide continue to be debated. Some experts believe that nitrogen dioxide acts, largely, as a surrogate or marker for other pollutants, for example fine particles, in the traffic-generated mixture; others believe that nitrogen dioxide at ambient concentrations is, *per se*, a toxicologically active pollutant and has significant effects on health. Much more work is needed in this area: it has serious implications for the setting of standards relating to ambient concentrations of nitrogen dioxide.

Carbon monoxide (a pollutant that is well known to produce lethal effects at high concentrations) has recently been shown by epidemiological studies to be associated with heart attacks and heart failure at current outdoor concentrations – a remarkable finding. Carbon monoxide may be acting as a marker for other pollutants in the ambient mixture, or at low concentrations it may have unexpected effects in sensitive subjects. Recent studies in volunteers who suffered from angina have shown that carboxyhaemoglobin concentrations as low as 2% are associated with a reduction in 'time to pain' and to significant depression of the ST segment of their electrocardiogram trace on exercise.

Sulphur dioxide was an important air pollutant in the days of coal smoke smogs in the United Kingdom. Concentrations have fallen and it no longer has an important direct effect of health at ambient concentrations in the United Kingdom. Sulphur dioxide, of course, contributes to the ambient aerosol by reactions which lead to the formation of sulphate-rich particles: that these have an effect on health as part of the fine ambient aerosol is very likely.

Effects on patients

Most people in the United Kingdom do not notice any effects of air pollutants on their health; at least this is true on most days of the year. Those who suffer from respiratory disorders, including asthma, may notice that their chests are 'tighter' on days when concentrations of pollutants are raised and should use their reliever medication inhalers appropriately. Those with cardiovascular disease are at some increased risk when levels of air pollutants are high but should not modify their medication, if any, without consulting their doctors. Further advice may be found on the web site of The Committee on the Medical Effects of Air Pollutants.

Carcinogenic air pollutants

Many well-recognized human carcinogens occur in ambient air, both outdoors and, often to a greater extent, indoors. Studies in UK homes have shown, for example, that concentrations of benzene indoors may exceed those outdoors. Motor vehicles generate benzene, 1,3-butadiene, and polycyclic aromatic hydrocarbons. High levels of arsenic may occur near metal smelting works. These carcinogens are genotoxic and thus no guarantee of safety can be provided at any level of exposure. All estimates of increased risk from carcinogenic air pollutants are based on mathematical extrapolation from studies, in animals or man, of increases in risk on exposure to high concentrations. The process is unlikely to be precise and the accuracy of the predictions cannot be ascertained. This has led regulators in the UK to adopt a pragmatic approach and to set standards for ambient concentrations at levels at which the risk is judged to be very small and not to attempt quantification of the effects. The WHO has published 'unit risk factors' that allow the risk to be estimated (expressed as an increase in risk of getting a specified cancer as a result of lifetime exposure to a unit concentration of the carcinogen). For example, lifetime exposure to benzene of $17\,\mu g/m^3$ is estimated to be associated with an increase of risk of 1 in 10 000. The unit risk at $1\,\mu g/m^3$ is estimated as 6×10^{-6}.

Indoor air pollution

All the pollutants discussed above, with the exception of ozone (which reacts rapidly with furnishings and fittings and disappears), occur indoors. Indoor concentrations are, in part, driven by outdoor sources as well as by specific indoor sources. Carbon monoxide and nitrogen dioxide are produced by fires and by cooking – peak levels

in kitchens of the latter are often higher than those commonly found outdoors. Recent work has led to concern about an association between nitrogen dioxide and respiratory infections, worsening of lung function in women with asthma, and increased sensitization and response to allergens. Long-term exposure to low levels of carbon monoxide is thought, by some, to cause lasting neurological effects. Exposure to smoke from the burning of biomass for cooking and space-heating is a major problem in some developing countries. Chronic obstructive pulmonary disease is associated with such exposures and other effects, including the induction of cataracts, have been reported.

Regulating indoor pollutant concentrations is difficult: fewer countries have produced standards for indoor air quality than for outdoor air quality. The need for regular maintenance of devices that can produce pollutants indoors, for carbon monoxide alarms and for constant vigilance on the part of doctors dealing with potentially poisoned patients is obvious.

Water and soil pollution

The quality of drinking water in developed countries is often accepted, unthinkingly, as high: it is assumed that the water is safe to drink. In many countries, however, such an assumption may be unwise because of microbiological and chemical contamination (Table 21.2). The former causes more disease than the latter and is

Table 21.2 Compounds that are of proved concerns as water and soil pollutants. See WHO reports in the references.

Arsenic
Arsenic is found in high concentrations in many countries including Argentina, Canada, Chile, China, Japan, Mexico, the Philippines and the United States. The recent discovery of arsenic concentrations at 70 times the national standard of 0.05 mg/L in West Bengal has highlighted this pollutant. Poisoning via water leads to evidence of chronic toxicity including melanosis, hyperkeratosis, and skin cancer. In West Bengal 200 000 people are reported to be suffering from arsenical skin lesions.

Nitrates
Nitrates leached from agricultural land may enter drinking water. The use of infant food prepared with such water can lead to poisoning because of methaemoglobin being produced by interaction between nitrite ions (produced from nitrate ions) and haemoglobin. The reaction is an oxidative one (ferrous iron in haemoglobin being converted to ferric iron in methaemoglobin) but the exact mechanism is unclear. In very young children cyanosis may occur. In 15 European countries 0.5–10% of the population may be exposed to nitrate levels in excess of the WHO standard of 50 mg/L.

Lead
Lead can be mobilized from pipes and solder joints, especially in areas with acidic water supplies ('soft water' areas). Lead is accumulated in the body and can damage the central nervous system. A number of studies have linked lead intake and a decreased intelligence quotient. Mercury and cadmium are examples of other metals that contaminate water supplies.

Fluoride
Fluoride is added to water in some countries to provide protection against tooth decay: effective protection is provided at levels of 0.5–1.0 mg/L. The margin between protective and toxic effects is unfortunately narrow, and effects ranging from dental fluorosis (mottling of enamel) to skeletal fluorosis occur in some areas. High levels of fluoride are found in parts of the Middle East, Africa, and North and South America.

covered in Chapter 19. Accidental contamination of water supplies occurs from time to time in all countries: in the United Kingdom the accidental contamination of water with aluminium sulphate in Camelford (Cornwall) in 1988 (Chapter 12) led to widespread complaints. The quality of water supplies is improving in many countries, but the rate of improvement is uneven. The WHO reported in 2010 that 874 million people still did not have access to improved (i.e. satisfactory) sources of drinking water. (WHO 2010). In some countries, including developed countries such as the United Kingdom, concern has been expressed about the possible impacts on health of so-called endocrine-disrupting chemicals.

Conclusion

Pollution of air, soil and water remains a problem in nearly all parts of the world. In developed countries air pollution tends to attract the greatest attention, and considerable efforts to control outdoor sources of air pollutants have been made. In developing countries both air and water pollution remain important problems, and a large effort will be needed before these are removed.

Further reading

Holgate ST, Samet JM, Koren HS, Maynard RL, eds. *Air Pollution and Health.* London, New York: Academic Press, 1999. *A comprehensive review of all aspects of air pollution*

Ayres J G, Harrison R M, Nichols G L, Maynard R L (eds) *Environmental Medicine.* Hodder Education, 2010. *A comprehensive review of the field.*

World Health Organization. *Air Quality Guidelines for Europe,* 2nd edn. WHO Regional Publications, European Series, No 91. Copenhagen: WHO, 2000. *An update of the original 1987 edition providing guidelines for 35 air pollutants*

World Health Organization. *Air Quality Guidelines, Global Update 2005. World Health Organization,* 2006. *A further very detailed update of evidence of effects on health of a limited range of air pollutant including a detailed account of indoor air pollution.*

World Health Organization. *Health and Environment in Sustainable Development. Five years after the Earth Summit.* Geneva: WHO, 1997. *A useful and wide ranging report*

Maynard RL, Howard CV (eds) *Particulate matter: properties and effects upon health.* Oxford: BIOS Scientific Publishers Ltd, 1999. *A collection of papers by leading research workers*

Department of Health. Committee on the Medical Effects of Air Pollutants. *Cardiovascular disease and Air pollution.* 2006. *A detailed review of recent evidence*

Department of Health. Committee on the Medical Effects of Air Pollutants. *Long-Term Exposure to Air Pollution: Effect on Mortality.* 2009. *A detailed review of recent evidence providing the basis for calculations of effects in the UK.*

World Health Organization. *International programme on chemical safety. Guidelines for drinking-water quality,* 2nd ed. Vol. 1. *Recommendations.* Geneva: WHO, 1993

World Health Organization. *International programme on chemical safety. Guidelines for drinking-water quality,* 2nd ed. Vol 2. *Health criteria and other supporting information.* Geneva: WHO, 1997. *These two reports contain detailed and invaluable accounts providing background material to the guidelines*

World Health Organization 2010: *Progress on Sanitation and Drinking Water–2010 Update*

CHAPTER 22

Global Health

Paolo Vineis

Imperial College of Science, Technology and Medicine, London, UK

OVERVIEW

- Global health has been defined as 'health problems, issues, and concerns that transcend national boundaries, may be influenced by circumstances or experiences in other countries, and are best addressed by co-operative actions and solutions'

- There are numerous and increasing examples of such 'boundary transcending problems', like the flow of migrant workers who suffer from specific health problems (including distress and mental health conditions)

- While some global health issues are well described, like the outbreaks of emerging or re-emerging infectious diseases (Box 22.1), little is known about others such as the massive exposure in low-income countries to environmental toxins such as arsenic, asbestos and air pollutants

- The health effects of climate change are yet to be accurately defined

- Some health problems are pandemic in nature, such as the current explosion of obesity and diabetes affecting both low- and high-income countries. The relative contribution of the various causes are still largely unknown; the new paradigm of 'built environment', incorporating notions of decreased physical exercise and outdoor activities due to changes in town planning – in addition to changes in food habits – has been proposed.

- Tobacco-related effects continue as the main example of premature death, disability and chronic disease due to a single cause, and are expected to increase in low-income countries if effective measures against the use of tobacco are not taken

- As the dramatic example of the effects of the drug thalidomide showed, it is important to identify early signals of negative impacts on health and rigorously assess their likely significance

What is global health?

Global health has been defined as 'health problems, issues, and concerns that transcend national boundaries, may be influenced by circumstances or experiences in other countries, and are best

ABC of Occupational and Environmental Medicine, Third Edition.
Edited by David Snashall and Dipti Patel.
© 2012 John Wiley & Sons Ltd. Published 2012 by John Wiley & Sons Ltd.

Box 22.1 Emerging and re-emerging infectious diseases

Emerging infectious diseases are those that have been recently discovered, have increased in humans over the past two decades, or threaten to increase in the future.

Re-emerging infections are infectious diseases which have increased (previously having diminished in incidence) because of ecological changes, public health decline, or development of drug resistance.

Six major factors have contributed to their emergence or re-emergence:

1 Changes in human demography and behaviour (e.g. immunosuppression, ageing population, migration, risky behaviours)
2 Advances in technology and changes in industry practices (e.g. air conditioning cooling towers, changes in food processing, changes in rendering)
3 Economic development and changes in land use patterns (encroachment on the tropical rainforests, conservation efforts, climate changes)
4 Dramatic increases in volume and speed of international travel and commerce of people, animals and foodstuffs
5 Microbial adaptation and changes
6 Breakdown of public health capacity to address infectious diseases.

In most instances, the emergence of a specific agent results from a complex interaction of several factors.

Examples of emerging and re-emerging infections are given in Chapter 20.

addressed by co-operative actions and solutions' (United States Institute of Medicine; see also Skolnick 2008). Interest in global health usually starts with the following observations.

- **There have been major improvements in health**. Average global life expectancy has increased from 50 to 67 years since 1960; smallpox has been eradicated and deaths from measles fell by 48%, from 871 000 in 1999 to an estimated 454 000 in 2004.
- **There are even larger disparities in health than before.** There are over 6 billion people in the world, 1 billion of whom can expect to lead a long and healthy life, but 5 billion are not so fortunate. For example, a child born in Japan has a life expectancy of 82 years, but one born in Swaziland will only live an average

of 32 years. Maternal mortality rates range from 830 per 100 000 births in African countries to 24 per 100 000 births in European countries.

- **Health and disease have no borders.** Health issues are not confined within national or regional borders. For example, an outbreak of severe acute respiratory syndrome in China in 2002 rapidly spread across the globe and within 8 months caused 8422 probable cases and 916 deaths in 29 countries. Control programmes need to be approached at an international level.

In the examples that follow all components of the definition above are fulfilled – these are health problems that not only 'transcend the boundaries' or have a worldwide dimension, but comprise issues that require concerted international action involving several institutions at different levels. Box 22.2 gives some additional information on the background global context.

Box 22.2 The global context: carrying capacity, biodiversity and policy responses

Carrying capacity

Man's activities of production and consumption affect not only our local environment but the environment of whole regions and the entire planet. Given the large scale of such activities in an increasingly globalized world, certain polluting or resource depleting activities that the carrying capacity of the local environment used to absorb now result in overload or contamination of global proportions. One of the best recognized examples in the twentieth century has been the devastating effect of acid rain on natural ecosystems whose ability to absorb and eliminate sulphuric acid was overwhelmed. The carrying capacity amounts to some 10 hectares for every person for the richest countries compared with only 2.5 hectares per person on a global average. Thus, on this and other measures there is not enough land to support the world's population at the level of consumption enjoyed by the most industrialized countries. Of course, there is no widespread enthusiasm to reduce levels of consumption. On the contrary, there are widespread aspirations to increase industrial production and employment and to reduce, or eliminate, poverty. Various attempts have been made to estimate how many people can comfortably and sustainably live on this planet, based on some reasonable compromise between the (low) current average standard of living and the high average in the richest countries. Realistic estimates based on food production, water usage, energy consumption and the integrated footprints fall mostly in the range of 3–5 billion people. With a world population of 6 billion and projected increases to at least 10 billion before any prospect of levelling off, the sustainable carrying capacity of the planet is already being exceeded.

Biodiversity

As pressure on land has increased in the past 100 years, the rate of extinction has accelerated. It is estimated that 20–50% of species present 100 years ago will have become extinct by 2100, with the rate of loss accelerating from now until then. Many species are lost as biodiverse tropical rainforests are depleted by clearance and burning. This has practical consequences on human health by affecting food and drugs. Medicines have been identified and developed from tropical plants, and pharmacological possibilities for numerous species have not been explored. In the case of food, we

have in the past relied on the cross-breeding of food crops with wild strains to maintain productivity and resistance to pests, and will no doubt need to continue to do this, whatever achievements arise from genetic modification in laboratories.

Policy responses

The examples in the text have been selected to illustrate the wide range of environmental impacts on health. Our choice of modes of transport has both local and global impacts. Our energy consumption has an impact via its contribution to global warming. Toxic chemicals in the environment may cause local problems or be bioaccumulating and thus contribute to remote risk. In a parallel manner, policy instruments for preventing adverse environmental impacts operate on various levels. At a global level international conventions play a major role, although the important and potentially expensive ones are the most difficult to get all parties to agree to and ratify. The Kyoto agreement on limiting climate change gases will remain in limbo as long as the major polluters refuse to ratify it. Regulation at national and, for the European Union, a European level is embodied in directives, regulations and policies such as, in the United Kingdom, the national ambient air quality standards (NAAQS). Local initiatives prompted by the Rio de Janeiro meeting on environment and development have become an important focus for both local authority initiatives and the involvement of civil society. The so-called La21, or Local Agenda 21, developed as an idea intended to catalyse local environmental initiatives. Finally, industrial undertakings by their very size can have large environmental impacts by virtue of employment or pollution, or make products which have significant environmental impacts. Responsible corporate and product stewardship can be implemented to seek to reduce adverse environmental (or environmental health) impacts. This may be represented by adherence within the worksite to quality standards such as the Eco-Management and Audit Scheme or ISO 14 000 environmental quality schemes, or the adoption of 'cradle to grave' product stewardship initiatives, ensuring that raw materials such as wood are derived from sustainable sources, recycling is maximized, and products are designed so that they can be recycled.

Bangladesh as an example

Bangladesh is often used as a case study because it exemplifies at least three health-related changes that are typical: massive migration (mainly of men) towards rich countries such as Dubai and Qatar; susceptibility to the effects of climate change, partly related to changes in economic scenarios; and recent spectacular improvements in infant mortality. The first two phenomena match the definition of global health, because they result from global changes that transcend the boundaries of the country, and require cooperative action to be addressed. In addition, they are relevant to the work of physicians, and occupational and public health specialists in high-income countries, because an increasing number of migrants or refugees escaping from poverty or the effects of climate change may seek their help The third, a rapid decrease in infant mortality, has been obtained thanks to local action. It is an impressive, world-wide phenomenon seen also in several other low-income countries (see video section at end of chapter).

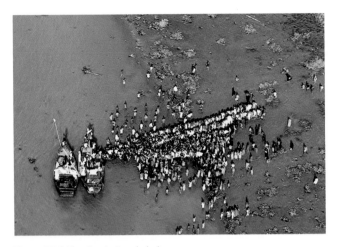

Figure 22.1 Flooding in Bangladesh.

According to the fourth assessment report by the Intergovernmental Panel on Climate Change (IPCC) there is 'high confidence' that marine and coastal ecosystems in South and South East Asia will be affected by sea-level rise, leaving a million or so people at risk from flooding (Figure 22.1), whereas future climate change is likely to have severe effects on agriculture and water security ('medium confidence'). The direct (short-term, i.e. hours or days) health risks from climate change are related to the physical hazards of floods, storms and associated infectious diseases. Less obvious or indirect (intermediate- and long-term, i.e. weeks to years) health risks are related to changes in food yields, population displacement as a result of sea-level rise and water shortages, mental health problems and other chronic diseases. The risk of malaria has been shown to be sensitive to variability in climate caused by the El Niño phenomenon in Central Asia, Africa and South America. Results, based on time-series analysis, suggest that the coupling between climate variability and cholera cycles has become stronger in recent decades.

The complexity of performing studies in a real-life climate change scenario is illustrated by the example of salt-water intrusion in Bangladesh. For decades, salinity levels in surface and ground water in coastal Bangladesh have been rising at unprecedented rates. Salt water from the Bay of Bengal has penetrated over 100 km along tributary channels, currently affecting 20 million people and 830 000 ha of arable land by increased salinity. This has raised serious public health concerns as various salt-related diseases have been reported in those areas, in particular hypertension and eclampsia of pregnancy. Also cholera outbreaks are occurring as a consequence of changes in water quality and temperature that facilitate the proliferation of *Vibrio cholerae*. Shrimp farming, which requires high levels of salt in pond water for cultivation, has increased in the same region and has become a major export industry, further worsening the ecological situation by substituting fresh water in rice fields with brackish water.

Although many of the factors are local to Bangladesh, climate change is obviously the effect of global changes. Bangladesh contributes almost zero CO_2 emissions compared to high-income countries (Figure 22.2), although it could be one of the first and main victims.

Tens of thousands of Bangladeshi workers migrate every year to the Middle East, where they live in very poor conditions and receive low salaries. The effects on health are considerable, particularly mental health. Depression and anxiety prevalence rates among migrants (refugees and labour migrants) may be linked – among other factors – to difficult financial conditions in the country of immigration. A systematic literature review conducted by Lindert and colleagues (2009) shows that the prevalence rates for depression were 20% among labour migrants versus 44% among refugees; for anxiety the estimates were 21% among labour migrants versus 40% among refugees (n = 24 051). Higher gross national product (GNP) in the country of immigration was related to a lower prevalence of symptom of depression and/or anxiety in labour migrants but not in refugees. The authors conclude that depression and/or anxiety in labour migrants and refugees require separate consideration, and that better economic conditions in the host country reflected by a higher GNP appear to be related to better mental health in labour migrants but not in refugees.

In conclusion, Bangladesh exemplifies the multifaceted changes occurring in many low-income countries, both negative and positive.

The global epidemic of tobacco-related diseases

Tobacco is a potent multisite carcinogen with a substantial worldwide impact, causing cancers of the lung, upper aerodigestive tract, pancreas, stomach, liver, lower urinary tract (renal pelvis and bladder), kidney and uterine cervix–also some forms of acute myeloid leukaemia. Both cigarette smoking and smoking other forms of tobacco, including bidi, pipe and cigars, can cause cancers in multiple organs. There is high coherence for causality between the epidemiological evidence and the mechanistic or biological evidence involving measurements of carcinogenic metabolites of tobacco compounds, the formation of chemical bonds with DNA, and the typical spectrum of gene mutations found in cancers developed by smokers.

The worldwide consequences of tobacco smoking are dramatic and are likely to worsen in the near future. Tobacco smoking is currently responsible for approximately 30% of cancer deaths in developed countries, and for an increasing proportion of the cancer deaths in developing countries. Furthermore, smoking causes more deaths from vascular, respiratory, and other diseases than it does from cancer. Of all lifetime users of tobacco, half will die because of their habit, and half of these individuals will die in middle age. If current smoking patterns persist, then in the twenty-first century there will be more than 1 billion deaths attributed to smoking. Figure 22.3 shows the projected numbers of deaths related to tobacco to 2030, overall in the world and in high-income and low–medium-income countries respectively. It is clear that all the increase is expected to occur in the latter if there is not drastic action to contain the penetration of tobacco sales into developing countries (see video section at end of chapter).

CO$_2$ emissions in 2002

Tonnes per capita

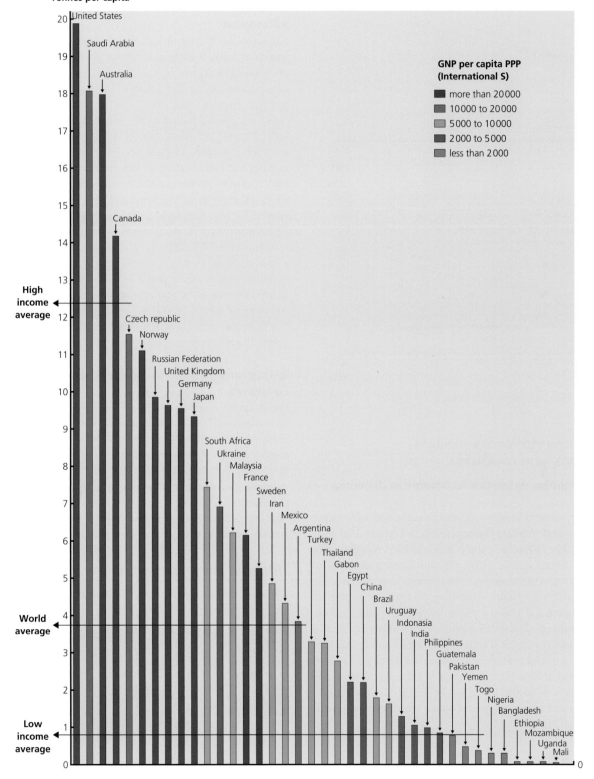

Figure 22.2 The contribution of different nations to CO$_2$ emissions, in tonnes per capita. *Source:* World Bank online database 2004.

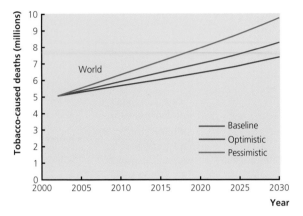

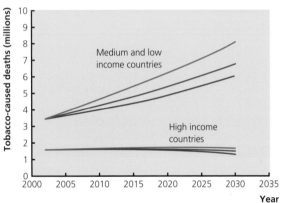

Figure 22.3 The global burden of tobacco.

Environmental contaminants in low-income countries

Environmental exposure to arsenic in drinking water

Chronic exposure to arsenic is known to cause non-melanocytic skin and internal tumours (lung, bladder) in humans, exhibiting dose-dependent effects. In a study assessing the potential burden of internal cancers due to arsenic exposure in Bangladesh, excess lifetime risks of death from liver, bladder and lung cancers using exposure distribution, death probabilities and cancer mortality rates from Bangladesh and dose-specific relative risk (RR) estimates from Taiwan have been calculated. Results indicate at least a doubling of lifetime mortality risks from such cancers attributable to exposure to arsenic in drinking water in Bangladesh. Overall, it has been estimated that at least 137 million people in the world, including the 70 million or so that reside in the Padma-Meghna plain in Bangladesh and adjoining parts of India, are exposed to arsenic through drinking water.

Biomass fumes

Biomass, including wood, crop residues and dung, is largely used for cooking and heating in developing countries, in addition to coal. The burning of these materials gives rise to heavy exposure, mainly indoors, to polycyclic aromatic hydrocarbons (PAHs) and other airborne carcinogens. It has been estimated by Vineis and Xun (2009) that tens of thousands of lung cancer deaths could

be prevented each year in developing countries, for example by increasing ventilation.

Aflatoxins

Aflatoxins are a class of toxic metabolites produced by certain species of fungi, including *Aspergillus flavus*, which can contaminate groundnuts, tree nuts and grains. Laboratory studies have demonstrated the carcinogenicity of aflatoxins in rodents, primates and fish. Hepatocellular carcinoma (HCC) has been observed in numerous species, indicating the liver as a primary target organ. HCC is one of the most common cancers worldwide with a large geographic variation in incidence. In a study of >18 000 people in Shanghai, individuals with both urinary aflatoxins and positive HBV (hepatitis B) status had a relative risk of 59 for developing HCC (aflatoxin alone was associated with a RR of 3.4, and HBV alone of 7.3, thus suggesting a strong interaction between the two). The number of people exposed to high levels of aflatoxin worldwide is unknown but it is likely to be at least 0.5 billion. If we assume a relative risk of ~5, then it follows that the number of preventable deaths from liver cancer would be at least 80% of the total of the 85 000 occurring every year in populations exposed in developing countries, i.e. 68 000 (85 000 has been estimated as half of all liver cancer deaths occurring in developing countries). Prevention could be effective by simple means, such as storing grain in dry conditions.

Waste landfill sites in developed and developing countries

Illegal landfill sites in developed countries cause exposure to carcinogens such as dioxins, polychlorinated biphenyls, arsenic, cadmium, nickel, PAHs and solvents (including benzene). Illegal landfill sites in developing countries are probably more common, more frequently polluted with toxic chemicals, and closer to dwellings than in developed countries. The Food and Agriculture Organization of United Nations (FAO) has estimated that 120 000 out of the 500 000 tonnes of toxic wastes produced in the world are actually stored in Africa.

Obesity: the example of the Pacific Islands

Obesity is now a dramatic reality in the Pacific Islands, and there are very high rates of diabetes (Figure 22.4). Although changes

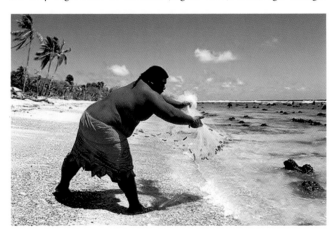

Figure 22.4 A common phenotype in Tonga.

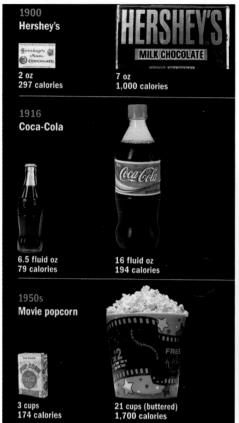

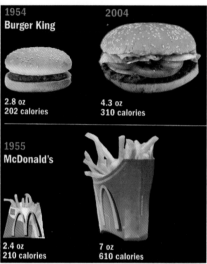

Figure 22.5 The increasing food portions from 1950s to 2000s.

in eating habits, including increasing portion size, are certainly playing a role (Figure 22.5 exemplifies the changes that occurred in portion sizes in the United States in a few decades), the story is obviously more complex. An example is the island of Nauru. This small Pacific island (with only 14 000 inhabitants) underwent incredibly rapid development in the 1970s because of the discovery of a guano deposit that was exploited to sell phosphates as fertilizer. Nauru's per capita income skyrocketed, becoming the highest in the world by the end of the decade. Increasing wealth was associated with a number of important social changes: overmining resulted in loss of arable land, and the diet changed from local fish and vegetables to imported unhealthy foods. Also, the islanders adopted a sedentary lifestyle. In 1975 the prevalence of diabetes was 34%, still in 2007 one of the highest in the world according to the International Diabetes Federation. Unfortunately overmining and mismanagement of investments led Nauru to bankruptcy, and now the inhabitants have to deal with an epidemic of obesity and diabetes from the standpoint of a poor country. Seventy-five per cent of hospital beds are occupied by patients with diabetes and its complications with only 10 physicians in the whole island.

The urban sprawl, the built environment and health

It seems that the current epidemic of obesity in the whole world is not entirely explained by changes in eating habits or a decline in physical activity. Although these changes certainly contribute, rising rates of obesity are not entirely accounted for by them. The likely explanation is a strong 'non-linear interaction' between different factors. A useful concept to address this interaction is that of '*the built environment*', defined as follows by the US National Institute of Environmental Health Sciences in 2004:

> **the built environment … encompasses all buildings, spaces and products that are created, or modified, by people. It includes homes, schools, workplaces, parks/recreation areas, greenways, business areas and transportation systems. … It includes land-use planning and policies that impact on our communities in urban, rural and suburban areas.**

At increasing speed, suburban areas are covering the world's surface: the so-called 'urban sprawl'. The implications for health are intuitive if we look at Figure 22.6. This shows how small towns have evolved in many parts of Europe and the world. The old town was compressed and had well-defined boundaries, and in fact the original design of many European towns was related to defence. Houses, shops and factories were close to each other and even in very recent times walking was the obvious way to move around. Now the town has expanded beyond the original boundaries, and the new design is mainly dominated by two conditioning factors: large supermarkets on the outskirts and the use of cars. Even when distances are not very large, the figure shows that it is inconvenient for a pedestrian to reach other places like shops or offices. The use of a car becomes a necessity.

Suburban Sprawl

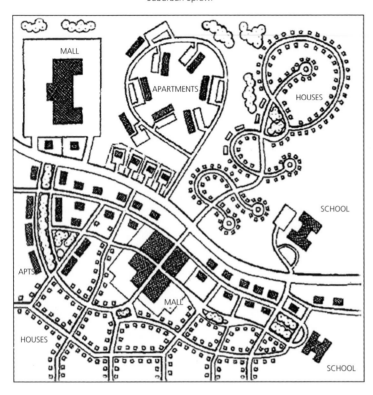

Traditional Neighborhood

Figure 22.6 Urban sprawl. From *Urban Sprawl and Public Health* by Howard Frumkin, Lawrence Frank, and Richard Jackson. Copyright © 2004 Howard Frumkin, Lawrence Frank, and Richard Jackson. Reproduced by permission of Island Press, Washington, DC.

The model of the urban sprawl is expanding from high-income to low-income countries. The relationships between obesity and the built environment have been studied in New York, using a methodology called geo-coding (GIS). Indicators such as *walkability indices* for urban and suburban territories have been developed, based on the urban design and the extent to which this allows pedestrian activities or requires the use of cars. Similarly, indicators of recreational activities have been developed such as extensions of parks, and the availability of healthy food. Investigating the relationships between these different indicators has demonstrated that low walkability, low access to public transportation, dependence on cars and low availability of healthy food were all associated with obesity, independent of socioeconomic status. The point here is that the built environment facilitates an accumulation and interaction of different risk factors.

Although much research has been conducted on the genetic origins of obesity, and some genetic variants that explain individual susceptibility have been detected, it is clear that the quick rise of obesity in all countries cannot be explained by genes. A much more promising research stream, at least in terms of public health, emerges from the concepts of non-linear interactions and urban sprawl in a globalized world.

Policy issues: the precautionary principle

The world is facing tremendous challenges related to globalization. It is clearly important to identify early signals of negative impacts, particularly from the public health perspective. Observing past changes may help to understand the consequences of rejecting early warnings. In the early 1960s Europe was affected by a severe epidemic of birth defects due to the use of the drug thalidomide in pregnancy. The United States had very few cases of limb defects from the drug because an officer of the US Food and Drug Administration delayed approval of the drug based on suspicion that cases were occurring. Both the officer and a doctor in Germany (who described as many as 4000 babies with malformations) received strong criticism because their findings were considered preliminary, and they had to face threats to their professional credibility.

The Precautionary Principle, which is included in European Directives and national laws, is based on two general criteria: (a) appropriate public action should be taken in response to limited, but plausible and credible, evidence of likely and substantial harm; (b) the burden of proof is shifted from demonstrating the presence of risk to demonstrating the absence of risk. Both good reasons for adopting the Principle (e.g. the impossibility of setting thresholds for carcinogenic exposures; long latent periods for many modern diseases; uncertainties about mechanisms of action; large-scale effects of new pollutants) and considerations of its limitations (e.g. what is the minimum level of suspicion that leads to precautionary action) The Precautionary Principle can be paralysing, as some examples suggest, as risks tend to be evaluated independently of benefits). One of the reasons for seriously considering early warnings is the limited understanding of many serious diseases probably influenced by environmental factors such as Alzheimer's and Parkinson's diseases, amyotrophic lateral sclerosis and many types of cancer. A coupling between sound science and the Precautionary Principle should help to more effectively protect people from environmental hazards. The interface between science and policy is in fact one of the most difficult challenges we have to face today, with the threats of conflicts, limited availability of food and water in large areas of the world, mass migrations and climate change. The role of international agencies is likely to need strengthening in the next few years.

References

Skolnick R. *Essentials of Global Health*. Sudbury: Jones and Bartlett, 2008. This is a clear introductory book to all aspects of global health

Further reading

Chen Y, Ahsan H. Cancer burden from arsenic in drinking water in Bangladesh. *Am J Public Health* 2004; 94: 741–744. *A classical paper on the epidemic of arsenic-related health effects in Bangladesh.*

IPCC 2007. *IPCC fourth assessment report*. Cambridge: Cambridge University Press, 2009. The report from a panel of eminent independent scientists on climate change and its effects

Lindert J, Ehrenstein OS, Priebe S, *et al*. Depression and anxiety in labor migrants and refugees–a systematic review and meta-analysis. *Soc Sci Med* 2009; 69: 246–257. *A complete systematic review on the mental problems of migrants and refugees*

Lovasi GS, Hutson MA, Guerra M, Neckerman KM. Built environments and obesity in disadvantaged populations. *Epidemiol Rev* 2009; 31: 7–20. *A systematic review of the relationships between built environment, deprivation and health*

McMichael AJ. *Human frontiers, environments and disease: past patterns, uncertain futures*. Cambridge: Cambridge University Press, 2001. A classical book on the projections of human demographics and health in the light of huge environmental changes including climate change

Vineis P, Alavanja M, Buffler P, *et al*. Tobacco and cancer: recent epidemiological evidence. *J Natl Cancer Inst* 2004; 96: 99–106. *A systematic synthesis of our recent knowledge on tobacco and cancer*

Vineis P, Xun W. The emerging epidemic of environmental cancers in developing countries. *Ann Oncol* 2009; 20: 205–212. *A systemic analysis of what is known about environmental carcinogens in developing countries*

Kriebel D, Tickner J, Epstein P, *et al*. The precautionary principle in environmental science. *Environ Health Perspect* 2001; 109: 871–876. *A seminal paper on the precautionary principle*

Patterson A, McLean C. Misleading and dangerous: the use of the precautionary principle in foreign policy debates. *Med Confl Surviv* 2010; 26: 48–67. *If applied outside environmental hazards the precautionary principle can be misleading*

Videos

A video on infant mortality in Bangladesh and other countries (Poor beat rich in MDG), from Gapminder: http://www.gapminder.org/videos/poor-beats-rich.

A video on worldwide CO2 emissions, from Gapminder: http://www.gapminder.org/videos/gapcasts/gapcast-10-energy.

A video on the lung cancer epidemic, from Gapminder: http://www.gapminder.org/videos/lung-cancer-statistics.

A video on obesity and the built environment, 'The weight of the world': http://www.nfb.ca/film/weight_of_the_world.

Index

Note: Page references in *italics* refer to Figures; those in **bold** refer to Tables and Boxes